2010
YEAR BOOK OF
SPORTS MEDICINE®

The 2010 Year Book Series

Year Book of Anesthesiology and Pain Management™: Drs Chestnut, Abram, Black, Gravlee, Lien, Mathru and Roizen

Year Book of Cardiology®: Drs Gersh, Cheitlin, Elliott, Gold, Graham, and Suri

Year Book of Critical Care Medicine®: Drs Dellinger, Parrillo, Balk, Dorman, Dries, and Zanotti-Cavazzoni

Year Book of Dermatology and Dermatologic Surgery™: Dr Del Rosso

Year Book of Diagnostic Radiology®: Drs Osborn, Abbara, Birdwell, Elster, Manaster, Oestreich, Offiah, Rosado de Christenson, and Walker

Year Book of Emergency Medicine®: Drs Hamilton, Bruno, Handly, Mullin, Quintana, and Ramoska

Year Book of Endocrinology®: Drs Schott, Apovian, Clarke, Eugster, Ludlam, Meikle, Ovalle, Schinner, Schteingart, and Toth

Year Book of Gastroenterology™: Drs Talley, Dempsey, Harnois, Lange, Pearson, Picco, Rombeau, and Scolapio

Year Book of Hand and Upper Limb Surgery®: Drs Yao and Steinmann

Year Book of Medicine®: Drs Barker, Berney, Garrick, Gersh, Khardori, LeRoith, Talley, and Thigpen

Year Book of Neonatal and Perinatal Medicine®: Drs Fanaroff, Benitz, Donn, Neu, and Papile

Year Book of Neurology and Neurosurgery®: Drs Klimo and Rabinstein

Year Book of Obstetrics, Gynecology, and Women's Health®: Drs Dungan and Shulman

Year Book of Oncology®: Drs Thigpen, Arceci, Bauer, Byhardt, Gordon, and Lawton

Year Book of Ophthalmology®: Drs Rapuano, Cohen, Flanders, Hammersmith, Milman, Myers, Nelson, Penne, Pyfer, Sergott, Shields, and Vander

Year Book of Orthopedics®: Drs Morrey, Beauchamp, Huddleston, Swiontkowski, and Trigg

Year Book of Otolaryngology-Head and Neck Surgery®: Drs Sindwani, Balough, Franco, Gapany, and Mitchell

Year Book of Pathology and Laboratory Medicine®: Drs Raab, Parwani, Bejarano, and Bissell

Year Book of Pediatrics®: Dr Stockman

Year Book of Plastic and Aesthetic Surgery™: Drs Miller, Gosain, Gurtner, Gutowski, Ruberg, Salisbury, and Smith

Year Book of Psychiatry and Applied Mental Health®: Drs Talbott, Ballenger, Buckley, Frances, Krupnick, and Mack

Year Book of Pulmonary Disease®: Drs Barker, Jones, Maurer, Raza, Tanoue, and Willsie

Year Book of Sports Medicine®: Drs Shephard, Cantu, Feldman, Jankowski, Khan, Lebrun, Nieman, Pierrynowski, and Rowland

Year Book of Surgery®: Drs Copeland, Behrns, Daly, Eberlein, Fahey, Huber, Mozingo, and Pruett

Year Book of Urology®: Drs Andriole and Coplen

Year Book of Vascular Surgery®: Drs Moneta, Gillespie, Starnes, and Watkins

2010

The Year Book of SPORTS MEDICINE®

Editor-in-Chief

Roy J. Shephard, MD (Lond), PhD, DPE

Professor Emeritus of Applied Physiology, Faculty of Physical Education and Health, University of Toronto, Toronto, Ontario, Canada

ELSEVIER
MOSBY

ELSEVIER
MOSBY

Vice President, Continuity Publishing: Kimberly Murphy
Editor: Ruth Malwitz
Production Supervisor: Donna M. Skelton
Electronic Article Manager: Jennifer C. Pitts
Illustrations and Permissions Coordinator: Dawn Vohsen

2010 EDITION

Composition by TnQ Books and Journals Pvt Ltd, India

Editorial Office:
Elsevier, Inc.
Suite 1800
1600 John F. Kennedy Boulevard
Philadelphia, PA 19103-2899

International Standard Serial Number: 0162-0908
International Standard Book Number: 978-0-323-06846-8

Associate Editors

Robert C. Cantu, MA, MD, FACS, FACSM

Clinical Professor of Neurosurgery, Boston University School of Medicine; Co-Director, Neurological Sports Injury Center at Brigham and Women's Hospital; Neurosurgery Consultant, Boston College Eagles and Boston Cannons Lacrosse Teams; Co-Director, Center for the Study of Traumatic Encephalopathy (CSTE), Boston University Medical Center, Boston, Massachusetts; Co-Founder and Chairman, Medical Advisory Board Sports Legacy Institute (SLI), Waltham, Massachusetts; Chairman, Department of Surgery, Chief, Neurosurgery Service, and Director, Service Sports Medicine, Emerson Hospital, Concord, Massachusetts; Adjunct Professor, Exercise and Sport Science, University of North Carolina; Medical Director, National Center for Catastrophic Sports Injury, Research, Chapel Hill, North Carolina

Debbie Ehrmann Feldman, PT, PhD

Assistant Research Professor, Division of Geriatric Medicine, University of Colorado, Denver, Colorado

Catherine M. Jankowski, PhD

Senior Instructor, Geriatric Medicine, University of Colorado Denver and Health Sciences Center, Denver, Colorado

Karim M. Khan, MD, PhD

Professor, Centre for Hip Health and Mobility, Vancouver Coastal Health Research Institute, and the University of British Columbia; Department of Family Practice, University of British Columbia, Vancouver, British Columbia, Canada

Connie Lebrun, MD

Clinical Director, Glen Sather Sports Medicine Clinic; Associate Professor, Faculty of Physical Education and Recreation, University of Alberta, Edmonton, Alberta, Canada

David C. Nieman, DrPH

Professor, Health and Exercise Science, Appalachian State University, Boone, North Carolina; Director, The Human Performance Laboratory, North Carolina Research Campus, Kannapolis, North Carolina

Michael R. Pierrynowski, PhD

Associate Professor, School of Rehabilitation Science and the Department of Kinesiology, McMaster University, Hamilton, Ontario, Canada

Thomas Rowland, MD

Professor of Pediatrics, Tufts University School of Medicine, Boston; and Chief, Pediatric Cardiology, Baystate Medical Center, Springfield, Massachusetts

Table of Contents

Journals Represented

Journals represented in this YEAR BOOK are listed below.

Academic Emergency Medicine
Acta Obstetricia et Gynecologica Scandinavica
Acta Paediatrica
Allergy
American Journal of Cardiology
American Journal of Clinical Nutrition
American Journal of Emergency Medicine
American Journal of Epidemiology
American Journal of Medicine
American Journal of Obstetrics and Gynecology
American Journal of Otolaryngology
American Journal of Preventive Medicine
American Journal of Sports Medicine
Annals of the Rheumatic Diseases
Archives of Internal Medicine
Archives of Pediatrics & Adolescent Medicine
Archives of Physical Medicine and Rehabilitation
Brain
Brain Research
British Journal of Cancer
British Journal of Sports Medicine
British Medical Journal
Cancer Epidemiology, Biomarkers & Prevention
Canadian Medical Association Journal
Chest
Circulation
Clinical Biomechanics
Clinical Endocrinology
Clinical Journal of Sport Medicine
Diabetes
Diabetes Care
European Heart Journal
European Journal of Echocardiography
European Respiratory Journal
Foot & Ankle International
Headache
Heart
Human Reproduction
Injury
International Journal of Cancer
International Journal of Cardiology
International Journal of Obesity
International Journal of Sports Medicine
Journal of Adolescent Health
Journal of Applied Physiology
Journal of Athletic Training
Journal of Bone Mineral Research

Journal of Cardiac Failure
Journal of Clinical Endocrinology & Metabolism
Journal of Clinical Oncology
Journal of Clinical Psychiatry
Journal of Clinical Rheumatology
Journal of Electrocardiology
Journal of Manipulative and Physiological Therapeutics
Journal of Pediatric Orthopaedics
Journal of Pediatrics
Journal of Sports Sciences
Journal of the American Geriatrics Society
Journal of the Neurological Sciences
Journal of Ultrasound in Medicine
Lancet
Laryngoscope
Maturitas
Medicine and Science in Sports and Exercise
Neurology
Neurosurgery
New England Journal of Medicine
Obstetrics & Gynecology
Orthopedics
Pediatrics
Pharmacotherapy
Proceedings of the National Academy of Sciences of the United States of America
Radiology
Skeletal Radiology
Sports Medicine
Stroke
The Clinical Journal of Pain
The Journal of the American Medical Association
The Journal of Bone and Joint Surgery
The Journals of Gerontology
The Spine Journal
Transfusion

Standard Abbreviations

The following terms are abbreviated in this edition: acquired immunodeficiency syndrome (AIDS), cardiopulmonary resuscitation (CPR), central nervous system (CNS), cerebrospinal fluid (CSF), computed tomography (CT), deoxyribonucleic acid (DNA), electrocardiography (ECG), health maintenance organization (HMO), human immunodeficiency virus (HIV), intensive care unit (ICU), intramuscular (IM), intravenous (IV), magnetic resonance (MR) imaging (MRI), ribonucleic acid (RNA), and ultrasound (US).

Note

The Year Book of Sports Medicine is a literature survey service providing abstracts of articles published in the professional literature. Every effort is made to assure the accuracy of the information presented in these pages. Neither the editors nor the publisher of the Year Book of Sports Medicine can be responsible for errors in the original materials. The editors' comments are their own opinions. Mention of specific products within this publication does not constitute endorsement.

To facilitate the use of the YEAR BOOK OF SPORTS MEDICINE as a reference tool, all illustrations and tables included in this publication are now identified as they appear in the original article. This change is meant to help the reader recognize that any illustration or table appearing in the YEAR BOOK OF SPORTS MEDICINE may be only one of many in the original article. For this reason, figure and table numbers will often appear to be out of sequence within the YEAR BOOK OF SPORTS MEDICINE.

Present Role of Maximal Oxygen Intake Measurements in Sports Medicine

Roy J. Shephard, MD (Lond), PhD, DPE

Faculty of Physical Education and Health, University of Toronto, Toronto, Ontario, Canada

Introduction

The measurement of maximal oxygen intake has been widely accepted as the best single measure of an individual's endurance fitness since the middle of the previous century.[1-4] Indeed, the concept that an individual's oxygen intake reaches a plateau in response to a progressive increase in work rate dates back to A.V. Hill and his associates.[5] A search of the HealthStar-Ovid.database for studies on maximal/maximum oxygen intake/uptake and maximal/maximum aerobic power/capacity reveals a total of some 4798 papers published over the past 60 years. During this period, authors have progressively developed a preference for the grammatically correct term "maximal" rather than "maximum" and the dimensionally correct term "power" (a rate of working) rather than "capacity" (the ability to sustain oxygen transport for a specified period). A vast literature covers potential techniques of measurement, the theoretical significance of observations, and practical applications of the data.

Nevertheless, one can still find occasional studies that question both the existence of an oxygen consumption plateau[6] and the practical value of such testing to the sports physician.[7,8] It thus seems useful to revisit the concept of maximal oxygen intake and to consider its practical value to the sports physician and the exercise scientist. The findings and recommendations of the International Biological Programme (IBP) Working Party provide an appropriate and authoritative starting point for the present discussion.[9]

Findings and Recommendations of the IBP Working Party

Noting the central importance of maximal oxygen intake to studies in sports medicine and exercise science, in the summer of 1966 the IBP convened a working party of the world's leading investigators with the mandate to determine the protocols most appropriate to a variety of field and laboratory situations.[9] Their detailed test recommendations still offer helpful guidance to investigators, particularly those who have found difficulty in demonstrating the classic plateau of oxygen consumption (an increase in oxygen consumption of less than 2 ml/[kg·min] in response to an increase of work rate). Among key requirements, subjects should be well motivated and familar with the laboratory and its equipment, and investigators should follow an appropriate and internationally standardized protocol. Expired gas should be collected using a low resistance, low dead space system, and analyses performed without systematic error. In the era of the IBP Working Party, the Douglas bag technique was used rather than a metabolic cart that includes "black box" calculations of uncertain validity; this approach avoided issues of technical accuracy, sampling time and uncertain methods of calculation that have dogged more recent investigators.[10]

The underlying data were derived from the most comprehensive investigation yet undertaken in the field of stress testing. The subjects were 24 men aged 20 to 40 years, ranging widely in initial fitness (maximal oxygen intake 30.6 to 69.1 ml/[kg·min]). Each participant performed 11 successive maximal oxygen intake tests over a 3-week period, using three different test modalities (treadmill, cycle ergometer, and step test) and both continuous and discontinuous test protocols according to a random block design. All subjects reached a clear oxygen consumption plateau with all three modes of exercise and both types of protocol, thus offering multiple test options to investigators. Nevertheless, on average, treadmill values were 4% higher than those for the step test and 7% higher than those for the cycle ergometer. Values over the 3-week study were highly reproducible but increased by about 1% per day in response to the training stimulus imposed by repeated maximal testing. However, it was also recognized that over a longer time frame, an individual's maximal oxygen intake could change by up to 20% in response to changes in health and training status.[11]

The final arterial lactate values in the IBP trial, although less than the 30 m/L reported after some types of athletic competition,[12] were nevertheless substantially higher than those achieved in some laboratories, for example, 13.7 ± 1.7 and 12.7 ± 2.2 mM/L for the discontinuous and continuous treadmill tests respectively. The IBP data clearly demonstrate that given well-motivated subjects and an appropriate test protocol, young adults consistently reach an oxygen consumption plateau.

Technical Problems in Defining an Oxygen Consumption Plateau

Technical considerations are commonly to blame when there have been difficulties in demonstrating a plateau.[13,14] Specific issues include an inappropriate choice of test protocol, activation of an inadequate muscle mass, a lack of motivation on the part of the subject and/or the observer, specific characteristics of the population tested, and the existence of pathological conditions that lead to a premature termination of effort by the subject or the observer.

Test Protocol

In keeping with other authors,[15-17] the IBP recommended that a maximal oxygen intake test should begin after a 5-minute "warm up" at exercise demanding 50% to 70% of maximal oxygen intake. However, this precaution has not always been observed.[9,18] The definitive test must also be of sufficient duration in order to demonstrate a plateau. The first of a series of discontinuous tests should begin at 110% of the maximal oxygen intake, as estimated from the warmup data; subsequent tests should be set at slightly higher or lower work rates, depending on the subject's response to the first bout of exercise. A duration of 2-6 minutes seems appropriate for discontinuous measurements.[19,20] If a continuous ramp-function protocol is chosen, effort should begin at 90% to 100% of the individual's estimated maximal value; small increments of work rate (treadmill speed and/or slope) are then made in each subsequent 1- to 2-minute interval. The total duration of a continuous test is ideally 8 to 12 minutes,[21] although if the final treadmill slope is not excessive, valid results have been obtained over exercise times varying from 7 to 26 minutes.[9,18] Studies failing to demonstrate a plateau have adopted excessively large increments in the intensity of effort; often the subjects concerned have become exhausted before reaching the exercise intensity where an oxygen consumption plateau is likely to be observed.

Muscle Mass

Activation of an adequate muscle mass is a second important prerequisite for reaching an oxygen consumption plateau. The IBP Working Party suggested that in the average subject, this condition was best satisfied during uphill treadmill running.[9] The muscle volume was less adequate when tests were performed on a standard cycle ergometer; effort was then constrained in part by factors such as peripheral vascular capacity and a local limitation of blood flow through strongly contracting muscles.[9,22–25]

Most categories of athlete have a sport-specific development of their musculature, and their maximal oxygen intake is best measured when they are undertaking actual or simulated sport (using, for instance, pool or flume measurements on a swimmer, and rowing ergometer or telemetric measurements from a boat in the case of an oarsperson).

The relative importance of central (cardiac) and peripheral (muscular) limitations during different forms of exercise has been highlighted by two main approaches. A comparison of single- versus two-leg ergometry.[26] shows that the peak oxygen consumption during one-leg exercise is substantially more than a half of that seen during two-leg effort; in other words, greater perfusion of the leg muscles is possible when most of the cardiac output is directed to a single limb. If the peak oxygen intake when breathing room air is compared with that seen when breathing a gas mixture containing 12% oxygen,[27] the adverse impact of the hypoxic mixture increases in proportion to the volume of active muscle, because with greater muscle involvement the individual's effort is progressively limited by central oxygen transport rather than peripheral factors.

Motivation

Perhaps the most critical element in any measurement of maximal oxygen intake is the motivation of the subject and the investigator. It is essential to push the test participant to ever greater effort in the face of discomfort and a feeling of impending collapse. As the work rate is increased, the cardiac output becomes insufficient to sustain the ever growing demands of both the skeletal muscles and other tissues. The IBP article (p 759) gives a dramatic description of the failing circulation: "subjects complained of nausea, breathlessness and chest pain, looked intensely cyanosed, and in some cases became unsteady on their legs."[9] As early investigators realized,[1] much depends on the individual's determination and sense of physical self-efficacy.[28,29] Thus, ratings of perceived exertion[30,31] and other multidimensional perceptions of fatigue help in deciding whether the subject has made a valid maximal effort.[32] A cursory examination of peak values for secondary criteria such as arterial lactate, respiratory gas exchange ratio and ratings of perceived exertion underlines the problem that motivation has been inadequate in studies where a plateau of oxygen consumption has not been observed.

Population Characteristics

The IBP team recognized that although there were no problems when testing young male subjects, it was more difficult to demonstrate consistent plateau values in other populations such as young children, sedentary women and the elderly.

Children

Some authors have reported a plateau of oxygen intake in as few as one half[24,33] or one third[24,33] of young children, the likelihood of successful testing being greatest in fit children. One training study found a similar increment of peak oxygen transport in subjects who failed to reach a plateau, although the results for such individuals had a poor reliability.[34] The IBP investigators had the wisdom to invite their representative sample of 47 prepubescent children to the laboratory for a preliminary familiarization session. A single maximal treadmill test was performed at a subsequent visit, and 35 of the 47 subjects then demonstrated a clear oxygen consumption plateau. These subjects made what was judged as either a strenuous (final arterial lactate 11.7 ± 2.0 mM/L in boys, 12.2 ± 3.5 mM/L in girls) or an average effort (8.1 ± 0.3 mM/L in boys, 8.0 ± 0.5 mM/L in girls), and their final oxygen consumption values showed no systematic deviation from the maxima predicted from submaximal data. Comparable final lactate levels were observed by Åstrand,[33] but peak lactates were much lower in some recent reports (for instance, 5.4-6.5 mM/L in one study).[34] In the remaining 12 children who participated in the IBP study, effort was judged as inadequate; their terminal arterial lactate concentrations were 6.7 mM/L or less, and their peak oxygen intake values were substantially less than predicted from submaximal testing.

Elderly Subjects

Some authors have found no difficulty in testing older adults. Shephard and Sidney[35] examined the ability of seniors as old as 83 years to undertake maximal oxygen intake testing. The usual criterion of an oxygen consumption plateau was well satisfied by 18 of 26 elderly men and 19 of 29 elderly women (respective plateau readings of 0.5 ± 1.8 and 0.8 ± 1.4 mL/[kg·min], and final arterial lactate readings of 12.3 ± 3.7 and 10.1 ± 2.2 mM/L. The 18 individuals who failed to reach a plateau could readily be distinguished by subjective ratings of the quality of effort, a lower peak heart rate, a lower respiratory gas exchange ratio, and a lower final arterial lactate concentration (6 to 7 mM/L). Moreover, about a half of the individuals thus identified were able to reach a plateau at their second attempt.[35]

CONCLUSIONS

In young children and elderly subjects, a minority of individuals fail to reach the usually accepted definition of an oxygen consumtion plateau. However, such individuals can be identified fairly readily by a subjective rating of their motivation and objective measures of the effort that they achieved, particularly the final arterial lactate concentration, but including also peak heart rate and respiratory gas exchange ratio.

Pathological Conditions

One study demonstrated an oxygen consumption plateau in 20 of 36 patients undergoing rehabilitation following myocardial infarction.[36] Nevertheless, in many patients with cardiovascular disease, maximal effort may be halted by warning symptoms or signs,[37] such as irregularities of heart rhythm, depression of the ST segment of the electrocardiogram, and an excessive rise or a fall of blood pressure before an oxygen consumption plateau has been attained. The value thus observed is termed a peak rather than a maximal oxygen intake. As discussed below, the information may still have clinical value, particularly when setting an appropriate exercise prescription for the patient concerned.

Theoretical Basis of Oxygen Consumption Plateau

An analysis of oxygen concentrations along the transport chain from the lungs to the mitochondria[38,39] suggests that the efforts of both endurance athletes and more sedentary individuals are normally limited by circulatory factors.[40,41] However, in some circumstances peripheral influences such as muscle capillarity, the diffusion of oxygen from the capillaries to the mitochondria, and even the ability of the mitochondria to utilize oxygen can become the main limiting factor.[42,43] Poor motivation, the learning of competitive tactics or a failure of cerebral blood flow can also lead to a central limitation of neuromuscular drive.[44,45]

If a large muscle volume is activated, as in uphill treadmill running, then the maximal blood flow to the peripheral tissues is certainly the primary constraint.[46,47] The dominance of circulatory factors is strongly supported by a mathematical analysis of conductances in the oxygen transport chain.[38] However, top-level athletes sometimes show ventilatory limitations, with a significant decrease of arterial oxygen saturation during maximal effort.[48,49] The restrictions imposed by a finite pulmonary diffusing capacity of some 600 $mL \cdot min^{-1}\ kPa^{-1}$ are exacerbated by exposure to high altitudes, and by any trend to pulmonary edema during prolonged effort.[50] On occasion, an endurance athlete may also be limited by an inadequate circulatory transport of oxygen or glucose to the motor cortex, with a resulting failure of the motoneurons.[41,51]

If the volume of active muscle is small (for example, during arm ergometry), the critical factor limiting an 8- to 12-minute bout of exercise becomes a local accumulation of lactate in the working muscles; this progressively hampers the resynthesis of ATP and creatine phosphate.[43] Finally, in self-paced or poorly motivated effort, limits may be imposed by the individual's willingness to activate the neurons of the motor cortex.[45] Particularly during prolonged effort, athletes deliberately hold effort over most of an event to a level that minimizes lactate accumulation in the active muscle.

Factors Limiting Cardiac Output

The plateauing of oxygen intake with increasing effort normally occurs at or near maximal steady-state heart rate. Stroke volume plateaus at a lower intensity of effort, and it may actually show some decline as peak effort is approached. If a relatively small muscle mass is activated, a further consideration is the ability of the peripheral vasculature to accept the available blood flow without provoking an excessive rise of blood pressure.

Heart Rate

Many authors have found a plateauing of heart rate either before[9,52] or immediately following a plateauing of oxygen consumption.[35,53–55] The reason for the ceiling of steady-state heart rates remains unclear. Substantially higher values can be reached for brief periods (for instance, during a ski turn). Lower maxima are seen both at altitude and in the elderly; this might seem to indicate an influence of local oxygen lack upon the myocardium, as suggested by A.V. Hill.[5] But against this hypothesis, the administration of oxygen does not bring peak heart rates to the levels seen in young adults at sea level. Possibly, problems of diastolic filling may be involved, or baroreceptor reflexes may be activated by rising pressures in the systemic and pulmonary circulation; prolonged exercise also reduces the heart rate response to catecholamines.[44]

Stroke Volume

Changes of cardiac stroke volume with exercise depend on the individual's posture. During supine exercise, there may be little increase over resting values; however, in the upright position stroke volume increases progressively until the individual reaches the optimal part of the Frank-Starling curve, commonly around 70% of maximal oxygen intake.[56] In young adults, the stroke volume may then continue relatively unchanged through to maximal effort,[57-59] but in elderly subjects, the stroke volume sometimes decreases as maximal effort is approached.[60] This could reflect a limitation of venous return and/or impaired venous filling at rapid heart rates,[61] or changes in myocardial contractility.[62]

Other Feedback and Feed-Forward Controls

A variety of feedback and feed-forward controls can sometimes limit maximal cardiac output, and thus the transport of oxygen and nutrients needed for aerobic activity. Plainly, the stroke volume diminishes if a lack of venous return or a slow relaxation of the ventricles restricts diastolic filling. At the opposite end of the spectrum, an excess of diastolic filling pushes the heart muscle beyond the optimum point on the Frank-Starling curve, with a resulting decrease in myocardial contractility. The ejection fraction may be diminished further by the rising systolic pressure. A further potential restraint is the resistance to myocardial distension imposed by the pericardium.[63]

The circulation is regulated against an excessive rise of either systemic or pulmonary blood pressure by feedback from the baroreceptors, with additional influences from the central vasomotor centers, the muscle pressor reflex and central blood volume receptors.[64,65]

As cardiac output reaches its limiting value, the supply of oxygen and glucose to the brain may become inadequate. This leads to a failure of muscle coordination, a reduction of neuromuscular drive, and ultimately a loss of consciousness.

Finally, if the volume of active muscle is small, an inadequate peripheral circulation leads to a progressive accumulation of lactate; this in turn causes muscular pain and further effort is inhibited because the resynthesis of ATP and creatine phosphate is compromised.

Practical Uses of Maximal Oxygen Intake Measurements in Sports Medicine and Exercise Science

The practical applications of maximal oxygen intake measurements include objective determinations of habitual physical activity and resulting levels of aerobic fitness, prescribing appropriate intensities of exercise and training, assessing responses to conditioning programs, evaluation of the aerobic demands of various sports and the condition of individual participants, determination of the ergogenic potential of various drugs and procedures, the monitoring of over-training and rehabilitation, and specific clinical applications such as the prediction of prognosis and defining safe levels of exercise for those with cardiorespiratory disease.

Habitual Physical Activity and Aerobic Fitness

Accurate determinations of habitual physical activity are a pre-requisite when assessing the current fitness of populations,[2,4,66] examining secular trends in their fitness and lifestyle,[67] looking at the effectiveness of various community and work-site health promotion initiatives[68,69] and determining possible relationships between physical activity and the risks of various types of chronic disease.[4,70] Aerobic power measurements are also important when examining the ability of people to engage in various types of physically demanding occupations at various ages; such information is frequently required in discussions of equal opportunity in employment.[71]

Unfortunately, available physical activity questionnaires are notoriously inaccurate, and simple activity measuring instruments such as pedometers and accelerometers also fail to capture many significant sources of energy expenditure.[72] For this reason, it is preferable to base most analyses on the individual's response to regular aerobic activity, as shown by the level of his or her maximal oxygen intake; associations with health outcomes such as all-cause mortality are much stronger for measurements of aerobic fitness than for more direct estimates of habitual activity.[73] When making an epidemiological study of a large group, it may be possible to use predictions of aerobic fitness, based on treadmill endurance time or the heart rate observed during submaximal effort; such measurements generally do not have a large systematic error, but the imprecision of individual estimates attenuates relationships between fitness and health outcomes or work tolerance.[4] Thus, for accurate analyses, it is important to use direct measurements of maximal oxygen intake.

Exercise Prescription

The intensity of exercise needed to develop aerobic fitness is commonly expressed as a percentage of the individual's maximal oxygen intake; 50% of maximum is an appropriate starting value for an elderly person,[74] but 60% to 70% of maximum is a usual prescription for a younger adult.[4]

When recommending exercise to an ostensibly healthy young person, it may be sufficient to specify the intensity of effort by using such simple surrogates as the heart rates observed during a progressive submaximal exercise test, or the ability to maintain a conversation during the prescribed activity.[4,37] However, a more precise knowledge of the stimulus is required when undertaking laboratory studies of training; it is then advisable to make direct measurements of each participant's maximal oxygen intake and thus to obtain accurate information on the relative intensity of effort that has been undertaken. Even exercise prescriptions based on direct determinations of maximal oxygen intake are hampered by measurement errors of 4% to 5%, and somewhat larger intraindividual variations in maximal aerobic power related to the current health of the individual.[11] Moreover, it may be difficult to translate the findings of laboratory exercise on a treadmill to a corresponding load during sport; problems often arise from large inter-individual differences in the oxygen cost of popular activities such as swimming. Thus, a laboratory prescription of the intensity of exercise usually requires fine-tuning, based on direct observations of heart rates and dyspnea under field conditions.

Training Response

In general, changes in maximal oxygen intake provide a valid indication of the group response to both training programs and any subsequent detraining.[75] However, when evaluating an elderly person or someone with chronic disease, the initial test may be halted prematurely because of nervousness on the part of the subject or the investigator; further, if confidence is greater at a second visit to the laboratory, the resultant increase in peak oxygen intake may exaggerate the true training response.[74]

When assessing an individual, it is important to recognize that the percentage error of the difference between paired maximal oxygen intake measurements ($\sqrt{[5^2] + [5^2]}$) is quite large relative to the likely training response (a 10% to 20% gain in maximal oxygen intake). Moreover, initial aberrant measurements tend to show a regression towards the mean if they are repeated.[76,77]

Evaluation of Athletes

The extent of inter-individual differences of physiological characteristics between top-level athletes in any given discipline is quite small, and the competitive outcome usually depends more on technique and motivation than on biology. The laboratory measurement of maximal oxygen intake thus contributes little to the selection process.[78] However, if a competitor has a low maximal oxygen intake relative to peers who are engaged in the same sport and at the same level of competition, then he or she may need to focus more specifically on aerobic training. A comparison of average maximal oxygen intake values between sport disciplines or between playing positions within a given discipline also provides a measure of the importance of oxygen transport to success in a given class of activity.[78]

Noakes has suggested that the measurement of maximal oxygen intake is unrealistic when assessing an athlete, because the intensity of effort on a laboratory treadmill is determined by the observer rather than the competitor.[8] However, this does not seem a valid objection. It is quite possible (and indeed desirable) to test the athlete for 8 to 12 minutes under self-paced and realistic conditions (for example, when cycling on rollers, swimming in a pool where a metabolic cart is pushed alongside the competitor, or rowing with telemetric transmission of data to the laboratory).[78] Pacing is certainly a key to success in many types of aerobic competition, and skilled competitors select a pace that avoids an excessive build-up of lactate until the final few seconds of their event.[4] But this practice does not negate the value of maximal oxygen intake measurements. Indeed, in longer events such as a marathon run, the fraction of the maximal oxygen intake that the athlete can sustain during several hours of activity is an important determinant of race outcome.[79]

Assessment of Potentially Ergogenic Drugs and Procedures

Demonstration that the maximal oxygen intake is unchanged after the administration of a potentially ergogenic drug such as a beta-agonist is helpful to international committees that must determine for competitors an acceptable range of medications, permitted dosages and routes of administration.[80] Accurate measurements of maximal oxygen intake are also invaluable when gauging the effects upon performance of exposure to unusual environments (for instance, competition at high altitude), optimal approaches to acclimatization,[81] and the value of specific adaptive regimens such as "living high, training low."[82]

Monitoring of Overtraining and Rehabilitation

Excessive training can lead to a decrease in an athlete's performance (over-reaching and over-training).[83] Performance statistics and psychological data provide the clearest evidence of such a problem,[84] but overtraining also leads to a progressive decrease in the athlete's maximal oxygen intake; a laboratory can use such data to monitor both the extent of the disorder and the course of recovery.

The immobility associated with a serious injury or illness also leads to a quite rapid decrease in aerobic power, and serial measurements of maximal oxygen intake are helpful in monitoring the recovery process.[75]

Clinical Applications

The measurement of maximal oxygen intake in itself has little diagnostic value, but it does provide a helpful index of the severity of various cardio-respiratory disorders, and the ability to sustain independent living as age advances.[85] Clinicians have become particularly interested in the potential of maximal aerobic power to indicate overall prognosis in conditions such as myocardial infarction, chronic heart disease and cardiac transplantation.[86,87] Whether making an immediate assessment or estimating long-term prognosis, the measurement of maximal oxygen intake is probably providing an assessment of myocardial health, which is a central determinant of outcome in chronic cardio-respiratory disease.

In many patients, the laboratory test may be limited by the onset of symptoms such as anginal pain, or the appearance of adverse signs such as abnormalities of heart rhythm or an excessive depression of the ST segment of the electrocardiogram. The measured value is then described as a peak rather than a maximal oxygen intake, although sometimes there may be little difference between the peak and a true plateau value, and the peak figure continues to indicate prognosis for the patient.[88]

It is important to ensure that clinical tests are not halted prematurely because of excessive anxiety on the part of the patient or the supervising physician. If anxiety is reduced at a second visit, a larger peak oxygen intake may exaggerate any training response. A preliminary familiarization visit to the laboratory contributes to a successful evaluation. If testing is well performed, it can define a safe upper limit to the intensity of effort that a patient should undertake, and indicate the response to rehabilitation.[89]

Conclusions

The measurement of maximal oxygen intake continues to offer a precision measure of oxygen transport, important in many areas of sports medicine and exercise science. Young adults should be tested using a progressive, activity-specific exercise protocol, carried to a plateau of oxygen consumption as specified by the International Biological Programme. Such data offer helpful assessments of current physical activity and aerobic fitness. The findings are fundamental to both the prescription of aerobic exercise and the evaluation of differences, whether between populations or in response to interventions such as a training program, environmental change or administration of ergogenic aids. In some clinical conditions, it is only possible to determine a peak oxygen intake. Nevertheless, limiting signs and symptoms can be noted. Myocardial function is an important determinant of peak oxygen intake, and peak values thus provide an important indication of prognosis in chronic cardiorespiratory disease.

References

1. Taylor HL, Buskirk ER, Henschel A. Maximal oxygen intake as an objective measure of cardio-respiratory performance. *J Appl Physiol.* 1955;8:73-80.
2. Shephard RJ. *Human Physiological Work Capacity.* Cambridge, UK: Cambridge University Press; 1978.
3. Shephard RJ. Tests of maximum oxygen intake. A critical review. *Sports Med.* 1984;1:99-124.
4. Shephard RJ. *Aerobic Fitness and Health.* Champaign, IL: Human Kinetics; 1994.
5. Hill AV, Long CN, Lupton H. Muscular exercise, lactic acid and the supply and utilization of oxygen. *Proc R Soc Lond B Biol Sci.* 1924-5;96/97:438-475. 84-138; 155-176.
6. Myers J, Walsh D, Buchanan N, et al. Can maximal cardiopulmonary capacity be recognized by a plateau in oxygen uptake? *Chest.* 1989;96:1312-1316.
7. Noakes TD. How did A.V. Hill understand the $\dot{V}O_{2max}$ and the "plateau phenomenon"? Still no clarity? *Br J Sports Med.* 2008;42:574-580.
8. Noakes TD. Testing for maximum oxygen consumption has produced a brainless model of human exercise performance. *Br J Sports Med.* 2008;42:551-555.
9. Shephard RJ, Allen C, Benade AJS, et al. The maximum oxygen intake. An international reference standard of cardiorespiratory fitness. *Bull World Health Organ.* 1968;38:757-764.
10. Macfarlane DJ. Automated metabolic gas analysis systems: a review. *Sports Med.* 2001;31:841-861.
11. Wright GR, Sidney KH, Shephard RJ. Variance of direct and indirect measurements of aerobic power. *J Sports Med Phys Fitness.* 1978;18:33-42.
12. Nielsen HB. pH after competitive rowing: the lower physiological range? *Acta Physiol Scand.* 1999;165:113-114.
13. Astorino TA, Willey J, Kinnahan J, Larsson SM, Welch H, Dalleck LC. Elucidating determinants of the plateau in oxygen consumption at $\dot{V}O_{2max}$. *Br J Sports Med.* 2005;39:655-660.
14. Bentley DJ, Newell J, Bishop D. Incremental exercise test design and analysis: implications for performance diagnostics in endurance athletes. *Sports Med.* 2007;37:575-586.
15. Taylor AH, Cable NT, Faulkner G, Hillsdon M, Narici M, Van Der Bij AK. Physical activity and older adults: a review of health benefits and the effectiveness of interventions. *J Sports Sci.* 2004;22:703-725.
16. Pirnay F, Petit JM, Bottin R, Deroanne R, Juchmes J, Belge G. Comparaison de deux méthodesde mésure de la consommation maximum d'oxygène. *Int Z Angew Physiol.* 1966;23:203-211.
17. Martin BJ, Robinson S, Wiegman DL, Aulick LH. Effect of warm-up on metabolic response to strenuous exercise. *Med Sci Sports.* 1975;7:146-149.
18. Midgley AW, Bentley DJ, Luttikholt H, McNaughton LR, Millet GP. Challenging a dogma of exercise physiology: does an incremental exercise test for valid $\dot{V}O_{2max}$ determination really need to last between 8 and 12 minutes? *Sports Med.* 2008;38:441-447.
19. Midgley AW, McNaughton LR, Carroll S. Physiological determinants of time to exhaustion during intermittent treadmill running at $\dot{V}O_{2max}$. *Int J Sports Med.* 2006;28:273-280.
20. Hill DW, Poole DC, Smith JC. The relationship between power and the time to achieve $\dot{V}O_{2max}$. *Med Sci Sports Exerc.* 2002;34:709-714.
21. Buchfuhrer MJ, Hansen JE, Robinson TE, Sue DY, Wasserman K, Whipp BJ. Optimizing the exercise protocol for cardiopulmonary assessment. *J Appl Physiol.* 1983;55:1558-1564.
22. Hoes M, Binkhorst RA, Smeekes-Kuyl A, Vissers AC. Measurement of forces exerted on a pedal crank during work on the bicycle ergometer at different loads. *Int Z Angew Physiol.* 1968;26:33-42.

23. Davies CTM. The contribution of leg (muscle plus bone) volume to maximal aerobic power output: the effects of anemia, malnutrition and physical activity. *J Physiol.* 1973;231:108P-109P.
24. Cumming GR, Friesen W. Bicycle ergometer measurement of maximal oxygen uptake in children. *Can J Physiol Pharmacol.* 1967;45:937-946.
25. Glassford RC, Bayford GH, Sedgwick AW, Macnab RB. Comparison of maximal oxygen uptake values determined by predicted and actual methods. *J Appl Physiol.* 1965;20:509-513.
26. Davies CTM, Sargeant AJ. Physiologic responses to one- and two-leg exercise breathing air and 45% oxygen. *J Appl Physiol.* 1974;36:142-148.
27. Shephard RJ, Bouhlel E, Vandewalle H, Monod H. Muscle mass as a factor limiting physical work. *J Appl Physiol.* 1988;64:1472-1479.
28. Tenenbaum G, Hall HK, Calcagnini N, Lange R, Freeman G, Lloyd M. Coping with physical exertion and negative feedback under competitive and self-standard conditions. *J Appl Soc Psychol.* 2001;31:1582-1626.
29. Midgley AW, McNaughton LR, Polman R, Marchant D. Criteria for determination of maximal oxygen uptake: a brief critique and recommendations for future research. *Sports Med.* 2007;37:1019-1028.
30. Borg GA. Perceived exertion. *Exerc Sport Sci Rev.* 1974;2:131-153.
31. Noble BJ, Robertson RJ. *Perceived Exertion.* Champaign, IL: Human Kinetics; 1996.
32. Hutchinson JC, Tenenbaum G. Perceived effort—Can it be considered Gestalt? *Psychol Sport Exerc.* 2006;7:463-476.
33. Åstrand PO. *Experimental Studies of Physical Working Capacity in Relation to Age and Sex.* Copenhagen: Munksgaard; 1952.
34. Cunningham DA, van Waterschoot BM, Paterson DH, Lefcoe M, Sangal SP. Reliability and reproducibility of maximal oxygen uptake measurement in children. *Med Sci Sports.* 1977;9:104-108.
35. Sidney KH, Shephard RJ. Maximum and submaximum exercise tests in men and women in the seventh, eighth, and ninth decades of life. *J Appl Physiol.* 1977;43:280-287.
36. Kavanagh T, Shephard RJ. Maximum exercise tests on "postcoronary" patients. *J Appl Physiol.* 1976;40:611-618.
37. American College of Sports Medicine. *ACSM's Guidelines for Exercise Testing and Prescription.* 6th ed. Philadelphia, PA: Lippincott, Williams & Wilkins; 2000.
38. Shephard RJ. The oxygen conductance equation. In: Shephard RJ, ed. *Frontiers of Fitness.* Springfield, IL: C.C. Thomas; 1971:129-164.
39. Wagner PD. Algebraic analysis of the determinants of $\dot{V}O_{2max}$. *Resp Physiol.* 1993;93:221-237.
40. Bassett DR, Howley ET. Maximal oxygen uptake: "classical" versus "contemporary" viewpoints. *Med Sci Sports Exerc.* 1997;29:591-603.
41. Secher NH. Cardiorespiratory limitations to performance. In: Maughan RJ, ed. *The Olympic Textbook of Science in Sport.* Chichester, UK: Wiley-Blackwell; 2009:307-323.
42. Harms CA. Effect of skeletal muscle demand on cardiovascular function. *Med Sci Sports Exerc.* 2000;32:94-99.
43. Stephens FB, Greenhaff PL. Metabolic limitations to performance. In: Maughan RJ, ed. *The Olympic Textbook of Science in Sport.* Chichester, UK: Wiley-Blackwell; 2009:324-339.
44. Wagner PD, Secher NH. Maximal exercise: is it centrally or peripherally limited?. In: Taylor NAS, Groeller H, McLennan P, eds. *Physiological Bases of Human Performance During Work and Exercise.* Edinburgh, Scotland: Elsevier; 2008:170-176.
45. Noakes TD, Crews H, Tucker R. The brain and fatigue. In: Maughan RJ, ed. *The Olympic Textbook of Science in Sport.* Chichester, UK: Wiley-Blackwell; 2009:340-364.

46. Andersen P, Saltin B. Maximal perfusion of skeletal muscle in man. *J Physiol.* 1985;366:233-249.
47. Rowell LB. *Human Cardiovascular Control.* New York, NY: Oxford University Press; 1993.
48. Dempsey JA, Wagner PD. Exercise-induced arterial hypoxemia. *J Appl Physiol.* 1999;87:1997-2006.
49. Nielsen HB, Boushel R, Madsen P, Secher NH. Cerebral desaturation during exercise reversed by O_2 supplementation. *Am J Physiol.* 1999;277:H1045-H1052.
50. Hanel B, Law I, Mortensen J. Maximal rowing has an acute effect on the blood-gas barrier in elite athletes. *J Appl Physiol.* 2003;95:1076-1082.
51. Dalsgaard MK. Fuelling cerebral activity in exercising man. *J Cereb Blood Flow Metab.* 2006;26:731-750.
52. Åstrand I. Aerobic work capacity. Its relation to age, sex and other factors. *Circulation Res.* 1960;20:211-217.
53. Cumming GR, Borysyk LM. Criteria for maximum oxygen intake in men over 40 in a population survey. *Med Sci Sports.* 1972;4:18-22.
54. Davies CTM. Limitations to the prediction of maximum oxygen intake from cardiac frequency measurements. *J Appl Physiol.* 1968;24:700-706.
55. Wyndham CH, Strydom NB, Maritz JS, Morrison JF, Peter J, Potgieter ZU. Maximum oxygen intake and maximum heart rate during strenuous work. *J Appl Physiol.* 1959;14:927-936.
56. Shephard RJ. *Physiology and Biochemistry of Exercise.* New York, NY: Praeger Publications; 1982.
57. González-Alonso J. Point: Stroke volume does/does not decline during exercise at maximal effort in healthy individuals. *J Appl Physiol.* 2006;104:275-276.
58. Beck KC, Lakesha NR, Bailey KR, Wood CM, Snyder EM, Johnson BD. Relationship between cardiac output and oxygen consumption during upright cycle exercise in healthy humans. *J Appl Physiol.* 2006;101:1474-1480.
59. Vella CA, Robergs RA. Non-linear relationships between central cardiovascular variables and •VO_2 during incremental cycling exercise in endurance-trained individuals. *J Sports Med Phys Fitness.* 2005;45:452-459.
60. Strandell T. Heart rate and work load at maximal working intensities in old men. *Acta Med Scand.* 1964;176:301-318.
61. Mortensen SP, Dawson EA, Yoshiga CC, et al. Limitations to systemic and locomotor limb muscle oxygen delivery and uptake during maximal exercise in humans. *J Physiol.* 2005;566:273-285.
62. Faulkner JA, Roberts DE, Elk RL, Conway J. Cardiovascular responses to submaximum and maximum effort cycling and running. *J Appl Physiol.* 1971; 30:457-461.
63. Noakes TD, Secher NH. Human performance and maximal aerobic power. In: Taylor NAS, Groeller H, McLennan P, eds. *Physiological Bases of Human Performance During Work and Exercise.* Edinburgh, Scotland: Elsevier; 2008.
64. Gallagher K, Fadel PJ, Strømstad M, et al. Effect of exercise pressor reflex activation on carotid baroreflex function during exercise in humans. *J Physiol.* 2001;533:871-880.
65. Ogoh S, Volianitis S, Nissen P, Wray DW, Secher NH, Raven PB. Carotid baroreflex responsiveness to head-up tilt induced central hypovolaemia: effect of aerobic fitness. *J Physiol.* 2003;551:601-608.
66. Tomkinson GR, Olds TS. *Pediatric Fitness: Secular Trends and Geographic Variability.* Basel, Switzerland: Karger Publications; 2007.
67. Shephard RJ, Rode A. *The Health Consequences of 'Modernization.' Evidence from Circumpolar Peoples.* London, UK: Cambridge University Press; 1996.
68. Shephard RJ. A critical analysis of work-site fitness programs and their postulated economic benefits. *Med Sci Sports Exerc.* 1992;24:354-370.
69. Shephard RJ. Effectiveness of training programs for prepubescent children. *Sports Med.* 1992;13:194-213.
70. Bouchard C, Shephard RJ, Stephens T. *Physical Activity, Fitness and Health.* Champaign, IL: Human Kinetics; 1994.

71. Shephard RJ. Assessment of occupational fitness in the context of human rights legislation. *Can J Sport Sci.* 1990;15:89-95.
72. Montoye HJ, Kemper HCG, Saris WHM, et al. *Measuring Physical Activity and Energy Expenditure.* Champaign, IL: Human Kinetics; 1996.
73. Blair SN, Kohl KW, Paffenbarger RS, Clark DG, Cooper KH, Gibbons LW. Physical fitness and all-cause mortality. A prospective study of healthy men and women. *JAMA.* 1989;262:2395-2401.
74. Shephard RJ. *Aging, Physical Activity and Health.* Champaign, IL: Human Kinetics; 1997.
75. Saltin B, Blomqvist G, Mitchell JH, et al. Response to exercise after bed rest and after training: a longitudinal study of adaptive changes in oxygen transport and body composition. *Circulation.* 1968;38:VII-1-VII-78.
76. Shephard RJ. Regression to the mean. A threat to exercise science? *Sports Med.* 2003;33:575-584.
77. Shephard RJ, Rankinen T, Bouchard C. Test-retest errors and the apparent heterogeneity of training response. *Eur J Appl Physiol.* 2004;91:199-203.
78. Shephard RJ, Åstrand P-O. *Endurance in Sport.* Oxford, UK: Blackwell Science; 2000.
79. Costill DL. Physiology of marathon running. *JAMA.* 1972;221:1024-1029.
80. Naranjo Orellana J, Centeno Prada RA, Carranza Márquez MD. Use of β_2 agonists in sport: are the present criteria right? *Br J Sports Med.* 2006;40:363-366.
81. Shephard RJ. Problems of high altitude. In: Shephard RJ, Åstrand PO, eds. *Endurance in Sport.* 2nd ed. Oxford, UK: Blackwell Science; 2000:614-627.
82. Levine BD, Stray-Gundersen J. "Living high-training low": effect of moderate altitude acclimatization with low altitude training on performance. *J Appl Physiol.* 1997;83:102-112.
83. Meeusen R. The overtraining syndrome. In: Schwellnus MP, ed. *Olympic Textbook of Medicine in Sport.* Chichester, UK: Wiley-Blackwell; 2008:138-159.
84. Verde T, Thomas S, Shephard RJ. Potential markers of heavy training in highly trained distance runners. *Br J Sports Med.* 1992;26:167-175.
85. Jones NL, Campbell EJM, Edwards R, Robertson DG. *Clinical Exercise Testing.* Philadelphia, PA: Saunders; 1975.
86. Kavanagh T, Hamm LF, Beyene J, et al. Usefulness of improvement in walking distance versus peak oxygen uptake in predicting prognosis after myocardial infarction and/or coronary artery bypass grafting in men. *Am J Cardiol.* 2008;101:1423-1427.
87. Kavanagh T, Mertens DJ, Hamm LF, et al. Peak oxygen intake and cardiac mortality in women referred for cardiac rehabilitation. *J Am Coll Cardiol.* 2003;42:2139-2143.
88. Day JR, Rossiter HB, Coats EM, Skasick A, Whipp BJ. The maximally attainable $\dot{V}O_2$ during exercise in humans: the peak vs. maximum issue. *J Appl Physiol.* 2003;95:1901-1907.
89. Shephard RJ. *Ischemic Heart Disease and Exercise.* London, UK: Croom Helm; 1981.

1 Epidemiology, Prevention of Injuries, Lesions of Head and Neck

Bicycle-related injuries in children: Disturbing profile of a growing problem

Klin B, Rosenfeld-Yehoshua N, Abu-Kishk I, et al (Assaf Harofeh Med Ctr, Zerifin, Israel)

Injury 40:1011-1013, 2009

Context.—We observed a changing pattern of bicycle-related injuries in children, with the focus changing from head trauma to thoracic and abdominal injuries, and a trend to increasingly severe injuries.

Objective.—To assess the changing injury pattern, and investigate the development of preventive measures to improve safety.

Design, Setting, and Participants.—Retrospective record review of 142 paediatric patients admitted to our Department of Paediatric Surgery between 1996 and 2005 following bicycle-related injuries. Clinical, laboratory, diagnostic, and therapeutic aspects were analysed. Additional information concerning children's bicycle-related injuries in Israel was obtained from the Gertner Institute (Israel National Center for Trauma and Emergency Medicine Research) and from Beterem (The National Center for Children's Safety & Health, the Safe Kids Israeli Chapter) National Report on Child Injuries in Israel 2006.

Main Outcome Measures.—The nature and severity of injuries were reviewed, and two 5-year periods compared—from 1996 to 2000 (53 children—Group 1), and from 2001 to 2005 (89 children—Group 2).

Results.—Head trauma was more common in the Group 1 patients (52.6% vs. 45.2%), but skull fractures and intracranial haemorrhage occurred more frequently in Group 2 (28.5% vs. 16.7%; 21.3% vs. 8.3%, respectively). Injury to the stomach or duodenum, kidneys and liver were all more common in Group 2. Splenic injury occurred with equal frequency in both groups, but more severe injuries were seen in Group 2. More children in Group 2 required intensive care (31% vs. 19.3%).

Conclusions.—There is a changing pattern of bicycle-related injuries in children, with chest and abdominal injuries dominating, and an increasing incidence of more severe injury. These findings are important in decision-making regarding preventive measures.

▶ This study from Israel showed a small decrease in incidence of head trauma—but greater severity—from bicycle accidents in a comparison of hospital admissions between 1996-2000 and 2001-2005. The article does not indicate how many had been wearing safety helmets. A major media campaign was initiated in 1997 in that country encouraging use of helmets, but legislation requiring their use was not passed until after this study period. So, in a sense, this study describes an untreated control group with which to contrast reductions in head injuries of up to 85% in other countries when helmet use was mandated. This much seems clear—cycle helmet regulations are effective for protecting the craniums of our children. However, and less optimistically, half of the accidents in this report involve serious trauma to locations other than the head. Cycle accidents are a serious business. As we encourage children to be more active—walking, cycling, running—we must increase efforts to assure the safety of these activities. For cycling that means not just passing and enforcing helmet regulations, but also by improving cycle safety education for youth and the general public alike.

T. Rowland, MD

Cheerleading-related injuries in the United States: A prospective surveillance study

Shields BJ, Smith GA (Nationwide Children's Hosp, Columbus, OH; Ohio State Univ College of Medicine, Columbus)

J Athl Train 4:567-577, 2009

Context.—Cheerleading injuries are on the rise and are a significant source of injury to females. No published studies have described the epidemiology of cheerleading injuries by type of cheerleading team and event.

Objective.—To describe the epidemiology of cheerleading injuries and to calculate injury rates by type of cheerleading team and event.

Design.—Prospective injury surveillance study.

Setting.—Participant exposure and injury data were collected from US cheerleading teams via the Cheerleading RIO (Reporting Information Online) online surveillance tool.

Patients or Other Participants.—Athletes from enrolled cheerleading teams who participated in official, organized cheerleading practices, pep rallies, athletic events, or cheerleading competitions.

Main Outcome Measure(s).—The numbers and rates of cheerleading injuries during a 1-year period (2006–2007) are reported by team type and event type.

Results.—A cohort of 9022 cheerleaders on 412 US cheerleading teams participated in the study. During the 1-year period, 567 cheerleading injuries were reported; 83% (467/565) occurred during practice, 52% (296/565) occurred while the cheerleader was attempting a stunt, and 24% (132/563) occurred while the cheerleader was basing or spotting 1 or more cheerleaders. Lower extremity injuries (30%, 168/565) and strains and sprains (53%, 302/565) were most common. Collegiate cheerleaders were more likely to sustain a concussion (P=.01, rate ratio [RR] = 2.98, 95% confidence interval [CI] = 1.34, 6.59), and All Star cheerleaders were more likely to sustain a fracture or dislocation (P=.01, RR = 1.76, 95% CI = 1.16, 2.66) than were cheerleaders on other types of teams. Overall injury rates for practices, pep rallies, athletic events, and cheerleading competitions were 1.0, 0.6, 0.6, and 1.4 injuries per 1000 athlete-exposures, respectively.

Conclusions.—We are the first to report cheerleading injury rates based on actual exposure data by type of team and event. These injury rates are lower than those reported for other high school and collegiate sports; however, many cheerleading injuries are preventable.

▶ Through our work with the National Center for Catastrophic Sports Injury Research with Dr Fred Mueller, we have published data that indicate the risk of catastrophic head and neck injury in cheerleading is higher than any other organized sport. Although it is difficult to get a precise denominator for just how many cheerleaders are actually flyers, it is estimated that the risk of catastrophic head and neck injury is 16 times higher for a flyer in cheerleading than in other sports of known high risk for head and neck injuries such as football, ice hockey, and gymnastics.

With regard to catastrophic injuries, the incidence seems to be higher when athletes were attempting stunts for which they had not been properly trained or supervised or spotted.

In this study, the authors—on the opposite side of information from observed reports and other publications—found that experience, qualifications, and training of cheerleading coaches did not seem to have an effect on cheerleading injury rates, nor did they find a lower injury rate when the cheerleaders were supervised by more experienced, trained, and qualified coaches.

Most findings in this article coincide with other published reports in cheerleading injury, namely that the lower extremity is the most frequently injured body part, with the ankle being the most often-injured body site. Strains and sprains were the most common types of injuries, and most injuries occurred during gymnastic maneuvers or partner stunts and pyramids.

Some of the limitations of this study are that only about half of the selected cheerleading groups enrolled in this online injury surveillance report participated in the study. Also, the reporters were usually not certified athletic trainers and, therefore, there can be some doubt as to the accuracy of the injury reported.

Overall, though, this was an interesting study that adds to the published information on the injury rates in this extremely high-risk activity—especially as it pertains to the flyer.

R. C. Cantu, MD, MA

Commotio Cordis and the Epidemiology of Sudden Death in Competitive Lacrosse

Maron BJ, Doerer JJ, Haas TS, et al (Hypertrophic Cardiomyopathy Ctr, Minneapolis, MN; et al)
Pediatrics 124:966-971, 2009

Objective.—Athletic field risks associated with blunt, nonpenetrating chest blows (commotio cordis) are receiving increasing attention, but the epidemiology of these events is incomplete.

Methods.—We assessed our Sudden Death in Young Athletes Registry, 1980–2008, to formulate a clinical profile of those sudden deaths attributed to commotio cordis (and other causes) occurring in competitive lacrosse, the most rapidly growing youth sport in the United States.

Results.—Twenty-three sudden deaths or cardiac arrests were identified in high school and college lacrosse participants. Ages were 18 ± 2 years; each athlete was male. Ten died after blunt precordial blows, including 4 goalies wearing commercially available chest protectors. Twelve others collapsed because of presumed or documented cardiovascular disease, including hypertrophic cardiomyopathy, long QT syndrome, mitral valve prolapse, or ruptured cerebral aneurysm. The mortality rate associated with lacrosse was 1.46 deaths per 100 000 person-years and was similar to that of other sports including baseball, basketball, football, and hockey. However, deaths attributed to commotio cordis were more frequent in lacrosse (0.63 deaths per 100 000 person-years) than in other sports ($P < .02$), with the exception of hockey.

Conclusions.—Sudden deaths in competitive lacrosse participants are rare and no more common than in most other sports. These catastrophic events were caused disproportionately by commotio cordis and included athletes wearing chest barriers, thereby underscoring the importance of developing effective chest protection to create a safer athletic environment for our youth.

▶ We've become much more aware of commotio cordis: the tragedy of youth collapsing and dying suddenly after being struck in the chest (usually with a ball). Experimental evidence suggests that these fatalities are essentially a matter of bad luck, the youngster's heart receiving this blow at a particularly sensitive period in the cardiac cycle, which triggers ventricular fibrillation. This study documents the frequency of such events during lacrosse play; other sports often involved are baseball and hockey. Fortunately, the incidence of such tragedies is very low (in this survey, 10 events in the United States over a period of 28 years). The bad news is that there seems to be no easy answer to preventing these tragedies. Some have advocated stronger chest protectors or reducing the weight of baseballs. What might work, or even be feasible, remains problematic.

T. Rowland, MD

Declining Incidence of Catastrophic Cervical Spine Injuries in French Rugby: 1996-2006

Bohu Y, Julia M, Bagate C, et al (Univ of Paris VI, France; Fédération Française de Rugby, Paris, France; et al)
Am J Sports Med 37:319-323, 2009

Purpose.—To investigate the incidence and the risk factors of catastrophic cervical spine injuries in French rugby.

Study Design.—Descriptive epidemiology study.

Methods.—The patients included had cervical spine injuries causing neurological disorder classified from the ASIA scale, grade A to D. A retrospective review of all cases that occurred between the 1996-1997 and the 2005-2006 seasons was made. Circumstances of the injuries and of the clinical outcome were collected by interview.

Results.—There were 37 cases of catastrophic cervical spine injuries in French rugby for the last 10 years. The incidence of the cervical spine injuries decreased during this period. The rates of injury were 2.1 per 100 000 players per year during the 1996-1997 season and 1.4 during the 2005-2006 season ($P < .01$). The scrum was a major cause of injury, accounting for 51.3% (19/37). The forwards represented 89.2% (33/37) of the injured players. The hookers were involved in 37.8% (14/37) of the cases. The measures of prevention with the modification of the rules of scrum and the creation of a medical certificate required for players to play in the front row must have been successful.

Conclusion.—The incidence of disabling cervical spine injuries in French rugby has decreased for the last 10 years, which is linked to the decreasing incidence of injuries in the scrum. This epidemiological study shows the effectiveness of the preventive measures on cervical spine injuries in French rugby players. A national register of catastrophic cervical spine injuries extends our epidemiological observations.

► This is a very interesting article for those who are afficionados of the game of rugby. The authors have done a retrospective review (by way of a structured interview) of all identified cases of catastrophic cervical spine injuries (CCSIs) in French rugby over a 10-year time span (1996-2006). They have categorized the injuries based on the American Spinal Injuries Association (ASIA) scale A to D and have also broken out the different age categories, phase of play, and position of the player. Without any information on the number of player hours, they used the number of registered players (obtained from the French Rugby Union) as the denominator to estimate the average yearly incidence of spinal injuries per 100 000 players. With this descriptive epidemiological design, they noted both an overall general decrease in incidence of CCSIs during this time period and a change in injury pattern following rule changes about scrums in French rugby at the beginning of the 2000-2001 season. This also included the institution of a rugby passport that specifies the capacity of the player to play in the front row, based on a medical examination confirming both skill and morphological capacity to compete in a scrum.

Some of the weaknesses of the study are identified by the authors in the discussion. There are other sources of potential bias, such as exclusion of players with head trauma or fatal injuries from the numerator. The statement in the Abstract under Results, "The measures of prevention...MUST have been successful," is a bit strong and technically not really right as cause and effect have not been proven. Nevertheless, this article provides a good description of the position of the players in the scrum and the most probable mechanism of cervical spine injury. It compares the data with that available from several other countries and correctly suggests that the most effective prevention is a public awareness campaign concerning all participants in rugby and that further prospective studies are necessary.

C. Lebrun, MD

Mountain Biking Injuries in Children and Adolescents

Aleman KB, Meyers MC (West Texas A and M Univ, Canyon)
Sports Med 40:77-90, 2010

Over the last decade, the sport of mountain biking has experienced extensive growth in youth participation. Due to the unpredictable nature of outdoor sport, a lack of rider awareness and increased participation, the number of injuries has unnecessarily increased. Many believe that the actual incidence of trauma in this sport is underestimated and is just the 'tip of the iceberg'. The most common mechanism of injury is usually attributed to downhill riding and forward falling. Although rare, this type of fall can result in serious cranial and thoraco-abdominal trauma. Head and neck trauma continue to be documented, often resulting in concussions and the possibility of permanent neurological sequelae. Upper limb injuries range from minor dermal abrasions, contusions and muscular strains to complex particular fracture dislocations. These are caused by attempting to arrest the face with an outstretched hand, leading to additional direct injury. Common overuse injuries include repeated compression from the handlebars and vibration leading to neurovascular complications in the hands. Along with reports of blunt abdominal trauma and lumbar muscle strains, lower extremity injuries may include various hip/pelvic/groin contusions, patellofemoral inflammation, and various muscle strains. The primary causes of mountain biking injuries in children and adolescents include overuse, excessive fatigue, age, level of experience, and inappropriate or improperly adjusted equipment. Additional factors contributing to trauma among this age group involve musculoskeletal immaturity, collisions and falls, excessive speed, environmental conditions, conditioning and fitness status of the rider, nonconservative behavioural patterns, and inadequate medical care. The limited available data restrict the identification and understanding of specific paediatric mountain biking injuries and injury mechanisms. Education about unnecessary risk of injury, use of protective equipment, suitable bikes and proper riding technique, coupled with attentive and proper behaviour, are encouraged to reduce unnecessary injury. This article provides information on the causation and risk factors associated with injury among young mountain bikers, and recommendations to minimize trauma and enhance optimal performance and long-term enjoyment in this outdoor sport.

▶ Participation in sports has to be undertaken with an understanding of the risks involved and how they might be minimized. It seems that the thrill of sport play and the challenges that it brings are often directly related to such risk. And with youth increasingly involved in the adult realm of highly competitive sport, we are encountering increasing concern regarding the safety of these activities for young people. Typically, the popularity of a particular sport escalates in the population well in advance of an understanding of the risks involved and, most particularly, of the proper education of participants. As a result, this study is timely. I do not think anyone would be astonished with the findings. Risk of injury is high in mountain biking in children, factors such as fatigue and inadequate preparation and equipment are identified, and we are in need of much better safety education for young people participating in this activity. Organizers of sport activities for children have a responsibility for not only promoting the growth of their sport but also assuring the safety of its young competitors.

T. Rowland, MD

No injuries, but plenty of pain? On the methodology for recording overuse symptoms in sports

Bahr R (Oslo Sports Trauma Res Ctr, Norway)

Br J Sports Med 43:966-972, 2009

Overuse injuries may represent as much of a problem as do acute injuries in many sports. This paper reviews key concepts related to the methodology for recording overuse symptoms. Results from the FIVB Volleyball Injury Study were used to compare two different recording methods. The aim of this paper was to provide recommendations on how standardised methodology can be developed to quantify overuse injuries in surveillance studies. Using beach volleyball data, a "traditional" cohort study approach using a time-loss injury definition suggested that injury risk was very low. In contrast, the data from a survey of past and present pain problems in the shoulder, knees and low back demonstrated that these were prevalent. The following recommendations are made: (1) studies should be prospective, with continuous or serial measurements

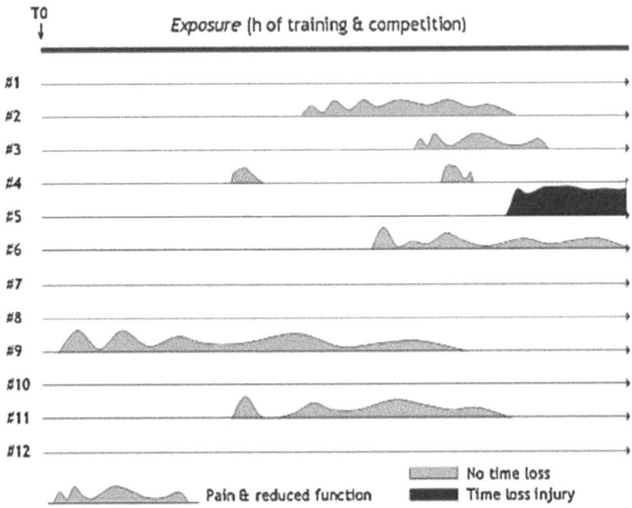

FIGURE 3.—Hypothetical example of results from a prospective cohort study on symptoms of pain and reduced function among 12 athletes followed for one season. Although a total of eight episodes with significant symptoms can be observed, only one of these would have been detected if a time loss definition of injury had been used. (Reprinted from Bahr R. No injuries, but plenty of pain? On the methodology for recording overuse symptoms in sports. *Br J Sports Med.* 2009;43:966-972, with permission from the BMJ Publishing Group.)

of symptoms; (2) valid and sensitive scoring instruments need to be developed to measure pain and other relevant symptoms; (3) prevalence and not incidence should be used to report injury risk; (4) severity should be measured based on functional level and not time loss from sports. In conclusion, new approaches are needed to develop more appropriate methodology to quantify overuse injuries in studies (Fig 3).

▶ This article looks at critical issues in sports medicine. It reflects a turning point in the study of the epidemiology of overuse injuries. Thus, it applies to researchers studying injuries such as tendinopathies, stress fractures, etc, as well as clinicians aiming to reduce the burden of these injuries.

Norway's Professor Roald Bahr, one of the pre-eminent injury prevention researchers, highlights that the current injury definition, focusing on time loss, is wholly inadequate for overuse injuries, which is well illustrated in Fig 3. A more appropriate method is to capture the periods of pain.

The 4 recommendations are as follows: (1) studies should be prospective, with continuous or serial measurements of symptoms; (2) valid and sensitive scoring instruments need to be developed to measure pain and other relevant symptoms; (3) prevalence and not incidence should be used to report injury risk; and (4) severity should be measured based on functional level and not time loss from sports.

These recommendations are immediately applicable to sports medicine epidemiology.

K. M. Khan, MD, PhD

Incidence, Risk, and Protective Factors of Mild Traumatic Brain Injury in a Cohort of Australian Nonprofessional Male Rugby Players

Hollis SJ, Stevenson MR, McIntosh AS, et al (Univ of Sydney, Australia; The Univ of New South Wales, Sydney, Australia; et al)

Am J Sports Med 37:2328-2333, 2009

Background.—Mild traumatic brain injury (mTBI) is an emerging public health issue in high-contact sports. Understanding the incidence along with the risk and protective factors of mTBI in high-contact sports such as rugby is paramount if appropriate preventive strategies are to be developed.

Purpose.—To estimate the incidence and identify the risk and protective factors of mTBI in Australian nonprofessional rugby players.

Study Design.—Cohort study; Level of evidence, 2.

Methods.—A cohort of 3207 male nonprofessional rugby players from Sydney, Australia, was recruited and followed over 1 or more playing seasons. Demographic information, history of recent concussion, and information on risk and protective factors were collected. The incidence of mTBI was estimated and the putative risk and protective factors were modeled in relation to mTBI.

Results.—The incidence of mTBI was 7.97 per 1000 player game hours, with 313 players (9.8%) sustaining 1 or more mTBIs during the study. Players who reported always wearing protective headgear during games were at a reduced risk (incident rate ratio [IRR], 0.57; 95% confidence interval [CI], 0.40-0.82) of sustaining an mTBI. In contrast, the likelihood of mTBI was almost 2 times higher among players who reported having sustained either 1 (IRR, 1.75; 95% CI, 1.11-2.76) or more mTBIs (IRR, 1.65; 95% CI, 1.11-2.45) within the 12 months before recruitment.

Conclusion.—Nonprofessional rugby has a high incidence of mTBI, with the absence of headgear and a recent history of mTBI associated with an increased risk of subsequent mTBI. These findings highlight that both use of headgear and the management of prior concussion would likely be beneficial in reducing the likelihood of mTBI among nonprofessional rugby players, who compose more than 99% of rugby union players in Australia.

▶ In the sports of rugby, soccer, and Australian rules football, sports-specific headgear has not been shown to significantly reduce the risk of concussion. Furthermore, biomechanical studies of the padded headgear that has recently been introduced in soccer and rugby have not shown the headgear significantly reduce acceleration forces as compared with helmet headgear in the sports of football, lacrosse, and hockey. For that reason the use of the soft headgear has been generally frowned upon for fear of falsely giving the sense of protection and perhaps leading the athlete to a more risk-taking style of play with regard to head injury.

This article is at odds with that reasoning as the authors found a reduced incidence of concussion in the athlete wearing the padded headgear. Assuming the biomechanical data are correct, this unexplained finding, which is at odds with previous studies, certainly warrants further study on the efficacy of padded headgear with regard to concussion incidence.

R. C. Cantu, MD, MA

Female soccer referees selected for the FIFA Women's World Cup 2007: survey of injuries and musculoskeletal problems

Bizzini M, Junge A, Bahr R, et al (FIFA Med Assessment and Res Centre (F-MARC), Zurich, Switzerland; Oslo Sports Trauma Res Centre (OSTRC), Norway; et al)

Br J Sports Med 43:936-942, 2009

Background.—Few studies have examined the physiology, training and more recently injury profile of the soccer referee, and these have involved almost exclusively male referees.

Purpose.—To analyse the frequency and characteristics of injuries and musculoskeletal problems in female referees selected for the FIFA Women's World Cup 2007.

Study Design.—Retrospective and prospective descriptive epidemiological study.

Methods.—During the preparation camps a few months before the FIFA Women's World Cup 2007, all 81 preselected female referees completed a questionnaire on injuries and musculoskeletal problems. During the final 32 matches of the tournament in China, all injuries, musculoskeletal problems and related treatment of the 36 officiating referees were documented.

Results.—Almost 50% of the referees reported having incurred at least one injury during their career that had led to time loss from the game. In the previous 12 months, 13 (16%) referees reported having sustained an injury and 64 (79%) reported musculoskeletal problems related to refereeing. During the World Cup and 14 (39%) referees incurred an injury and 17 (33%) were treated for musculoskeletal problems. The commonest location of injuries and problems were hamstrings, quadriceps, calf and ankle. The prospectively collected data found an incidence of 34.7 match injuries per 1000 match hours (95% CI 4.2 to 65.1).

Conclusion.—Top-level female referees are exposed to an even greater risk of injury and/or musculoskeletal problems related to officiating than are male referees. Considering the growth of women's soccer, injury prevention programmes should be specifically developed for female referees.

▶ The growth of women's soccer in recent years has brought attention to the paucity of data on injuries in female soccer referees. The exercise intensity of male and female soccer players is equivalent at the level of Federation Internationale de Football Association (FIFA) World Cup. Because the referees' exercise intensity is dictated by the players' intensity, it is reasonable to assume that female referees must maintain a high level of exercise intensity during match play. In this study, retrospective injury data were collected by questionnaire from 81 female World Cup referees attending FIFA preparation camps. Prospective injury data were collected in 36 of these referees selected to officiate the 2007 World Cup matches in China. Training and match injuries were reported for the last match officiated in the previous year and the entire career. Prospective injury data were collected by the World Cup medical team during the 2-week pretournament training session and the 20-day tournament schedule. Additionally, the injury data in female referees were also compared with that of male FIFA World Cup referees obtained in 2006. In the year before the World Cup, the average (±SD) workload of the female referees was 2.8 ± 1.2 matches per week and 7.5 ± 3.1 hours of training per week. Over the entire career, about 50% of referees sustained injuries, and all resulted in at least a 2-week absence from soccer. About half of the injuries occurred during match play, with the other half occuring during training. The most common injuries were musculoskeletal and headache. Surprisingly, during World Cup competition, more than 70% of injuries or problems treated were not related to previously reported injuries. The gender comparison revealed that females had shorter careers than males, similar training volume in the year before the World Cup, but about 4 times the injury rate of males. The injury locations most often reported (calf, hamstring, and ankle) were similar in men and women. These data suggest that female referees are more prone to injury and more likely to experience a new injury during World Cup officiating than their male counterparts, perhaps because female referees are not receiving adequate training guidance. Improved preparation of female referees for World Cup officiating should be a priority of FIFA.

C. M. Jankowski, PhD

Pediatric Tree House–Related Injuries Treated in Emergency Departments in the United States: 1990–2006

Randazzo C, Stolz U, Hodges NL, et al (The Ohio State Univ, Columbus; Univ of Arizona, Tucson; The Res Inst at Nationwide Children's Hosp, Columbus, OH)

Acad Emerg Med 16:235-242, 2009

Objectives.—The objective was to describe the epidemiology of tree house–related injuries in the United States among children and adolescents.

Methods.—The authors conducted a retrospective analysis using data from the National Electronic Injury Surveillance System for patients ≤19 years who were treated in an emergency department (ED) for a tree house-related injury from 1990 through 2006.

Results.—An estimated 47,351 patients ≤19 years of age were treated in EDs for tree house–related injuries over the 17-year study period. Fractures were the most common diagnosis (36.6%), and the upper extremities were the most commonly injured body part (38.8%). The odds of sustaining a head injury were increased for children aged <5 years. Falls were the most common injury mechanism (78.6%) and increased the odds of sustaining a fracture. Falls or jumps from a height ≥10 feet occurred in 29.3% of cases for which height of the fall/jump was recorded. Boys had significantly higher odds of falling or jumping from a height of ≥10 ft than girls, and children 10 to 19 years old also had significantly higher odds of falling or jumping from a height of ≥10 feet, compared to those 9 years old and younger. The odds of hospitalization were tripled if the patient fell or jumped from ≥10 feet and nearly tripled if the patient sustained a fracture.

Conclusions.—This study examined tree house–related injuries on a national level. Tree house safety deserves special attention because of the potential for serious injury or death due to falls from great heights, as well as the absence of national or regional safety standards. The authors provide safety and prevention recommendations based on the successful standards developed for playground equipment.

▶ In our zeal to provide recreational facilities for our children, we shouldn't forget the risks for injury that might be incurred. backyard trampolines have already received a great deal of attention in this regard. In this article we see evidence of a rather extraordinary number of injuries associated with every child's dream—their own treehouse, safe from parents. It turns out, however, that a treehouse is not so safe. In fact, a good amount of the treehouse-related injuries reported in this survey were of serious—and even potentially life-threatening—nature. Because one might assume that the treehouses involved were not constructed by the child alone, the responsibility obviously falls on parents to assure that recreational equipment and facilities they provide for their children are safe. Physicians, too, should add this counsel to their long list of safety recommendations for the families under their care.

T. Rowland, MD

Comprehensive warm-up programme to prevent injuries in young female footballers: cluster randomised controlled trial

Soligard T, Myklebust G, Steffen K, et al (Oslo Sports Trauma Res Centre, Norway; et al)

BMJ 337:a2469, 2008

Objective.—To examine the effect of a comprehensive warm-up programme designed to reduce the risk of injuries in female youth football.

Design.—Cluster randomised controlled trial with clubs as the unit of randomisation.

Setting.—125 football clubs from the south, east, and middle of Norway (65 clusters in the intervention group; 60 in the control group) followed for one league season (eight months).

Participants.—1892 female players aged 13-17 (1055 players in the intervention group; 837 players in the control group).

Intervention.—A comprehensive warm-up programme to improve strength, awareness, and neuromuscular control during static and dynamic movements.

Main Outcome Measure.—Injuries to the lower extremity (foot, ankle, lower leg, knee, thigh, groin, and hip).

Results.—During one season, 264 players had relevant injuries: 121 players in the intervention group and 143 in the control group (rate ratio 0.71, 95% confidence interval 0.49 to 1.03). In the intervention group there was a significantly lower risk of injuries overall (0.68, 0.48 to 0.98), overuse injuries (0.47, 0.26 to 0.85), and severe injuries (0.55, 0.36 to 0.83).

Conclusion.—Though the primary outcome of reduction in lower extremity injury did not reach significance, the risk of severe injuries, overuse injuries, and injuries overall was reduced. This indicates that a structured warm-up programme can prevent injuries in young female football players.

Trial registration.—ISRCTN10306290 (Fig 2).

▶ The "11 + structured" soccer warm-up program was developed to prevent lower extremity injuries in young players, particularly female athletes because of their high rate of anterior cruciate ligament injury. In this randomized controlled study, 93 youth soccer clubs, including nearly 1900 girls, completed either the structured 20-min warm-up program or the usual training over a competitive season. The intervention comprised light intensity running intervals, stretching, and strength, plyometric, and balance exercises, followed by higher intensity running intervals that incorporated soccer-specific directional changes. This final segment of each training session was focused on proper

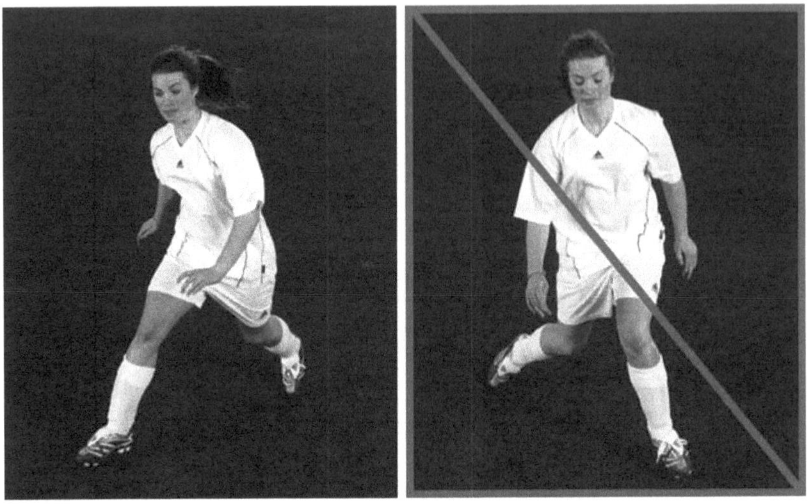

FIGURE 2.—Example of running exercise illustrating key objectives of all running, jumping, cutting, and landing exercises: core stability and correct lower extremity alignment. Left: correct technique; right: incorrect technique with pelvic tilt and knee valgus alignment to right. (Reprinted from Soligard T, Myklebust G, Steffen K, et al. Comprehensive warm-up programme to prevent injuries in young female footballers: cluster randomised controlled trial. *BMJ*. 2008;337:a2469.)

biomechanical technique and awareness of control during standing, running, planting, cutting, jumping, and landing to avoid excessive knee valgus (Fig 2). Although the study was slightly underpowered due to a greater than expected dropout rate, the intention-to-treat results were quite promising. The intervention warm up resulted in significantly fewer injuries and serious injuries. There was a tendency for all categories of injuries, except ankle injuries, to be lower in the intervention clubs. Within the intervention clubs, the risk of injury was 35% lower in the athletes with the best compliance compared with athletes with intermediate compliance (49 vs 23 sessions completed). The authors suggested that interventions such as "11+" should be implemented with younger soccer athletes who have not yet established basic motor patterns.

C. M. Jankowski, PhD

Comprehensive warm-up programme to prevent injuries in young female footballers: cluster randomised controlled trial

Soligard T, Myklebust G, Steffen K, et al (Oslo Sports Trauma Res Centre, Norway; et al)

BMJ 337:a2469, 2009

Objective.—To examine the effect of a comprehensive warm-up programme designed to reduce the risk of injuries in female youth football.

Design.—Cluster randomised controlled trial with clubs as the unit of randomisation.

Setting.—125 football clubs from the south, east, and middle of Norway (65 clusters in the intervention group; 60 in the control group) followed for one league season (eight months).

Participants.—1892 female players aged 13-17 (1055 players in the intervention group; 837 players in the control group).

Intervention.—A comprehensive warm-up programme to improve strength, awareness, and neuromuscular control during static and dynamic movements.

Main Outcome Measure.—Injuries to the lower extremity (foot, ankle, lower leg, knee, thigh, groin, and hip).

Results.—During one season, 264 players had relevant injuries: 121 players in the intervention group and 143 in the control group (rate ratio 0.71, 95% confidence interval 0.49 to 1.03). In the intervention group there was a significantly lower risk of injuries overall (0.68, 0.48 to 0.98), overuse injuries (0.47, 0.26 to 0.85), and severe injuries (0.55, 0.36 to 0.83).

Conclusion.—Though the primary outcome of reduction in lower extremity injury did not reach significance, the risk of severe injuries, overuse injuries, and injuries overall was reduced. This indicates that a structured warm-up programme can prevent injuries in young female football players.

Trial Registration.—ISRCTN10306290.

▶ This is a crucially important article, and it may be one of the 10 most important articles published in 2009. Why do I say that? Because of the importance of the outcome measures lower limb injuries, and because of the prevalence of the sport—young women's soccer, and because I believe this program is readily translatable. The intervention is intended to be part of the football warm-up. The exercise program is available on the *BMJ* Web site and through the international football federation (FIFA) and the Oslo Sports Trauma Research Center (OSTRC) sites already. Thus, it has tremendous penetration even before it is picked up in sports medicine textbooks. The magnitude of the effect size can be seen in Fig 4 in the original article; the warm-up exercise program prevents all injuries and severe injuries (which includes anterior cruciate ligament [ACL] injuries). Note that the study was not powered for ACL injuries; nevertheless, this is a major landmark study in sports medicine.

K. M. Khan, MD, PhD

Comprehensive warm-up programme to prevent injuries in young female footballers: cluster randomised controlled trial

Soligard T, Myklebust G, Steffen K, et al (Oslo Sports Trauma Res Centre, Oslo, Norway; et al)

BMJ 337:a2469, 2008

Objective.—To examine the effect of a comprehensive warm-up programme designed to reduce the risk of injuries in female youth football.

Design.—Cluster randomised controlled trial with clubs as the unit of randomisation.

Setting.—125 football clubs from the south, east, and middle of Norway (65 clusters in the intervention group; 60 in the control group) followed for one league season (eight months).

Participants.—1892 female players aged 13-17 (1055 players in the intervention group; 837 players in the control group).

Intervention.—A comprehensive warm-up programme to improve strength, awareness, and neuromuscular control during static and dynamic movements.

Main Outcome Measure.—Injuries to the lower extremity (foot, ankle, lower leg, knee, thigh, groin, and hip).

Results.—During one season, 264 players had relevant injuries: 121 players in the intervention group and 143 in the control group (rate ratio 0.71, 95% confidence interval 0.49 to 1.03). In the intervention group there was a significantly lower risk of injuries overall (0.68, 0.48 to 0.98), overuse injuries (0.47, 0.26 to 0.85), and severe injuries (0.55, 0.36 to 0.83).

Conclusion.—Though the primary outcome of reduction in lower extremity injury did not reach significance, the risk of severe injuries, overuse injuries, and injuries overall was reduced. This indicates that a structured warm-up programme can prevent injuries in young female football players.

Trial Registration.—ISRCTN10306290.

▶ There exist a good number of traditional activities and interventions in competitive sport that are considered to either help prevent injuries or improve performance. For most of these, there is actually little or no scientific backing to support or refute their usefulness. As a result, studies such as this one are greatly welcomed. The investigators have attempted to verify what has always been considered prudent—a structured period of activities that might be expected to reduce the rate of soccer injuries. Perhaps it is a bit disappointing that the reduction in the number of injuries did not reach statistical significance, but at least a favorable trend was observed. This study, too, serves as a good model for investigations that could be conducted in other sport activities. That this study addressed uniquely females reminds us, as well, that the effectiveness of interventions in reducing sports injury rates could be gender dependent.

T. Rowland, MD

Development and Preliminary Validation of the Injury-Psychological Readiness to Return to Sport (I-PRRS) Scale

Glazer DD (Endicott College, Beverly, MA)

J Athl Train 44:185-189, 2009

Context.—Only a few scales measure confidence within sport; however, these scales are insufficient to measure confidence after athletic injuries. Therefore, better measures are needed to determine the psychological readiness of injured athletes to return to sport participation.

Objective.—To develop a scale that measures the psychological readiness of injured athletes to return to sport participation and to provide preliminary evidence of reliability and validity for the scale.

Design.—The Delphi method was used to develop the Injury-Psychological Readiness to Return to Sport scale (I-PRRS). Two 1-way analyses of variance with repeated measures and 6 Pearson product moment correlations were computed to help validate the scale.

Setting.—Athletic training clinics at 3 National Collegiate Athletic Association (NCAA) schools.

Patients or Other Participants.—Four certified athletic trainers (ATs) and professors of Commission on Accreditation of Athletic Training Education-accredited athletic training programs and 3 NCAA Division III coaches made up a panel of experts that participated in the Delphi portion of the study to develop the I-PRRS. In the second part of the study, 22 injured athletes, who missed a minimum of 1 week of practice, from 3 NCAA schools in Divisions II and III were surveyed along with their respective ATs. The injured athletes and ATs participated in the validation of the I-PRRS.

Main Outcome Measure(s).—The injured athlete completed the Profile of Mood States (POMS) short form and the I-PRRS shortly after injury, before returning to the first practice, before returning to competition, and immediately after competition. The respective AT completed the I-PRRS before and after competition. The I-PRRS is a 6-item scale that measures the psychological readiness of injured athletes to return to sport, and the POMS short form is a 30-item scale that measures mood states. I added the negative moods of the POMS and subtracted the positive moods of the POMS to calculate a Total Mood Disturbance (TMD) score.

Results.—The I-PRRS scores were negatively correlated with the TMD scores of the POMS short form at all 4 time intervals, showing concurrent validity. The I-PRRS scores were lowest after injury, increased before practice, increased again before competition, and had no change after competition. The I-PRRS as completed by the athlete and respective AT was positively correlated both before and after practice, demonstrating external validity.

Conclusions.—Preliminary evidence for reliability and validity of the I-PRRS was demonstrated. The I-PRRS can be a beneficial tool for ATs to assess an athlete's psychological readiness to return to sport participation after injury.

▶ It is well understood that after an athlete incurs an injury there is always a period of physical healing and often a period of psychological readiness to return as well. It is also true that depending upon the injury, the physical and the psychological may not reach return-to-play status at the same time. This is especially true if the athlete has suffered a career threatening injury or a serious injury such as a brain or spinal cord injury. If the athlete is not psychologically ready to play, it is probable that the athlete will not play as well as possible and may well be at greater risk of injury. It goes without saying therefore that in making return-to-play decisions, it would be useful to know of the psychological readiness of the athlete. This article seeks to validate a psychological readiness return-to-sport test, and suggests its use for athletic trainers.

The usefulness of this test will need to be validated by others, but certainly suggests that such adoption and use and validation or invalidation would be appropriate. However, it is also a fact that many athletes, especially after severe spine or head injuries or career threatening knee or other injuries, really do not have complete ability to block out the previous injury and risk of future injury until they have been back at their sport for a considerable period of time. If passing such a psychological return-to-play test were to be mandated before returning, it is probable that many athletes would be out a much greater period of time than they currently are.

R. C. Cantu, MD, MA

The Potential for Brain Injury on Selected Surfaces Used by Cheerleaders

Shields BJ, Smith GA (The Res Inst at Nationwide Children's Hosp, Columbus, OH)

J Athl Train 44:595-602, 2009

Context.—Although playground surfaces have been investigated for fall impact attenuation, the surfaces that cheerleaders use have received little attention.

Objective.—To determine (1) the critical height for selected surfaces used by cheerleaders at or below which a serious head impact injury from a fall is unlikely to occur, (2) the critical heights for non–impact-absorbing surfaces for comparison purposes, and (3) the effect of soil moisture and grass height on g_{max} (which is defined as the multiple of g [acceleration due to gravity at the earth's surface at sea level: ie, 32.2 feet$\cdot$s$^{-1}\cdot$s^{-1}] that represents the maximum deceleration experienced during an impact) and the Head Injury Criterion (HIC) at the critical height for a dry grass surface.

Design.—Observational study.

Settings.—A local cheerleading gym, indoor locations within the authors' institution, and various outdoor locations.

Main Outcome Measure(s).—g_{max}, HIC, and critical height.

Results.—Critical heights for the surfaces tested ranged from 0.5 ft (0.15 m) for concrete and vinyl tile installed over concrete to more than 11 ft (3.35 m) for a spring floor. Increases in grass height and soil moisture resulted in an increase in the critical height for grass surfaces. Only spring floors and 4-in (0.10-m)–thick landing mats placed on traditional foam floors had critical heights greater than 10.5 ft (3.20 m), thus providing enough impact-absorbing capacity for performance of 2-level stunts.

Conclusions.—The potential for serious head impact injuries can be minimized by increasing the shock-absorbing capacity of the surface, decreasing the height from which the person falls, or both. Cheerleaders and cheerleading coaches should use the critical heights reported in this study to compare the relative impact-absorbing capacities of the various surfaces tested, with critical height as an indicator of the impact-absorption capacity of the surface. The findings of this study can be used to select the most appropriate surface for the type of maneuver to be performed, based on the maximum height expected to be achieved by the cheerleader(s) during execution of the maneuver. Cheerleaders should not perform maneuvers at heights that exceed the critical height for the surface on which they are performing.

▶ Data collected by the National Center for Catastrophic Sports Injury Research has shown that the flier in cheerleading stunts is by far and away the most risky activity for sustaining a catastrophic head or spine injury. Most of those accidents occurred when a flier was not properly caught and dismounted with their head striking the underlying surface. Many of these injuries were sustained when the underlying surface was an inappropriately hard surface such as a gymnasium floor.

This is the first study that investigates the role of playground surfaces in attenuating fall impacts for cheerleaders, and makes recommendations as to what activities should be carried out on which surfaces.

The recommendations are that only when a 4-inch-thick landing mat is provided over foam floors is there sufficient impact absorption for the safe performance of two level cheerleading stunts. Therefore, if such protection in terms of an impact-absorbing surface is not able to be provided, 2-level stunts and tosses should be avoided, and cheerleading activities should be restricted to chants, dances, and tumbling routines. Pyramids, partner stunts, and tosses should be avoided.

While this article addresses a very important topic and its results are intuitively what one would anticipate, the actual calculation of risk for head and spine injuries involves factors beyond simple measuring of g-max acceleration forces. With regard to head injury, in addition to g-forces other factors not taken into consideration by this study include rotational acceleration, impact duration, impact location, multiplicity of impacts, as well as gender and age. Therefore, while this research is an excellent starting point, additional studies both with regard to head and spine injuries, as well as other types of injuries, are needed.

R. C. Cantu, MD, MA

Generalizability Theory Analysis of Balance Error Scoring System Reliability in Healthy Young Adults

Broglio SP, Zhu W, Sopiarz K, et al (Univ of Illinois at Urbana-Champaign)
J Athl Train 44:497-502, 2009

Context.—An assessment of postural control is commonly included in the clinical concussion evaluation. Previous investigators have demonstrated learning effects that may mask concussion-induced balance decrements.

Objective.—To establish the test-retest reliability of the Balance Error Scoring System (BESS) and to provide recommendations that account for known learning effects.

Design.—Test-retest generalizability study.

Setting.—Balance research laboratory.

Patients or Other Participants.—Young adults (n = 48) free from injuries and illnesses known to affect balance.

Intervention(s).—Each participant completed 5 BESS trials on each of the assessment dates, which were separated by 50 days.

Main Outcome Measure(s).—Total score of the BESS was used in a generalizability theory analysis to estimate the overall reliability of the BESS and that of each facet. A decision study was completed to estimate the number of days and trials needed to establish clinical reliability.

Results.—The overall reliability of the BESS was G = 0.64. The test-retest reliability was improved when male (0.92) and female (0.91) participants were examined independently. Clinically acceptable reliability (greater than 0.80) was established when 3 BESS trials were administered in a single day or 2 trials were administered at different time points.

Conclusions.—Learning effects have been noted in individuals with no previous exposure to the BESS. Our findings indicate that clinicians should consider interpreting the mean score from 3 BESS administrations on a given occasion for both normative data comparison and pretest and posttest design. The multiple assessment technique yields clinically reliable scores and provides the sports medicine practitioner with accurate data for clinical decision making.

▶ Sport-related concussion is frequently seen in both contact and collision sports. It is commonly known that there does not have to be a loss of consciousness (LOC) for a concussion to have occurred, rather there is an array of related signs and symptoms that can be readily assessed by the practitioner. Research is ongoing regarding the optimal methods of assessing readiness to return to play, but it is accepted that concussion has large negative effects on measures of self-reported symptoms, neurocognitive functioning, and postural control. Each aspect of such a test battery can provide useful information to supplement the clinical examination.

This article assesses the generalizability of the Balance Error Scoring System (BESS)—a tool that has been developed to measure postural stability without need for expensive equipment or extensive training. As improved balance (ie, fewer errors) can be seen with multiple administrations of the BESS, it is important to distinguish learning effects from true clinically significant change (ie, from baseline to postconcussion scores).

The design of this study allows for interpretation of both the reliability of the baseline measure (single test administration reliability) and the difference over the season (stability) of the trait. Through somewhat sophisticated statistical methods (generalizability theory analysis), the results have added to current knowledge of the test's psychometric properties. Specifically, when the test is administered on a single occasion (eg, a postmorbid or postconcussion assessment only), the mean score from 3 administrations is necessary to obtain a stable measure of balance performance with an acceptable reliability in both males and females. When the test is administered over 2 days and another source of variability is taken into consideration, the BESS only needs to be administered twice at each session, with averaging of the scores from both days. Practically speaking, the former strategy would be the most efficient and useful (either when comparing the score with baseline values or with normative data) to be used in clinical decision making. Another group has recommended that the postconcussion assessment on the BESS differ from baseline by at least 4 points to be considered clinically meaningful.[1]

The only caveat, however, for the usefulness of the findings in this study is that the currently recommended Sport Concussion Assessment Tool (SCAT2), as detailed elsewhere,[2] only uses 1 repetition of each of the test conditions and does not call for balance assessment on both firm and compliant surfaces as does the BESS. Therefore, such a study should be repeated under the conditions that are most commonly used at present in the clinical assessment of concussion.

C. Lebrun, MD

References

1. Reimann BL, Guskiewicz KM, Shields EW. Relationship between clinical and forceplate measures of postural stability. *J Sport Rehabil.* 1999;8:71-82.
2. McCrory P, Meeuwisse W, Johnston K, et al. Consensus statement on Concussion in Sport 3rd International Conference on Concussion in Sport held in Zurich, November 2008. *Clin J Sport Med.* 2009;19:185-200.

Concussion in Professional Football: Animal Model of Brain Injury—Part 15

Viano DC, Hamberger A, Bolouri H, et al (Natl Football League, NY; Univ of Gothenburg, Sweden)

Neurosurgery 64:1162-1173, 2009

Objective.—A concussion model was developed to study injury mechanisms, functional effects, treatment, and recovery. Concussions in National Football League football involve high-impact velocity (7.4–11.2 m/s) and rapid change in head velocity (ΔV) (5.4–9.0 m/s). Current animal models do not simulate these head impact conditions.

Methods.—One hundred eight adult male Wistar rats weighing 280 to 350 g were used in ballistic impacts simulating 3 collision severities causing National Football League-type concussion. Pneumatic pressure accelerated a 50g impactor to velocities of 7.4, 9.3, and 11.2 m/s at the left side of the helmet-protected head. A thin layer of padding on the helmet controlled head acceleration, which was measured on the opposite side of the head, in line with the impact. Peak head acceleration, ΔV, impact duration, and energy transfer were determined. Fifty-four animals were exposed to single impact, with 18 each having 1, 4, or 10 days of survival. Similar tests were conducted on another 54 animals, which received 3 impacts at 6-hour intervals. An additional 72 animals were tested with a 100g impactor to study more serious brain injuries. Brains were perfused, and surface injuries were identified.

Results.—The 50g impactor matches concussion conditions scaled to the rat. Impact velocity and head ΔV were within 1% and 3% of targets on average. Head acceleration reached 450g to 1750g without skull fracture. The test is repeatable and robust. Gross pathology was observed in 11%, 28%, and 33% of animals in the 7.4-, 9.3-, and 11.2-m/s single impacts, respectively. At 7.4 m/s, a single diameter area of less than 0.5 mm of fine petechial hemorrhage occurred on the brain surface in the parenchyma and meninges nearest the point of impact. At higher velocities, there were larger areas of bleeding, sometimes with subdural hemorrhage. When the 50g impactor tests were examined by logistic regression, greater energy transfer increased the probability of injury (odds ratio, 5.83; $P = 0.01$), as did 3 repeat impacts (odds ratio, 4.72; $P = 0.002$). The number of survival days decreased the probability of observing injury (odds ratio, 0.25 and 0.11 for 4 and 10 days, respectively, compared with 1 day). The 100g impactor produced more severe brain injuries.

Conclusion.—A concussion model was developed to simulate the high velocity of impact and rapid head ΔV of concussions in National Football League players. The new procedure can be used to evaluate immediate and latent effects of concussion and more severe injury with greater impact mass.

▶ When Pellman, Viano, and colleagues published their data on concussions in the National Football League (NFL) in this same journal, only 25 out of the 787 total concussions could be calculated because of the need for 2 camera angles showing 10 yards of markers on the field. The great majority of concussions that occurred in areas other than the open field, therefore, did not have forces calculated. Those calculations in which the forces could be calculated were all open field, and all were of an unusually high impact in which the player that did not see the ball coming in every case sustained a concussion inflicted by the player who was making a helmet tackle. These forces are therefore representative of the highest of G-forces and are not representative of most sustained concussions.

We know from subsequent research using the hit technology of accelerometers mounted in the helmets with G-forces telemetried to the sideline that most concussions recorded are surprisingly at relatively modest G-forces, and that consistently high G-forces do not necessarily correlate with a concussion. Therefore, I believe that this animal model based only on these extremely high-force impacts from the NFL study is a model that is flawed as these forces exceed what is necessary to produce a concussion.

R. C. Cantu, MD, MA

Concussion in Professional Football: Morphology of Brain Injuries in the NFL Concussion Model—Part 16

Hamberger A, Viano DC, Säljö A, et al (Univ of Göteborg, Sweden; Natl Football League, NY)

Neurosurgery 64:1174-1182, 2009

Objective.—An animal model of concussions in National Football League players has been described in a previous study. It involves a freely moving 300-g Wistar rat impacted on the side of the head at velocities of 7.4 to 11.2 m/s with a 50-g impactor. The impact causes a 6% to 28% incidence of meningeal hemorrhages and 0.1- to 0.3-mm focal petechiae depending on the impact velocity. This study addresses the immunohistochemical responses of the brain.

Methods.—Twenty-seven tests were conducted with a 50-g impactor and velocities of 7.4, 9.3, or 11.2 m/s. The left temporal region of the helmet-protected head was hit 1 or 3 times. Thirty-one additional tests were conducted with a 100-g impactor. Diffuse axonal injury in distant regions of the brain was assessed with immunohistochemistry for NF-200, the heaviest neurofilament subunit, and glial fibrillary acidic protein, an intermediate filament protein in astrocytes. Hemorrhages were analyzed by unspecific peroxidase. There were 10 controls.

Results.—A single impact at 7.4 and 9.3 m/s velocity with the 50-g impactor causes minimal neuronal injury and astrocytosis. Repeat impacts with 11.2 m/s velocity and more than 9.3-m/s impacts with 100 g cause diffuse axonal injury and distant injury bilaterally in the cerebral cortex, the subcortical, the white matter, the hippocampus CA1, the corpus callosum, and the striatum, as indicated by NF-200 accumulation in neuronal perikarya 10 days after impact. It also causes reactive astrocytosis in the midline regions of the cerebral cortex and periventricularly. Regions with erythrocyteloaded blood capillaries indicated brain edema in regions of the cerebral cortex, the brainstem, and the cerebellum.

Conclusion.—When the immunohistochemical results are extrapolated to professional football players, concussions result in no or minimal brain injury. Repeat impacts at higher velocity or with a heavier mass impactor cause extensive and distant diffuse axonal injury. Based on this model, the threshold for diffuse axonal injury is above even the most severe conditions for National Football League concussion.

▶ In a previous companion article in *Neurosurgery* I indicated the limitation of the National Football League (NFL) concussion data in terms of the ability to only record 25 out of 787 concussions, and how each of these impacts were rather unique and were of a very high change in velocity/acceleration load type. I will not dwell on those limitations in this article.

The major limitation of this research has been honestly presented by the authors themselves in a limitation section. They readily admit that the scaling for the forces comparing forces that a rat brain would sustain would be equal to what a human brain would tolerate have not been corroborated or validated by any previous brain research. It is very probable that any errors in the assumption would be greatly magnified by this scaling, and therefore to draw direct correlations from this small rodent work and what may or may not be received by the human brain, I believe is somewhat speculative.

R. C. Cantu, MD, MA

Effects of a Symptom-Free Waiting Period on Clinical Outcome and Risk of Reinjury After Sport-Related Concussion

McCrea M, Guskiewicz K, Randolph C, et al (Waukesha Memorial Hosp, WI; Univ of North Carolina at Chapel Hill; Loyola Univ Med School, Maywood, IL; et al)

Neurosurgery 65:876-882, 2009

Objective.—This study is the first to investigate the influence of a symptom-free waiting period (SFWP) on clinical outcome and risk of repeat injury after sport-related concussion.

Methods.—This was a prospective, nonrandomized study of 16 624 player seasons from 1999 to 2004, including a cohort of 635 concussed high school and college athletes grouped on the basis of an SFWP or no SFWP observed after their concussion. Clinical outcome in symptoms, cognitive functioning, and postural stability 45 and 90 days postinjury was compared with preinjury baseline. Data on SFWP and same-season repeat concussion were recorded.

Results.—An SFWP was observed in 60.3% of cases. There were no significant differences between the SFWP and no SFWP groups in acute injury characteristics or clinical outcome with respect to symptom recovery or postinjury performance on formal neuropsychological and balance testing. Most repeat concussions (79.2%) occurred within 10 days of the initial injury. The rate of repeat concussion was actually higher in the SFWP group (6.49%) than the no SFWP group (0.90%) ($P < 0.005$), but the repeat concussion subgroup's SFWP was 2.82 days shorter (95% confidence interval, 0.61–5.03; $P < 0.01$) and these athletes resumed participation 3.55 days sooner (95% confidence interval, 0.06–7.04; $P < 0.05$) than those in the SFWP group in which there was no repeat concussion.

Conclusion.—Our findings suggest that an SFWP did not intrinsically influence clinical recovery or reduce risk of a repeat concussion. The overall risk of same-season repeat concussion seems to be relatively low, but there may be a period of vulnerability that increases risk of repeat concussion during the first 7 to 10 days postinjury. Further study is required to investigate this preliminary finding and help determine whether this risk can be reduced further with specific injury-management strategies.

▶ Large, multicenter prospective studies have the advantage of large numbers of individuals studied and, therefore, a relatively large number of whatever the injury in question is as well. The disadvantage of a large multicenter study is that there are many people filling out the forms and making the diagnoses who may not all be on the same page in terms of accuracy. The advantage of a single-center study is that the observers should all be of the same accuracy in making and recording the injury, but of course the total number of injuries would be far lower.

There is inherently no logic as to why a group of individuals with a symptom-free wait period should not have a better clinical outcome than a group with no symptom-free wait period, assuming that the symptom-free wait period was significantly long and that it truly was an asymptomatic status that the individual had. The data in which almost all the repeat injuries happened was in the first 10 days after returning, and suggests to me that these individuals probably were never free of symptoms at the time that they were allowed to return. The symptom-free wait period as a group was returned to play in less than 1 week after their concussion, and those that did not have a symptom-free wait period were returned in a far shorter period of time. I do not know whether it was the accuracy of the reporting or whether it was that the symptom-free wait period was inadequately short (less that a week), but I would suspect that if a true meaningful symptom-free wait period were compared with no symptom-free wait period that the statistics would be different. This is a study in need of others to be done to see if the same findings are found.

R. C. Cantu, MD, MA

Head impact severity measures for evaluating mild traumatic brain injury risk exposure

Greenwald RM, Gwin JT, Chu JJ, et al (Simbex, Lebanon, NH)

Neurosurgery 62:789-798, 2008

Objective.—The aims of this study were to quantify the sensitivity of various biomechanical measures (linear acceleration, rotational acceleration, impact duration, and impact location) of head impact to the clinical diagnosis of concussion in United States football players and to develop a novel measure of head impact severity combining these measures into a single score that better predicts the incidence of concussion.

Methods.—On-field head impact data were collected from 449 football players at 13 organizations (n = 289,916) using in-helmet systems of six single-axis accelerometers. Concussions were diagnosed by medical staff and later associated with impact data. Principal component analysis and a weighting coefficient based on impact location were used to transform correlated head impact measures into a new composite variable, weighted principal component score (wPCS). The predictive power of linear acceleration, rotational acceleration, head injury criterion, and wPCS was quantified using receiver operating characteristic curves. The null hypothesis, that a measure was no more predictive than guessing, was tested (alpha = 0.05). In addition, receiver operating characteristic curves for wPCS and classical measures were directly compared to test the hypothesis that wPCS was more predictive of concussion than were classic measures (alpha = 0.05).

Results.—When all of the impacts were considered, every biomechanical measure evaluated was statistically more predictive of concussion than guessing ($P < 0.005$). However, for the top 1 and 2% of impacts based on linear acceleration, a subset that consisted of 82% of all diagnosed concussions, only wPCS was significantly more predictive of concussion than guessing ($P < 0.03$); when compared with each other, wPCS was more predictive of concussion than were classical measures for the top 1 and 2% of all of the data ($P < 0.04$).

Conclusion.—A weighted combination of several biomechanical inputs, including impact location, is more predictive of concussion than a single biomechanical measure. This study is the first to the authors' knowledge to quantify improvements in the sensitivity of a biomechanical measure to incidence of concussion when impact location is considered.

▶ The National Football League published data from reconstructed impacts of 25 concussions out of a total of 747 concussions that predicted if a g-force of 99 grams was exceeded, then 75% of such impacts would result in a cerebral concussion. This article that includes data from over a quarter of a million impacts refutes that finding. With impacts exceeding 99 grams the incidence of reported concussion was under 1%. Clearly, sustaining a cerebral concussion is a more complex phenomenon than simply measuring linear acceleration forces. These authors suggest that a higher predictability of when a concussion is sustained might be obtained by assessing multiple factors, such as linear acceleration, rotational acceleration, duration of impact, and location of impact.

The most frequent location of impact was the frontal region of the helmet with the side and top a close second. Although this data suffers from the fact that athletes may have been playing through concussive episodes that went unrecognized, it clearly indicates much more work is needed before we understand why hits of moderate g-force may result in a concussion whereas hits of a higher g-force do not.

In addition to the 4 factors cited by these authors, other factors such as multiplicity of hits in close proximity as suggested by Guskiewicz may play a significant role in determining when a concussion is sustained. Also, gender and age are other factors that may need to be considered as well.

R. C. Cantu, MD, MA

History of multiple self-reported concussions is not associated with reduced cognitive abilities

Bruce JM, Echemendia RJ (Univ of Missouri-Kansas City; Psychological and Neurobehavioral Associates, Inc, State College, PA)

Neurosurgery 64:100-106, 2009

Objective.—The long-term impact of sports-related concussion is uncertain. Several studies using traditional neuropsychological measures have found a relationship between a previous history of concussion and reduced cognitive abilities. In contrast, studies using computerized neuropsychological measures have typically found no relationship between concussion history and cognition. In the present study, we examined the association between a self-reported concussion history and cognition using traditional and computer-based neuropsychological tests.

Methods.—A computerized neuropsychological battery was administered to a sample of 858 collegiate male athletes. Of this sample, 298 athletes reported a history of concussion. A traditional neuropsychological battery was administered to a separate sample of 479 male collegiate athletes, 187 of whom reported a history of concussion. Finally, both a computerized and a traditional neuropsychological battery were administered to a third distinct sample of 175 male collegiate athletes, 57 of whom reported a history of concussion. Concussion history was assessed via self-report. None of the athletes had been concussed in the 6 months before testing.

Results.—No significant association was found between self-reported concussion history and performance on either computerized or traditional neuropsychological tests.

Conclusion.—Findings suggest that athletes who report a distant history of concussion have minimal enduring neurocognitive deficits. Given conflicting findings in the literature, prospective studies that attempt to identify moderating factors are necessary to help determine who is at risk for long-term cognitive difficulties after concussion.

▶ Whether a history of previous concussion(s) affects results on computer-based neuropsychological testing or traditional neuropsychological tests remains controversial. This study on college males with no learning disabilities or a concussion in the previous 6 months found, with either none or one or more self-reported diagnosed concussions, that the results were the same.

Because of the possible inaccuracies with self-report data, this study has obvious limitations. The most severe limitation, however, is in not recording the severity of concussions in those who had them. All concussions are not created equal. Those with signs and symptoms that require weeks or months to clear, especially cognitive symptoms, are more likely to have more serious cognitive problems with further concussions in my clinical experience of over 40 years. It would therefore have been of major interest to know if any of the group with previous concussion(s) had severe concussions with symptoms lasting a week or more.

I agree with the authors that the potentially deleterious effects of repeated concussions warrant further study, and also that ideally the concussion history will not be from self-report and that concussion severity will be obtained.

R. C. Cantu, MD, MA

Retropharyngeal Tendinitis May be More Common Than We Think: A Report on 45 Cases Seen in Danish Chiropractic Clinics

Hviid C, Salomonsen M, Gelineck J, et al (Private practice of chiropractic, Aarhus C, Denmark; Private practice of family medicine, Galten, Denmark; Aarhus Univ Hosp, Denmark; et al)

J Manipulative Physiol Ther 32:315-320, 2009

Objective.—This study presents information from 45 cases of retropharyngeal tendinitis that were collected in Danish chiropractic clinics.

Methods.—A practicing Danish chiropractor collected cases of retropharyngeal tendinitis from colleagues who were members of the Danish Society of Chiropractic and Clinical Biomechanics. Only cases where a patient history of acute severe neck pain, cervical stiffness, and dysphagia were considered, and these were supplemented with imaging in the form of x-rays, computed tomography, or magnetic resonance imaging scans. All cases were reviewed independently by the chiropractor and a medical radiologist with a specialty in musculoskeletal disorders before acceptance into this case series.

Results.—Forty-five cases fulfilled the inclusion criteria and were included in this review. Sixteen of these were recruited from a single chiropractic practice. Nineteen were males and 26 were females with an average age of 48 years. All but 2 patients had the characteristic depositions of calcium hydroxyapatite in the tendon of the longus colli muscle, and the average diameter of the retropharyngeal space was 8.1 mm.

Conclusions.—Patients presenting with a triad of acute severe neck pain, stiff neck, and dysphagia may have retropharyngeal tendinitis. This condition may be a more common than previously thought among patients presenting with acute neck pain in the primary health care sector.

▶ Although this is not a systematic prevalence study, it does underscore the existence of what was thought of as a relatively uncommon condition (and is possibly more prevalent than previously thought), retropharyngeal tendinitis. This diagnosis should be considered for patients who present with acute severe neck pain, stiff neck, and dysphagia, and can be diagnosed using standard radiographs. It is a self-limiting condition. It is unknown whether treatment with spinal manipulation or nonsteroidal anti-inflammatory drugs are effective. It appears that, once diagnosed, reassurance and symptomatic relief of pain should be used.

D. E. Feldman, PT, PhD

Amateur boxing and risk of chronic traumatic brain injury: systematic review of observational studies

Loosemore M, Knowles CH, Whyte GP (Northwick Park Hosp, Harrow, UK; Royal London Hosp; Liverpool John Moores Univ)

Br J Sports Med 42:564-567, 2008

Objective.—To evaluate the risk of chronic traumatic brain injury from amateur boxing.

Setting.—Secondary research performed by combination of sport physicians and clinical academics.

Design, data sources, and methods.—Systematic review of observational studies in which chronic traumatic brain injury was defined as any abnormality on clinical neurological examination, psychometric testing, neuroimaging studies, and electroencephalography. Studies were identified through database (1950 to date) and bibliographic searches without language restrictions. Two reviewers extracted study characteristics, quality, and data, with adherence to a protocol developed from a widely recommended method for systematic review of observational studies (MOOSE).

Results.—36 papers had relevant extractable data (from a detailed evaluation of 93 studies of 943 identified from the initial search). Quality of evidence was generally poor. The best quality studies were those with a cohort design and those that used psychometric tests. These yielded the most negative results: only four of 17 (24%) better quality studies found any indication of chronic traumatic brain injury in a minority of boxers studied.

Conclusion.—There is no strong evidence to associate chronic traumatic brain injury with amateur boxing.

▶ I am suggesting that this article be included because the subject matter is extremely important, and yet neither this article nor any other article has answered the question clearly whether there is a significant risk of chronic traumatic brain injury in amateur boxing. Whereas this article reviewed all studies after 1950 regarding the risk of chronic traumatic brain injury from amateur boxing, the quality of almost all the studies was so low that no definitive conclusions could be drawn. Chronic traumatic encephalopathy findings can occur years and even decades after the brain trauma that caused them ceased to be occurring. Virtually all of these studies were flawed, in that there was not a long period of follow-up. Thus, while the authors conclude that there is no "strong evidence to associate chronic traumatic brain injury with amateur boxing," I believe that the studies done to date simply do not adequately address the question in a class A evidence way, and therefore the answer is not known in terms of the relative risk of chronic traumatic encephalopathy in amateur boxers. This is a question that needs to be addressed in a double blinded, randomized study that not only looks at amateur boxers while active in their career, but also looks at them a decade or more later.

R. C. Cantu, MD, MA

The Role of Concussion History and Gender in Recovery From Soccer-Related Concussion

Colvin AC, Mullen J, Lovell MR, et al (Mount Sinai Med Ctr, NY; Univ of Pittsburgh Med Ctr, PA)

Am J Sports Med 37:1699-1704, 2009

Background.—This study was designed to investigate differences in recovery in male and female soccer athletes.

Hypotheses.—Soccer players with a history of concussion will perform worse on neurocognitive testing than players without a history of concussion. Furthermore, female athletes will demonstrate poorer performance on neurocognitive testing than male athletes.

Study Design.—Cohort study (prognosis): Level of evidence, 2.

Methods.—Computer-based neuropsychological testing using reaction time, memory, and visual motor-speed composite scores of the ImPACT test battery was performed postconcussion in soccer players ranging in age from 8 to 24 years (N = 234; 141 females, 93 males). A multivariate analysis of variance was conducted to examine group differences in neurocognitive performance between male and female athletes with and without a history of concussion.

Results.—Soccer players with a history of at least 1 previous concussion performed significantly worse on ImPACT than those who had not sustained a prior concussion ($F = 2.92$, $P = .03$). In addition, female soccer players performed worse on neurocognitive testing ($F = 2.72$, $P = .05$) and also reported more symptoms ($F = 20.1$, $P = .00001$) than male soccer players. There was no significant difference in body mass index between male and female players ($F = .04$, $P = .85$).

Conclusion.—A history of concussion and gender may account for significant differences in postconcussive neurocognitive test scores in soccer players and may play a role in determining recovery. These differences do not appear to reflect differences in mass between genders and may be related to other gender-specific factors that deserve further study.

▶ The role of age, gender, and previous concussion history remains controversial in terms of predicting recovery after a concussion. There are considerable studies that would suggest having sustained a previous concussion or two would have no role on recovery. Most of those studies involved multiple sports and often a mixed, male and female, composition. This study attempted to look at soccer alone and attempted to answer the question whether gender and/or a previous concussion influenced recovery. The sole tool used was Immediate Post-concussion Assessment and Cognitive Assessment, Pittsburgh, Pennsylvania (ImPACT) testing. The study suggested that one previous concussion or being female was statistically associated with a poor recovery.

In my opinion this study suffers from 3 major design flaws. First, only the neuropsychological test battery was used, and therefore, because a neurologic examination including detailed balance testing was not incorporated, we do not know if these athletes really had recovered from their concussion at the time they were tested.

A second significant flaw is that the group that had sustained a previous concussion was tested earlier, by a mean of 3 days, than the group that had sustained no previous concussions. This clearly gave the group with no previous concussions a longer time to recover from their current, first concussions and therefore a better outcome.

The major design flaw of this study, however, is that baseline data was not obtained for any of the test groups; rather they were compared with specific normative groups based on age and gender. I believe this is a serious design flaw as, especially, with people of high intelligence, comparing them to other than their own baseline can be quite imprecise.

R. C. Cantu, MD, MA

Head Impacts During High School Football: A Biomechanical Assessment

Broglio SP, Sosnoff JJ, Shin S, et al (Univ of Illinois at Urbana-Champaign; et al)

J Athl Train 44:342-349, 2009

Context.—Little is known about the impact biomechanics sustained by players during interscholastic football.

Objective.—To characterize the location and magnitude of impacts sustained by players during an interscholastic football season.

Design.—Observational design.

Setting.—On the field.

Patients or Other Participants.—High school varsity football team (n = 35; age = 16.85 ± 0.75 years, height = 183.49 ± 5.31 cm, mass = 89.42 ± 12.88 kg).

Main Outcome Measure(s).—Biomechanical variables (linear acceleration, rotational acceleration, jerk, force, impulse, and impact duration) related to head impacts were categorized by session type, player position, and helmet impact location.

Results.—Differences in grouping variables were found for each impact descriptor. Impacts occurred more frequently and with greater intensity during games. Linear acceleration was greatest in defensive linemen and offensive skill players and when the impact occurred at the top of the helmet. The largest rotational acceleration occurred in defensive linemen and with impacts to the front of the helmet. Impacts with the highest-magnitude jerk, force, and impulse and shortest duration occurred in the offensive skill, defensive line, offensive line, and defensive skill players, respectively. Top-of-the-helmet impacts yielded the greatest magnitude for the same variables.

Conclusions.—We are the first to provide a biomechanical characterization of head impacts in an interscholastic football team across a season of play. The intensity of game play manifested with more frequent and intense impacts. The highest-magnitude variables were distributed across all player groups, but impacts to the top of the helmet yielded the highest values. These high school football athletes appeared to sustain greater accelerations after impact than their older counterparts did. How this finding relates to concussion occurrence has yet to be elucidated.

▶ The most intriguing part of this study is not the results per se, but rather the report of technology that promises to provide critically important information on head impacts in high school football players. It comes as no surprise that such stresses are extremely forceful. The next step will be to determine the quantitative relationships of such factors to concussion outcomes. Such information would be very useful in the design of football helmets, but, perhaps more specifically, could help determine when individual players are receiving head impacts that would be potentially dangerous. The findings do support current regulations and practices, which are designed to prevent using the top of the helmet in tackling and blocking. It was also of interest in this study that linear acceleration from impacts was greater in high school players than that reported in collegiate competitors, an explanation for which is not clear.

T. Rowland, MD

Characteristics of a Mild Head Injury Subgroup With Extreme, Persisting Distress on the Rivermead Postconcussion Symptoms Questionnaire

Kirsch NL, de Leon MB, Maio RF, et al (Univ of Michigan, Ann Arbor; et al)
Arch Phys Med Rehabil 91:35-42, 2010

Objective.—To examine baseline variables and identify characteristics of participants with extremely high reports of symptoms (ie, outliers) 12 months after mild head injury (MHI).

Design.—A prospective cohort study of MHI with and without loss of consciousness (LOC) and/or posttraumatic amnesia (PTA) recruited from and interviewed at the emergency department (ED), with a follow-up telephone interview at 12 months.

Setting.—Level II community hospital ED.

Participants.—Participants (n = 58) with MHI and LOC less than or equal to 30 minutes and/or PTA less than 24 hours and participants (n = 173) with MHI but no PTA/LOC. Inclusion criteria: age greater than or equal to 18 years, less than or equal to 24 hours after injury, Glasgow Coma Scale score greater than or equal to 13, and discharge from the ED. Fourteen (6%) participants had extremely high scores on the Rivermead Postconcussion Symptoms Questionnaire (RPQ).

Main Outcome Measures.—RPQ and questions on health services use and litigation.

Results.—Characterizing the outlier cases are prior head injury, preinjury disability, history of substance use, unemployment, and elevated somatic symptoms at the ED. At 12 months, outliers had higher use of health services and litigation.

Conclusions.—The existence of a subgroup with a distinctive pattern of baseline characteristics in combination with elevated somatic symptoms at the time of presentation to the ED suggests that further taxonomic distinctions may be warranted for the MHI population, each requiring appropriately targeted interventions for addressing symptomatic complaints.

▶ As one who manages hundreds of concussion patients yearly, over a third of whom have postconcussion syndrome and, thus, signs and symptoms over 3 months after a concussion, I read this study with particular interest. I also read it with a critical eye to know whether the findings fit with my personal experience. My concussion patients are primarily athletes, most of whom are motivated to return to play and, thus, are not a perfect match for this emergency room cohort. However, not all the concussion patients I see are athletes, and not all the athletes I see, especially aging professional athletes with eroding skills, are necessarily eager to return.

What I found compelling about this group with mild head injuries with symptoms at 12 months after injury is that there was a substantial worsening of reported symptoms. This would suggest that a non-neuropathological brain injury mechanism is operable on a neurophyschological basis, and some, if not a complete, resolution of symptoms would be expected. Thus, it is no surprise that a previous history of unemployment, disability, alcohol, or drug abuse suggesting psychological or psychosocial factors was present in the outliers group with symptoms at 12 months. The other 2 factors—a history of previous head injury and high somatic symptom score on initial presentation—could be in a learned or neuropathological basis, as some could have incipient chronic traumatic encephalopathy. The outlier group deserves further study, and I recommend this article as a good primer.

R. C. Cantu, MD, MA

Current Sport-Related Concussion Teaching and Clinical Practices of Sports Medicine Professionals

Covassin T, Elbin R III, Stiller-Ostrowski JL (Michigan State Univ, East Lansing)

J Athl Train 44:400-404, 2009

Context.—Various consensus and position statements recommend a multifaceted approach when diagnosing a possible concussion. The effectiveness of these materials depends largely on their content being disseminated to educators and to those in the clinical setting.

Objective.—To identify the concussion management methods and guidelines currently taught in the athletic training classroom and clinical settings and to track the dissemination of the Vienna guidelines throughout the educational curriculum.

Design.—A 17-question Internet survey.

Setting.—A Web link was e-mailed to the program directors and certified athletic trainers holding educational positions in athletic training at 300 accredited programs in the United States.

Patients or Other Participants.—513 program directors and athletic trainers.

Main Outcome Measure(s).—Survey questions addressed education level, years of certification, employment setting, concussion assessment and return-to-play guidelines used in the clinical setting and the classroom, and clinical and teaching preferences for existing position statements and concussion grading systems. The Vienna guidelines' "simple" and "complex" definitions of concussions were provided with the return-to-play stepwise approach.

Results.—The National Athletic Trainers' Association position statement was the most widely used method of assessing, managing (61%), and making return-to-play decisions (47%) among participants. More than half of participants (66%) had never heard of the Vienna guidelines. After reading the Vienna guidelines' definitions and return-to-play criteria, nearly three-fourths of participants agreed with them. In addition, 68% said that they would use them, and 84% reported that they would teach them to students.

Conclusions.—The majority of program directors and certified athletic trainers used a multidimensional approach to assess and manage a concussion. The National Athletic Trainers' Association position statement and

Vienna guidelines were underused in both the classroom and clinical settings.

▶ This article suffers from all of the inherent problems with survey response research, especially when only a third of the potential participants responded. Because the article dealt only with athletic trainers, it is not surprising that most the athletic trainers overwhelmingly indicated that they primarily use the National Athletic Trainers' Association Position Statement for assessing and managing concussions (61%) and making return to play decisions (41%).

Less than 15% of respondents used the Vienna guidelines, which were not promulgated particularly to athletic trainers but rather all athletic medical disciplines. This study did find an increase in use of neuropsychological testing compared with previous years, but it still is not used by most athletic trainers.

This is an interesting study with regard to the current teaching of sports medicine athletic training professionals, but it really is confined just to that discipline. It therefore is of limited value to other athletic medical disciplines.

R. C. Cantu, MD, MA

Brain function decline in healthy retired athletes who sustained their last sports concussion in early adulthood

De Beaumont L, Théoret H, Mongeon D, et al (Centre de recherche en neuropsychologie et cognition, Canada; Département de Kinésiologie, Canada)

Brain 132:695-708, 2009

Recent studies have shown that the detrimental effects of sports concussions on cognitive and motor function may persist up to a few years post-injury. The present study sought to investigate the effects of having sustained a sports concussion more than 30 years prior to testing on cognitive and motor functions. Nineteen healthy former athletes, in late adulthood (mean age = 60.79; SD = 5.16), who sustained their last sport-related concussion in early adulthood (mean age = 26.05; SD = 9.21) were compared with 21 healthy former athletes with no history of concussion (mean age = 58.89; SD = 9.07). Neuropsychological tests sensitive to age-related changes in cognition were administered. An auditory oddball paradigm was used to evoke P3a and P3b brain responses. Four TMS paradigms were employed to assess motor cortex excitability: (i) resting motor threshold; (ii) paired-pulse intracortical inhibition and intracortical facilitation; (iii) input/output curve and (iv) cortical silent period (CSP). A rapid alternating movement task was also used to characterize motor system dysfunctions. Relative to controls, former athletes with a history of concussion had: (i) lower performance on neuropsychological tests of episodic memory and response inhibition; (ii) significantly delayed and attenuated P3a/P3b components; (iii) significantly prolonged CSP and (iv) significantly reduced movement velocity (bradykinesia). The finding that the P3, the CSP as well as neuropsychological and motor indices were altered more than three decades post-concussion provides evidence for the chronicity of cognitive and motor system changes consecutive to sports concussion.

▶ It is well known that repetitive concussive and subconcussive brain forces can lead to chronic traumatic encephalopathy in susceptible individuals. In our Center for the Study of Traumatic Encephalopathy at Boston University School of Medicine we have now studied the brains of nearly 20 deceased former National Football League (NFL) football players; we found that most of the players with chronic traumatic encephalopathy were lineman who had a low number of recognized concussions and probably a very high number of subconcussive blows. This substantiates the belief that it is total brain trauma that leads to this condition, not simply the number of concussions sustained.

These authors looked at a group of athletes who had sustained concussions and another group of athletes who apparently had no concussions with a detailed neuropsychological assessment, including auditory-evoked potentials some 30 years after their athletic careers had terminated. They found evidence of a significant difference in terms of the neuropsychological test between the concussed groups that performed more poorly than the nonconcussed group.

Articles that talk about concussions without any knowledge of the severity of the concussion as defined by the duration of symptoms, however, tends to lump concussions as all being equal. We know this is not the case, as concussions that have symptoms lasting many months are obviously more severe than concussions where the clinical symptoms last for a very brief period of time. Also, concussions that are incurred very close together probably have a more deleterious effect than concussions incurred years apart.

This is a very interesting article that used a methodology not in the clinical mainstream of neuropsychology. It is nonetheless a very thought-provoking article, and one that I especially sure will be cited in future articles pointing to the effect of concussions and their possible long-standing effects on cognition.

R. C. Cantu, MD, MA

Brain Injury Forces of Moderate Magnitude Elicit the Fencing Response

Hosseini AH, Lifshitz J (Univ of Kentucky, Lexington, KY)

Med Sci Sports Exerc 41:1687-1697, 2009

Introduction.—Traumatic brain injury is heterogeneous, both in its induction and ensuing neurological sequelae. In this way, medical care depends on accurately identifying the severity of injury-related forces. Clinically, injury severity is determined by a combination of the Glasgow Coma Scale, length of unconsciousness, posttraumatic amnesia, and persistence of neurological sequelae. In the laboratory, injury severity is gauged by the biomechanical forces and the acute suppression of neurological reflexes. The present communication describes and validates the "fencing response" as an overt indicator of injury force magnitude and midbrain localization to aid in injury identification and classification.

Methods.—Using YouTube™, the Internet video database, videos were screened for head injury resulting in unconsciousness and documented for the fencing response. Adult male rats were subjected to midline fluid percussion brain injury at two severities, observed for acute neurological reflexes and the midbrain evaluated histopathologically.

Results.—Tonic posturing (fencing response) has been observed to precede convulsions in sports injuries at the moment of impact, where extension and flexion of opposite arms occurs despite body position or gravity. Of the 35 videos identified by an impact to the head and period of unconsciousness, 66% showed a fencing response at the moment of impact, regardless of the side of impact, without ensuing convulsion. Similarly, diffuse brain-injured rats demonstrate a fencing response upon injury at moderate (1.9 atm, 39/44 animals) but not mild severity (1.1 atm, 0/19 animals). The proximity of the lateral vestibular nucleus to the cerebellar peduncles makes it vulnerable to mechanical forces that initiate a neurochemical storm to elicit the neuromotor response, disrupt the blood–brain barrier, and alter the nuclear volume.

Conclusions.—Therefore, the fencing response likely indicates neurological disturbance unique from convulsion associated with mechanical forces of moderate magnitude imparted on the midbrain and can assist in guiding medical care after injury.

▶ This article attempts to correlate the forces that are associated with a loss of consciousness that elicits either the fencing or posturing response during the period of unconsciousness. This has been rather extensively previously reviewed in the neurologic and sports medicine literature, especially by Paul McCrory, and was included in the published document of the International Conference on Concussion in Sports Prague 2004 in the *British Journal of Sports Medicine*. It has long been thought to represent a brain stem response to the concussive injury and to not be associated with epilepsy or the likelihood for posttraumatic epilepsy. One interesting feature of this article is that the authors actually visualized knock-out episodes on YouTube and found that the fencing response, when carefully looked for, occurred in two-third of those individuals rendered unconscious.

Using a fluid percussion model of brain injury and looking at brain injuries sustained by rodents at mild and moderate forces, they found that the fencing reflex was usually not seen with the mild forces and was seen routinely with moderate forces.

These authors attempted therefore to correlate this fencing response with concussion to a concussion that would fall into the complex or moderate concussion as defined by the Prague statement.

I believe that because the definitions of simple and complex concussion have been rescinded by the Zurich document, that correlation is no longer valid. Perhaps the take away message from this article of greatest interest is that the fencing response is often missed unless it is carefully looked for, and that it occurs in a higher incidence of cases than previously thought. Furthermore, the extended arm does not appear to be related to the side of the head that received the blow. The fact that it does not represent epilepsy or the chance for epilepsy has been previously documented and is not new.

R. C. Cantu, MD, MA

Immediate Post-Concussion Assessment and Cognitive Testing (ImPACT) Practices of Sports Medicine Professionals

Covassin T, Elbin RJ III, Stiller-Ostrowski JL, et al (Michigan State Univ, East Lansing; et al)
J Athl Train 44:639-644, 2009

Context.—Computerized neurocognitive testing is becoming popular among clinicians evaluating sport-related concussions across all levels of sport. Baseline neurocognitive testing has been recommended to provide more accurate representation of the preconcussion cognitive status of individual athletes. However, little is known about the use of baseline neurocognitive testing in concussion assessment and management.

Objective.—To examine implementation and practice trends of sports medicine professionals using baseline neurocognitive testing at the high school and collegiate levels.

Design.—Quantitative survey research.

Setting.—Online survey.

Patients or Other Participants.—Certified athletic trainers (ATs) from approximately 1209 US institutions listed on the ImPACT Web site were recruited. A total of 399 ATs completed the survey, for a response return rate of 32.7%.

Main Outcome Measure(s).—Survey questions addressed educational level, years of certification, employment setting, percentage of athletes baseline tested, and accuracy of baseline tests. Other items addressed post-concussive neurocognitive testing protocols and scenarios for return-to-play decisions based on neurocognitive testing.

Results.—Nearly all ATs (94.7%) administered baseline computerized neurocognitive testing to their athletes. However, only 51.9% examined these baseline tests for validity. The majority of ATs indicated that they administer baseline neurocognitive tests most frequently to football players (88.4%), followed by women's soccer players (78.8%) and men's soccer players (71.2%). Nearly all respondents (95.5%) stated that they would not return a symptomatic athlete to play if the athlete's neurocognitive scores were back to baseline. However, when asked if they would return an athlete who is symptom free but who scores below his or her baseline, 86.5% responded *no*, 9.8% responded *yes*, and 3.8% indicated that it *depended on the importance of the competition*.

Conclusions.—The use of baseline testing, baseline testing readministration, and postconcussion protocols among ATs is increasing. However, the

ATs in this study reported that they relied more on symptoms than on neurocognitive test scores when making return-to-play decisions.

▶ This article purports to sample the use of immediate post-concussion assessment of cognitive testing (ImPACT) by sports medicine professionals. Although certified athletic trainers are sports medicine professionals, the term also includes team physicians, and many physician and neuropsychologist sports medicine professionals as well. Therefore, as only certified athletic trainers were surveyed, this article really more correctly should have been titled "ImPACT practices of certified athletic trainers."

Although the fact that 95% used baseline testing was assuring and commendable, the fact that barely half the certified athletic trainers used the tool properly presents awareness of a problem. Only 52% of those studied examined baseline tests for validity. This means the accuracy of the test could have been seriously flawed by sandbagging the baseline.

It was commendable that the trainers used their own symptom assessment ahead of the ImPACT when making return to play decisions with nearly all trainers saying they would not return a symptomatic athlete to play. Although it is very commendable that athletic trainers used a symptom checklist and neuro-cognitive testing in making return to play decisions, a neurological examination, other than for balance testing, was not mentioned. A complete neurological examination that is normal, not just balance testing, should be a part of any return to play decision making after a concussion.

R. C. Cantu, MD, MA

Sport concussion assessment tool: baseline values for varsity collision sport athletes

Shehata N, Wiley JP, Richea S, et al (Univ of Calgary, Canada; et al)
Br J Sports Med 43:730-734, 2009

Objective.—To determine baseline symptom and neurocognitive norms for non-concussed and previously concussed varsity athletes using the sport concussion assessment tool (SCAT).

Study Design.—Descriptive cohort study.

Setting.—University of Calgary.

Subjects.—260 male and female university football, ice hockey and wrestling athletes over three seasons (2005–7).

Methods.—A baseline SCAT was completed during preseason medical evaluation. Subjects were grouped as follows: all participants, men, women, never concussed (NC) and previously concussed (PC).

Main Results.—The mean age of participants was 20.5 years (range 17–32). In total, 41.2% of all athletes had a total post-concussion symptom scale (PCSS) score of 0. The mean baseline PCSS scores were as follows: all participants 4.29; men 3.52; women 6.39; NC 3.75 and PC 5.25. The five most frequently reported symptoms for all athletes were fatigue/low energy (37% of subjects), drowsiness (23%), neck pain (20%), difficulty concentrating (18%) and difficulty remembering (18%). The median immediate recall score was 5/5 for all groups. Women scored a median of 5/5 on delayed recall, whereas all remaining groups scored a median of 4/5. Months in reverse order were successfully completed by 91.6% of subjects. All participants, women and PC scored a median of 6 on reverse digits, whereas men and NC scored a median of 5.

Conclusions.—The mean SCAT baseline PCSS score was approximately 5, although just under half of the athletes scored 0. Female athletes scored better on tests of neurocognitive function. PC athletes scored better than NC athletes on all neurocognitive tests except delayed five-word recall.

▶ When the proceedings of the second International Conference on Concussion in Sport held in Prague in 2004 were published in 2005, they included a sports concussion assessment tool (SCAT). The SCAT was designed primarily for the sideline assessment of concussion and was formed by incorporating the best features of several existing sideline assessment tools such as the SAC into this more robust tool. Although the SCAT is a paper neurocognitive assessment tool involving a postconcussion symptom scale and 3 cognitive tests, it was never meant to replace computer or formal neuropsychological testing. It was also not validated at the time it was published.

The purpose of this study on 260 male and female varsity college athletes, grouped into previous concussion and no previous concussion groups, was to determine SCAT baseline norms and to study subgroup differences for men and women who had no previous concussion history and those who did have a previous concussion history. The fact that the mean postconcussion symptom score was higher in women (6.39) than men (3.52) is consistent with recent literature. The fact that postconcussion athletes scored better on all cognitive tests than those with no previous concussion is unexpected and raises serious questions about the sensitivity of the test.

R. C. Cantu, MD, MA

A novel technique for treating auricular hematomas in mixed martial artists (ultimate fighters)

Roy S, Smith LP (Univ of Miami, FL)

Am J Otolaryngol 31:21-24, 2010

Purpose.—This study aimed to describe a "bolsterless" technique for managing auricular hematomas in professional fighters.

Methods.—Eight auricular hematomas were drained under local anesthesia by incising along an anatomical auricular crease. After evacuation of the hematoma and copious irrigation, the resultant skin flap was replaced in anatomical position, and through-and-through absorbable mattress sutures were used to secure the flap in place. Incision sites were

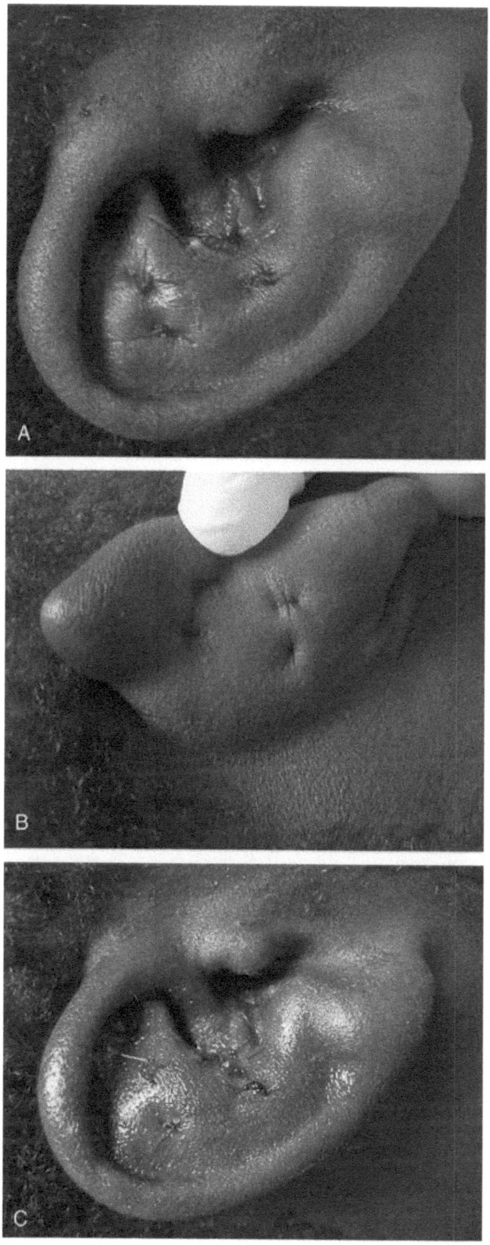

FIGURE 2.—(A) Anterior view of an extensive hematoma after incision and drainage and mattress suture placement. The incision is placed parallel to a natural skin crease. (B) Posterior auricular view after mattress suture placement after incision and drainage of an extensive auricular hematoma. (C) One week after bolsterless treatment of an auricular hematoma reveals no evidence of recurrence with an excellent cosmetic outcome. (Reprinted from Roy S, Smith LP. A novel technique for treating auricular hematomas in mixed martial artists (ultimate fighters). *Am J Otolaryngol.* 2010;31:21-24, with permission from Elsevier.)

left open and dressed with antimicrobial ointment. No bolsters were placed. The patients were given 1 week of oral antibiotic therapy.

Results.—All 8 hematomas resolved without further intervention. All 8 ears returned to their preinjury cosmetic state. Fighters were able to return to training within a week of the initial injury. No postoperative infections or other complications were noted.

Conclusions.—In contrast to wrestlers, mixed martial artists (also called "ultimate fighters") do not routinely wear protective head gear. As a result, they are at increased risk of recurrent auricular hematomas, often resulting in severe auricular deformities (cauliflower ear). These patients are anxious to return to training and fighting, and are reluctant to wear a bolster after repair. At their urging, we agreed to attempt this bolsterless technique. Although 2 patients in this series already had a significant cauliflower ear before being treated for the current hematoma, in all cases the auricle returned to its preinjury condition. Bolsterless treatment using mattress sutures and cosmetically placed incisions represents a successful technique for management of auricular hematomas in this population (Fig 2).

▶ Auricular hematomas are common in many competitive contact and combative type sports, such as rugby, wrestling, and judo. With the advent and increasing popularity of professional mixed martial artists (MMA) or ultimate fighters, there is another large population at risk for these injuries, particularly as they do not wear protective gear for the head or ear. If not properly managed, recurrent trauma to the pinnae can result in the cosmetic deformity of cauliflower ear. Many methods for evacuation of the blood and closure of the dead space are used, usually using either bolsters or pressure bandages—both of which make it difficult to continue with training and competition. Others have described the use of tincture of benzoin or plaster of Paris to create a hard mold inside the ear crease. Some have even sewn in a button or a specially cut piece of flexible plastic. All of these procedures require follow-up by a physician to remove the extra part of the dressing. With the technique illustrated in this article, even patients who are noncompliant and/or lost to follow-up can have a satisfactory outcome and return almost immediately to their physical activity.

C. Lebrun, MD

2 Other Musculoskeletal Injuries

Higher Opioid Doses Predict Poorer Functional Outcome in Patients with Chronic Disabling Occupational Musculoskeletal Disorders

Kidner CL, Mayer TG, Gatchel RJ (PRIDE Res Found, Dallas, TX)
J Bone Joint Surg Am 91:919-927, 2009

Background.—Opioids are frequently used for the postoperative treatment of chronic disabling occupational musculoskeletal disorders. In many such cases, long-term opioid use persists because of patient requests for ongoing pain relief. Little is known about the relationship between chronic opioid use and functional recovery in these patients.

Methods.—A total of 1226 patients with a chronic disabling occupational musculoskeletal disorder were consecutively admitted into an interdisciplinary functional restoration program. They were divided into two groups: 630 patients who reported no opioid use at the time of admission (No group) and 596 patients who reported some opioid use at the time of admission (Yes group). The 516 patients for whom daily opioid doses could be determined were further divided into four subgroups: Low (<30 mg, n = 267), Medium (31 to 60 mg, n = 112), High (61 to 120 mg, n = 78), and Very High (>120 mg, n = 59). During the initial weeks of treatment, patients consented to be weaned from all opioid medications. In addition, the patients were assessed before and after rehabilitation with regard to self-reported measures of pain, function, and depression and were analyzed for change. One year after the termination of treatment, socioeconomic outcomes were assessed to measure work and financial status, healthcare utilization, and recurrent injury-associated pain.

Results.—A higher post-injury opioid dose was associated with a greater risk of program noncompletion, which was anticipated because of the requirement that patients taper opioids. High opioid use was significantly related to important socioeconomic outcomes, such as lower rates of return to work and work retention as well as higher healthcare utilization ($p \leq 0.05$ for all). Moreover, at one year after treatment, the group reporting the highest opioid use was 11.6 times as likely to be receiving Social

Security Disability Income/Supplemental Security Income as compared with the group reporting no opioid use at the time of admission into the program.

Conclusions.—Chronic opioid use beginning after a work-related injury is a predictor of less successful outcomes for patients whose final treatment intervention is an interdisciplinary functional restoration program. Higher dose levels are associated with progressively greater indemnity and medical costs for ongoing disability. Physicians involved in the treatment of chronic disabling occupational musculoskeletal disorders should be aware of problems associated with permitting long-term opioid use in patients with a disabling occupational disorder.

▶ This is a large cohort study that has important clinical implications. The investigators followed 1226 patients with chronic occupational musculoskeletal disorders who were admitted to a rehabilitation program and determined that those who were taking opioids tended to have worse outcomes. Those who had higher opioid use had lower rates of completion of the rehabilitation program (a prerequisite of the rehabilitation program was agreement to be weaned off the medication). One year postrehabilitation, 88% of those who took opioids returned to work versus 94% of those who did not take these medications. Further, work retention rates (percentage of those who were still at work) were significantly higher for those who did not take opioids (85% vs 69%). Also, 30% of those who took opioids sought treatment from a new provider (mostly related to finding providers who would agree to restart the opioid prescription). There was a dose-response relationship: those persons who were higher users of opioids tended to have worse outcomes. All these analyses considered only those persons who completed the rehabilitation program—implying that perhaps the associations with opioid use may be even stronger than those reported (if we assume that noncompleters of the program had worse outcomes). This study has important clinical implications: prolonged opioid use does not seem advisable for patients with chronic musculoskeletal pain.

D. E. Feldman, PT, PhD

Mechanotherapy: how physical therapists' prescription of exercise promotes tissue repair

Khan KM, Scott A (Univ of British Columbia, Vancouver, Canada)

Br J Sports Med 43:247-251, 2009

Mechanotransduction is the physiological process where cells sense and respond to mechanical loads. This paper reclaims the term "mechanotherapy" and presents the current scientific knowledge underpinning how load may be used therapeutically to stimulate tissue repair and remodelling in tendon, muscle, cartilage and bone. The purpose of this short article is to answer a frequently asked question "How precisely does exercise promote tissue healing?" This is a fundamental question for clinicians who prescribe exercise for tendinopathies, muscle tears, non-inflammatory arthropathies and even controlled loading after fractures. High-quality randomised controlled trials and systematic reviews show that various forms of exercise or movement prescription benefit patients with a wide range of musculoskeletal problems. But what happens at the tissue level to promote repair and remodelling of tendon, muscle, articular cartilage and bone? The one-word answer is "mechanotransduction", but rather than finishing there and limiting this paper to 95 words, we provide a short illustrated introduction to this remarkable, ubiquitous, non-neural, physiological process. We also re-introduce the term "mechanotherapy" to distinguish therapeutics (exercise prescription specifically to treat injuries) from the homeostatic role of mechanotransduction. Strictly speaking, mechanotransduction maintains normal musculoskeletal structures in the absence of injury. After first outlining the process of mechanotransduction, we provide well-known clinical therapeutic examples of mechanotherapy–turning movement into tissue healing.

▶ I have a competing interest on this article as I was one of the authors, but I feel justified to comment on it because I have been invited to speak about this topic at many conferences, including the ACSM's Sutton Lecture (2009). The purpose of the article is to connect the basic science of mechanotransduction-cellular response to loading, with the clinical phenomenon of tissue responding to rehabilitation. The article argues that strengthening, per se, is unlikely to be the ultimate process that stimulates cellular repair; it is the process of mechanotransduction that is stimulated by strengthening that likely promotes healing. We reproduce a key figure to illustrate this here (Fig in the original article). The precise dose of mechanotransduction needed is not understood at the cellular level in tendon. In bone, animal studies suggest that certain frequencies of stimulus, with rest periods, are superior to large numbers of stimuli.

K. M. Khan, MD, PhD

Effect of taping on the shoulders of Australian football players

Bradley T, Baldwick C, Fischer D, et al (Univ of New South Wales, Sydney, Australia; St George Crows Sydney AFL Club, Australia)

Br J Sports Med 43:735-738, 2009

Background.—Taping of the shoulder is common in many sports, particularly Australian football, a contact sport that often involves marking (catching) the ball overhead and has a high incidence of shoulder instability.

Hypothesis.—Taping of the shoulder reduces glenohumeral joint laxity and improves proprioception without impairing function.

Study Design.—Crossover study design.

Methods.—33 male players aged 18–31 years were recruited from a local Australian football club. The dominant shoulder of each player was tested with and without taping in a randomised fashion by an examiner blinded to the presence or absence of taping. The tests were (1) inferior glenohumeral joint laxity (the Orthopaedic Research Institute laxometer), (2) shoulder joint position sense accuracy using an optical tracking system, and (3) handballing accuracy.

Results.—The methods for testing laxity and joint position sense had good intraobserver reliability and sensitivity. All subjects tolerated the taping and testing. Glenohumeral joint laxity ($p = 0.75$), joint position sense ($p = 0.56$) and handballing accuracy ($p = 0.6$) were not changed by taping.

Conclusions.—Taping of the shoulder joint in uninjured and non-symptomatic Australian football players in a pattern that attempted not to restrict their range of overhead movement did not significantly affect the accuracy of joint position sense, inferior laxity or handball accuracy.

Clinical relevance.—These data suggest that taping of the shoulder is unlikely to decrease the incidence of injury—specifically dislocation—of the shoulder in Australian football players.

▶ Shoulder instability is a common problem in many overhead sports, including Aussie rules football. Apparently, taping of the shoulder joint, even in asymptomatic uninjured players, is frequently done to ostensibly enhance proprioception and prevent excessive movement of the humeral head. This well-designed, single-blinded, crossover study uses a single physical therapist and taping

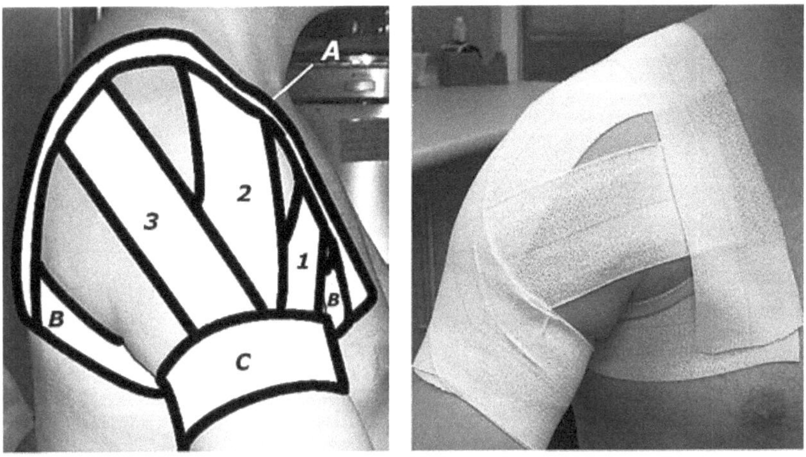

(a) (b)

FIGURE 1.—Taping pattern of rigid strapping tape. (a) A, first anchor; B, second anchor; C, third anchor; 1, first support strip; 2, second support strip; 3, third support strip. (b) Taping pattern of elastic overwrapping. (Reprinted from Bradley T, Baldwick C, Fischer D, et al. Effect of taping on the shoulders of Australian football players. *Br J Sports Med.* 2009;43:735-738, with permission from the BMJ Publishing Group.)

procedure (Fig 1), several previously validated measures of inferior shoulder laxity, joint position sense, and a functional assessment of the accuracy of a common skill—handballing a regulation Australian football through the center hole of a commercial Auskick canvas target. (Although the at-risk position for anterior shoulder dislocation is in an abducted, externally rotated position, and due to anterior instability, the authors have shown earlier[1] that inferior translation is enhanced in shoulders that have had an anterior dislocation.) In this population of 33 asymptomatic male players, taping had no significant effect on shoulder function, position sense, or inferior laxity. Further studies looking at symptomatic shoulder, taping under tension, and/or the use of the new Kinesio taping techniques are warranted.

C. Lebrun, MD

Reference

1. Sein ML, Appleyard RC, Walton JR, Bradley T, Murrell GA. Reliability testing of a new shoulder laxometer to assess inferior glenohumeral joint translation. *Br J Sports Med.* 2008;42:178-182.

Radial extracorporeal shockwave treatment compared with supervised exercises in patients with subacromial pain syndrome: single blind randomised study

Engebretsen K, Grotle M, Bautz-Holter E, et al (Ullevaal Univ Hosp, Oslo, Norway; Univ of Oslo; et al)
BMJ 339:b3360, 2009

Objective.—To compare the effectiveness of radial extracorporeal shockwave treatment with that of supervised exercises in patients with shoulder pain.

Design.—Single blind randomised study.

Setting.—Outpatient clinic of physical medicine and rehabilitation department in Oslo, Norway.

Participants.—104 patients with subacromial shoulder pain lasting at least three months.

Interventions.—Radial extracorporeal shockwave treatment: one session weekly for four to six weeks. Supervised exercises: two 45 minute sessions weekly for up to 12 weeks.

Primary Outcome Measure.—Shoulder pain and disability index.

Results.—A treatment effect in favour of supervised exercises at 6, 12, and 18 weeks was found. The adjusted treatment effect was −8.4 (95% confidence interval −16.5 to −0.6) points. A significantly higher proportion of patients in the group treated with supervised exercises improved—odds ratio 3.2 (1.3 to 7.8). More patients in the shockwave treatment group had additional treatment between 12 and 18 weeks—odds ratio 5.5 (1.3 to 26.4).

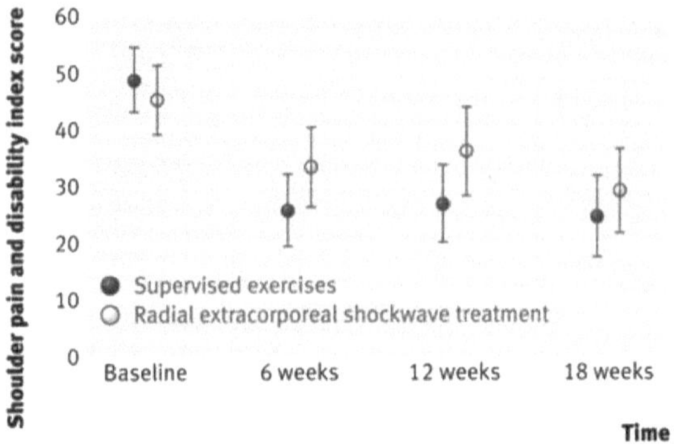

FIGURE 2.—Mean shoulder pain and disability index scores with 95% confidence intervals for supervised exercises and radial extracorporeal shockwave treatment. (Reprinted from Engebretsen K, Grotle M, Bautz-Holter E, et al. Radial extracorporeal shockwave treatment compared with supervised exercises in patients with subacromial pain syndrome: single blind randomised study. *BMJ*. 2009;339:b3360.)

Conclusion.—Supervised exercises were more effective than radial extracorporeal shockwave treatment for short term improvement in patients with subacromial shoulder pain.

Trial Registration.—Clinical trials NCT00653081.

▶ This is a well-documented randomized controlled trial that supports the benefit of supervised exercise for subacromial pain syndrome over that of radial extracorporeal shockwave treatment. Although there were no differences for pain, function, active range of motion, and use of medications, the supervised exercise group did better in terms of the main outcome: the shoulder pain and disability index (SPADI) score, as well as return to work. There was improvement in the score on the SPADI in both groups (Fig 2), although the supervised exercise group had a higher degree of improvement and more in this group achieved a reduction in SPADI score exceeding the smallest detectable difference of 19.6 points. Although there was no placebo group, the authors argue that previous research indicated that supervised exercise is superior to placebo; however, they do admit that previous research found no difference between sham and shockwave treatment. Nevertheless, it does appear that supervised exercises are superior to radial extracorporeal shockwave treatment for short-term improvement in persons with shoulder pain.

D. E. Feldman, PT, PhD

Impact of Cycling on Hip Subluxation in Children With Spinal Cord Injury

Johnston TE, Betz RR, Lauer RT (Shriners Hosps for Children, Philadelphia, PA)

J Pediatr Orthop 29:402-405, 2009

Background.—Hip subluxation is common in children with spinal cord injury, especially in those younger than 10 years. The effects of standing with functional electrical stimulation (FES) on hip subluxation have been studied in these children. However, FES cycling is now available to children with spinal cord injury, but the effect of this intervention on hip subluxation has not been studied.

Methods.—Hip migration indices were measured before and after a 6-month program of FES cycling, passive cycling, or electrical stimulation exercise without cycling performed 3 times per week. During cycling, children were positioned to avoid hip adduction and internal rotation to decrease potential stress on the hip.

Results.—There were no changes in the hip migration indices for children in any group after participating in the study.

Conclusions.—These findings suggest that the 3 interventions used in this study may be safe for the hip, provided that the hips are positioned to avoid adduction and internal rotation while cycling.

Level of Evidence.—Randomized controlled trial, level 2.

► The authors of this randomized trial state that cycling in a controlled fashion (ie, no hip adduction or internal rotation allowed) does not increase hip subluxation in children with spinal cord injuries. However, this study may be underpowered to test this relationship (10 children in each of the 3 intervention groups: controlled functional electric stimulation cycling; passive cycling; and electrical stimulation alone). Furthermore, there is no information regarding compliance with the cycling protocol (which was done at home under parental supervision and assistance) and it is unknown if these children actually completed the program as required. Because of these issues, I would hesitate to endorse the authors' conclusions. I would consider this a pilot study that suggests that controlled cycling may be a safe activity for children with spinal cord injury. To their credit, the authors do describe the interventions well and the measurement of hip migration indices. Replication of the project with a larger group of children may be indicated.

D. E. Feldman, PT, PhD

Cost-Effectiveness of Accelerated Perioperative Care and Rehabilitation After Total Hip and Knee Arthroplasty

Larsen K, Hansen TB, Thomsen PB, et al (Regional Hosp Holstebro, Denmark)
J Bone Joint Surg Am 91:761-772, 2009

Background.—Accelerated perioperative rehabilitation protocols following total hip and knee arthroplasties are currently being implemented worldwide, but the cost-effectiveness of these protocols from a societal perspective is not known. We compared the cost-effectiveness of an accelerated perioperative care and rehabilitation protocol with that of a more standard protocol for patients treated with total hip and knee arthroplasty.

Methods.—A cost-effectiveness study was undertaken as a study piggybacked on a randomized clinical trial comparing early outcomes of an accelerated and intensive postoperative rehabilitation regimen with those of a more standard rehabilitation protocol. We assessed eighty-seven patients (forty-two who received the standard protocol and forty-five who received the accelerated protocol) for a total of twelve months. Costs from the time of the patient's visit immediately before the operation to one year postoperatively were calculated with use of activity-based costing analysis. Postoperative quality-adjusted life-years (QALYs) were calculated from validated patient diaries and questionnaires at fifteen time points. The primary objective was to determine whether one intervention was dominant over the other during a twelve-month period or, if neither was dominant, to determine the incremental cost-effectiveness ratio.

Results.—The result of the randomized clinical trial showed the accelerated intervention to be effective, with a reduction in the length of the hospital stay and a gain in health-related quality of life at the three-month follow-up time point. The cost-effectiveness study showed the accelerated protocol to be significantly less expensive than the standard protocol ($p = 0.036$), with an average reduction in cost of 18,880 Danish kroner (95% confidence interval, 1899 to 38,152) (approximately US $4000). Patients treated with the accelerated protocol following hip arthroplasty had an additional average gain of 0.08 QALY (95% confidence interval, 0.02 to 0.15) compared with the patients who received the standard protocol ($p = 0.006$); this led to a 98% dominance of the accelerated protocol over the standard protocol. No significant or clinically relevant difference in the numbers of QALYs associated with the two protocols was observed for the patients treated with knee arthroplasty.

Conclusions.—An accelerated perioperative care and rehabilitation protocol can be both cost-saving and clinically more effective after total hip arthroplasty, whereas it can be cost-saving with no observed significant difference in effect, from a societal perspective, after knee arthroplasty.

▶ This study confirms that an accelerated intervention rehabilitation protocol is more cost-effective than a standard protocol for persons treated with hip or knee replacement surgery. The accelerated intervention includes a group information session before hospital admission, 1 nurse in charge (as opposed to several in the standard group) of a specialized multidisciplinary team of nurses, occupational therapists, and physiotherapists, nutrition screening, and focus on daily consumption of 1.5 L fluid and 2 protein beverages, mobilization started on the day of surgery (as opposed to the next day), and intensive mobilization (8 hrs daily vs 4 in the standard group). An original randomized trial demonstrated that the accelerated protocol reduced length of hospital stay and improved health related quality of life. This study assessed 1-year outcomes from a societal perspective, relating incremental costs of the 2 interventions to the incremental effect in quality-adjusted life years. The accelerated intervention was more cost-effective from a societal perspective for patients who underwent hip arthroplasty. It was also less costly for those who underwent knee arthroplasty, although there was no significant difference in effect for these persons. Based on this study as well as previous research that demonstrate better outcomes for patients, the authors' conclusion that these accelerated protocols should be instituted seems warranted.

D. E. Feldman, PT, PhD

Home Training, Local Corticosteroid Injection, or Radial Shock Wave Therapy for Greater Trochanter Pain Syndrome

Rompe JD, Segal NA, Cacchio A, et al (OrthoTrauma Evaluation Ctr, Mainz, Germany, Univ of Iowa; Ospedale "San Salvatore" di L'Aquila, Italy)
Am J Sports Med 37:1981-1990, 2009

Background.—There are no controlled studies testing the efficacy of various nonoperative strategies for treatment of greater trochanter pain syndrome.

Hypothesis.—The null hypothesis was that local corticosteroid injection, home training, and repetitive low-energy shock wave therapy produce equivalent outcomes 4 months from baseline.

Study Design.—Randomized controlled clinical trial; Level of evidence, 2.

Methods.—Two hundred twenty-nine patients with refractory unilateral greater trochanter pain syndrome were assigned sequentially to a home training program, a single local corticosteroid injection (25 mg prednisolone), or a repetitive low-energy radial shock wave treatment. Subjects underwent outcome assessments at baseline and at 1, 4, and 15 months. Primary outcome measures were degree of recovery, measured on a 6-point Likert scale (subjects with rating completely recovered or much improved were rated as treatment success), and severity of pain over the past week (0-10 points) at 4-month follow-up.

Results.—One month from baseline, results after corticosteroid injection (success rate, 75%; pain rating, 2.2 points) were significantly better than those after home training (7%; 5.9 points) or shock wave therapy (13%; 5.6 points). Regarding treatment success at 4 months, radial shock wave therapy led to significantly better results (68%; 3.1 points) than did home training (41%; 5.2 points) and corticosteroid injection (51%; 4.5 points). The null hypothesis was rejected. Fifteen months from baseline, radial shock wave therapy (74%; 2.4 points) and home training (80%; 2.7 points) were significantly more successful than was corticosteroid injection (48%; 5.3 points).

Conclusion.—The role of corticosteroid injection for greater trochanter pain syndrome needs to be reconsidered. Subjects should be properly informed about the advantages and disadvantages of the treatment options, including the economic burden. The significant short-term superiority of a single corticosteroid injection over home training and shock wave therapy declined after 1 month. Both corticosteroid injection and home training were significantly less successful than was shock wave therapy at 4-month follow-up. Corticosteroid injection was significantly less successful than was home training or shock wave therapy at 15-month follow-up.

▶ This study provides evidence that radial shock wave therapy and home exercise are both effective in the long term for greater trochanter pain syndrome. This study has a lot of positive features. First, the authors are very specific regarding inclusion criteria for persisting lateral hip pain or probable trochanteric bursitis. Second, the treatment procedures are also extremely well described, including the exact instructions for home exercises. Third, the follow-up was for 15 months, which is substantial for these types of studies. Limitations are well described by the authors, in particular the fact that there was no placebo group that could have provided data on the spontaneous course of greater trochanter pain syndrome. Finally, the authors' conclusion is well founded; they recommend that corticosteroid injection should be used with caution for this condition because there are high recurrence rates after 1 month. Furthermore, use of radial shock wave therapy or home exercises may depend on available resources, because in the long term there were no significant differences between the 2 types of treatment.

D. E. Feldman, PT, PhD

Adolescent Anterior Cruciate Ligament Reconstruction: A Retrospective Analysis of Quadriceps Strength Recovery and Return to Full Activity After Surgery

Wells L, Dyke JA, Albaugh J, et al (Children's Hosp of Philadelphia, PA)

J Pediatr Orthop 29:486-489, 2009

Background.—This study was intended to provide quantitative assessment of quadriceps muscle recovery in adolescent athletes after anterior cruciate ligament (ACL) reconstruction.

Methods.—Quadriceps peak torque values from 55 athletes who underwent ACL reconstruction were analyzed. The mean age of the patients was 15.93 ± 1.65 years (40 girls, 15 boys). Isokinetic data were obtained using the Biodex System 3. Quadriceps muscle recovery was defined as achieving ≥85% peak torque for side-to-side comparison.

Results.—Time-to-quadriceps muscle recovery was as follows: 15% by the end of 3 months, 11% by 4 months, 13% by 5 months, and 20% by 6 months. Overall, 32 patients (59%) achieved ≥85% quadriceps strength within 6 months of their surgery date. Of those patients, 16 (50%) patients returned to full activity within 6 months of the date of surgery. Sex was not found to be a significant difference in regard to strength outcomes.

Conclusions.—Quadriceps muscle recovery is one criterion considered when allowing return to unrestricted activities after ACL reconstruction.

On the basis of results of this study, middle and high school age athletes have the ability to regain the necessary quadriceps muscle strength required to return to sport within 6 months.

Significance.—Using objective measures of quadriceps muscle return after ACL reconstruction can pinpoint timing of recovery, aid in specific training of deficient muscle groups, and guide return-to-play recommendations for those treating athletes with ACL reconstruction.

▶ Athletes are always eager to return to action after knee ligament surgery. This study provides useful information in guiding team physicians as they make decisions and counsel young competitors. In particular, these investigators focus on measures of quadriceps function. Perhaps it should be noted that only half of these athletes could return to full activity within 6 months of their surgery. That these data can be gained from 55 athletes who are, on the average, only 16 years of age attests to the intensity of sports play by young athletes and the stresses that are placed on knee structures in today's sports competition. This report, which includes mostly female athletes, reminds us of the particular susceptibility of teenage girls for knee ligament injuries. Continued efforts to understand the reason for gender differences in anterior cruciate injuries should remain a high priority for future researchers.

T. Rowland, MD

Gait mechanics after ACL reconstruction: implications for the early onset of knee osteoarthritis

Butler RJ, Minick KI, Ferber R, et al (Univ of Evansville, IN; Univ of Calgary, Alberta, Canada)

Br J Sports Med 43:366-370, 2009

Background.—Individuals who sustain a rupture of the anterior cruciate ligament (ACL) are at an increased risk for developing early-onset knee osteoarthritis (OA). The mechanism behind the early onset of the disease is still unknown. Knee OA progression has been previously examined by calculating the internal knee-abduction moment during gait. However, knee-joint moments have not been examined in individuals after ACL reconstruction as a potential mechanism for disease progression in early knee OA.

Objective.—To determine if individuals who have undergone ACL reconstruction exhibit altered gait mechanics that may be associated with knee OA progression.

Methods.—In total, 17 people who had previously undergone ACL reconstruction were enrolled in the study. A matched control group was recruited for comparison. All participants underwent gait analysis at an intentional walking speed to examine variables previously associated with knee OA progression, primarily the internal peak knee-abduction moment, during gait. One way ANOVAs were performed to examine

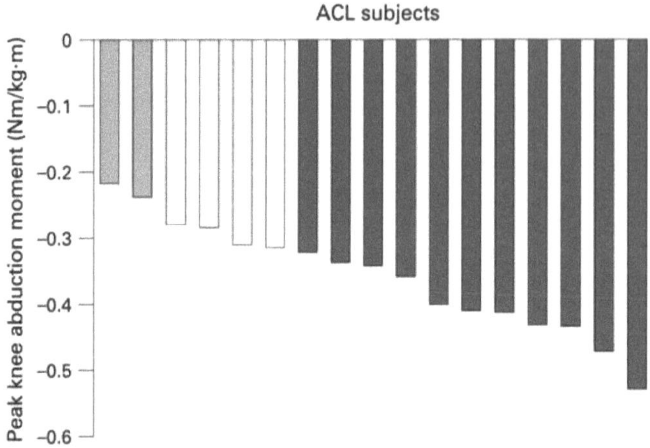

FIGURE 3.—Peak knee-abduction moment values for all subjects in the ACL group (grey bars represent individuals >1 SEM below mean value for controls, white bars represent individuals within 1 SEM of mean value for controls and the hatched bars represent individuals >1 above mean value for controls). (Reprinted from Butler RJ, Minick KI, Ferber R, et al. Gait mechanics after ACL reconstruction: implications for the early onset of knee osteoarthritis. *Br J Sports Med.* 2009;43:366-370, with permission from the BMJ Publishing Group.)

differences in gait mechanics between the two groups. All joint moments were calculated as internal moments.

Results.—The peak knee-abduction moment was increased by 21% in the ACL compared with the control group ($p = 0.04$). No other differences were seen in frontal plane knee or hip mechanics.

Conclusion.—It seems that individuals who have undergone ACL reconstruction exhibit an increased peak knee-abduction moment that may establish a potential mechanism of the earlier onset of knee OA in this population (Fig 3).

▶ Approximately half of those individuals who sustain an anterior cruciate ligament (ACL) injury will develop early onset osteoarthritis (OA). Because it is known that increased loading of the knee's medial compartment is an important predictor of OA progression, these authors hypothesized that individuals who have undergone ACL reconstruction would have a greater medial knee loading and are therefore at risk of developing medial compartment early onset OA. The authors report findings to support their hypothesis. Interestingly, the study had 2 patients who had significantly smaller medial knee loads compared with gender, age, activity, and body mass index matched controls (Fig 3). The authors suggest that these 2 patients are at risk for lateral compartment early onset OA. This is important clinically because the conservative interventions for patients with knee OA, wedged foot orthoses, and knee braces, are designed to reduce medial knee loads. Knowing that a postACL reconstruction patient presents with a reduced medial knee loading pattern suggests that the standard foot orthoses and knee braces would actually accelerate the lateral compartment early onset OA progression.

M. R. Pierrynowski, PhD

Management of Tendinopathy

Rees JD, Maffulli N, Cook J (Defence Med Rehabilitation Centre, Surrey, UK; Keele Univ School of Medicine, Staffordshire, UK; Deakin Univ, Melbourne, Victoria, Australia)

Am J Sports Med 37:1855-1867, 2009

Overuse disorders of tendons, or tendinopathies, present a challenge to sports physicians, surgeons, and other health care professionals dealing with athletes. The Achilles, patellar, and supraspinatus tendons are particularly vulnerable to injury and often difficult to manage successfully. Inflammation was believed central to the pathologic process, but histopathologic evidence has confirmed the failed healing response nature of these conditions. Excessive or inappropriate loading of the musculotendinous unit is believed to be central to the disease process, although the exact mechanism by which this occurs remains uncertain. Additionally, the location of the lesion (for example, the midtendon or osteotendinous junction) has become increasingly recognized as influencing both the pathologic process and subsequent management.

The mechanical, vascular, neural, and other theories that seek to explain the pathologic process are explored in this article. Recent developments in the nonoperative management of chronic tendon disorders are reviewed, as is the rationale for surgical intervention. Recent surgical advances, including minimally invasive tendon surgery, are reviewed. Potential future management strategies, such as stem cell therapy, growth factor treatment, and gene transfer, are also discussed.

▶ This is a well-written and comprehensive review of tendinopathies by 3 genuine leaders in the field. The authors review the pathogenesis debate concisely and begin to focus on the management of tendinopathy. They endorse that eccentric exercise has the best evidence as a first-line treatment, and they appropriately raise questions about the use of routine but unproven treatments such as corticosteroids at the lateral elbow.

This is an ideal article for a resident or fellow in orthopedics to read. It really will save them lots of time. The authors are open-minded about tendinopathy surgical results (ie, there is no hard sell that surgery is the answer). Importantly, they draw attention to the important clinical issue of the anatomical location of Achilles region pain—midportion or insertional. These pathologies have very different prognosis—the insertional condition is worse!

K. M. Khan, MD, PhD

Supervised exercise therapy versus usual care for patellofemoral pain syndrome: an open label randomised controlled trial

van Linschoten R, van Middelkoop M, Berger MY, et al (Erasmus Univ Med Centre, Rotterdam, Netherlands; et al)

BMJ 339:b4074, 2009

Objective.—To assess the effectiveness of supervised exercise therapy compared with usual care with respect to recovery, pain, and function in patients with patellofemoral pain syndrome.

Design.—Open label randomised controlled trial.

Setting.—General practice and sport physician practice.

Participants.—Patients with a new episode of patellofemoral pain syndrome recruited by their general practitioner or sport physician.

Interventions.—The intervention group received a standardised exercise programme for 6 weeks tailored to individual performance and supervised by a physical therapist, and were instructed to practise the tailored exercises at home for 3 months. The control group were assigned usual care, which comprised a "wait and see" approach of rest during periods of pain and refraining from pain provoking activities. Both the intervention group and the control group received written information about patellofemoral pain syndrome and general instructions for home exercises.

Main Outcome Measures.—The primary outcomes were self reported recovery (7 point Likert scale), pain at rest and pain on activity (0-10 point numerical rating scale), and function (0-100 point Kujala patellofemoral score) at 3 months and 12 months follow-up.

Results.—A total of 131 participants were included in the study: 65 in the intervention group and 66 in the control group. After 3 months, the intervention group showed better outcomes than the control group with regard to pain at rest (adjusted difference −1.07, 95% confidence interval −1.92 to −0.22; effect size 0.47), pain on activity (−1.00, −1.91 to −0.08; 0.45), and function (4.92, 0.14 to 9.72; 0.34). At 12 months, the intervention group continued to show better outcomes than the control group with regard to pain (adjusted difference in pain at rest −1.29, −2.16 to −0.42; effect size 0.56; pain on activity −1.19, −2.22 to −0.16; effect size 0.54), but not function (4.52, −0.73 to 9.76). A higher proportion of patients in the exercise group than in the control group reported recovery (41.9% *v* 35.0% at 3 months and 62.1% *v* 50.8% at 12 months), although the differences in self reported recovery between the two groups were not statistically significant. Predefined subgroup analyses revealed that patients recruited by sport physicians (n = 30) did not benefit from the intervention, whereas those recruited by general practitioners (n = 101) showed significant and clinically relevant differences in pain and function in favour of the intervention group.

Conclusion.—Supervised exercise therapy resulted in less pain and better function at short term and long term follow-up compared with usual care in patients with patellofemoral pain syndrome in general practice. Exercise therapy did not produce a significant difference in the rate of self reported recovery.

Trial Registration.—ISRCTN83938749.

▶ This article is of particular importance because patellofemoral pain is the most common presentation in sports medicine. The article builds on previous randomized control trials (RCTs) that have shown the effectiveness of exercise therapy[1,2] by comparing the exercise program with usual care. Thus, in this study, the control group received some static exercises the way a general practitioner (GP) may prescribe them.

Importantly, there were significant positive benefits from the physiotherapy at both 3 and 12 months. Interestingly, patients' "self-perception" of cure (total recovery) did not differ between groups. However, there are reasons why this may have occurred (including the definition of "total cure").

The bottom line from this excellent study is that physiotherapy exercise prescription does benefit patients with patellofemoral pain. Doctors should be prescribing it.

K. M. Khan, MD, PhD

References

1. Crossley K, Bennell K, Green S, Cowan S, McConnell J. Physical therapy for patellofemoral pain: a randomized, double-blinded, placebo-controlled trial. *Am J Sports Med.* 2002;30:857-865.
2. Collins N, Crossley K, Beller E, Darnell R, McPoil T, Vicenzino B. Foot orthoses and physiotherapy in the treatment of patellofemoral pain syndrome: randomised clinical trial. *BMJ.* 2008;337:a1735.

Evaluation of anterior talofibular ligament injury with stress radiography, ultrasonography and MR imaging

Oae K, Takao M, Uchio Y, et al (Shimane Univ School of Medicine, Japan; Teikyo Univ, Tokyo, Japan; et al)

Skeletal Radiol 39:41-47, 2010

Objective.—The purpose of this study was to clarify the efficacy of stress radiography (stress X-P), ultrasonography (US), and magnetic resonance (MR) imaging in the detection of the anterior talofibular ligament (ATFL) injury.

Methods.—Thirty-four patients with ankle sprain were involved. In all patients, Stress X-P, US, MR imaging, and arthroscopy were performed. The arthroscopic results were considered to be the gold standard. The imaging results were compared with the arthroscopic results, and the accuracy calculated.

Results.—Arthroscopic findings showed ATFL injury in 30 out of 34 cases. The diagnosis of ATFL injury with stress X-P, US, MR imaging were made with an accuracy of 67, 91 and 97%. US and MR imaging

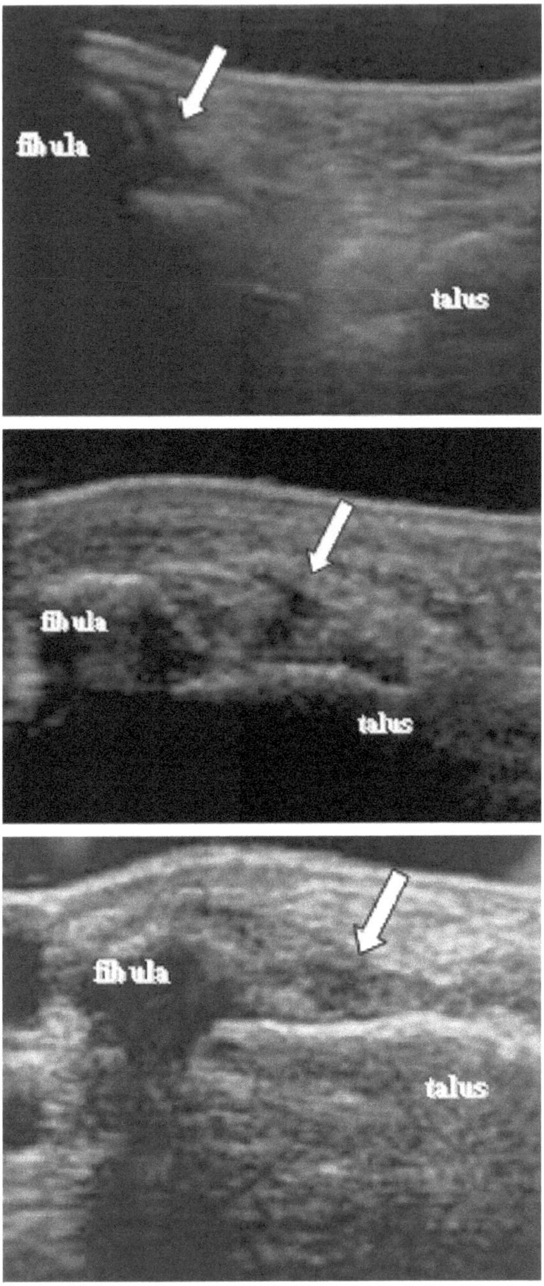

FIGURE 2.—Sonographic appearance of the ATFL. Hypoechoic lesion is seen in the disrupted site of the ligament. *Top*: at the attachment to the fibula; *middle*: at the mid-substance; *below*: at the attachment to the talus. (With kind permission from Springer Science+Business Media: Oae K, Takao M, Uchio Y, et al. Evaluation of anterior talofibular ligament injury with stress radiography, ultrasonography and MR imaging. *Skeletal Radiol*. 2010;39:41-47.)

demonstrated the same location of the injury as arthroscopy in 63 and 93%.

Conclusion.—We have clarified the diagnostic value of stress X-P, US, and MR imaging in diagnosis of ATFL injury. We obtained satisfactory results with US and MR imaging.

▶ Ankle sprains are commonly seen in sport medicine practice. Injuries to the anterior talofibular ligament (ATFL) are the most frequent, occurring primarily through an inversion mechanism. Although most of these are successfully treated with conservative therapy, some of the more severe cases require surgical management and, therefore, more precise and accurate assessment of the amount of damage. Clinical examination (by the anterior drawer and talar tilt tests) is sometimes limited in acute cases, secondary to pain and swelling; while in chronic conditions, it becomes more important to make the correct diagnosis before planning surgery. This study is interesting in that it compares the diagnostic accuracy of stress radiography (stress X-P) with ultrasonography (US) and magnetic resonance (MR) imaging in the detection of ATFL injury to the gold standard of arthroscopic findings in 34 consecutive patients. However, the lateral stress X-P views only evaluated anterior translation with the aid of the stress-testing device Telos (Telos, Griesheim, Germany), measuring the amount of anterior displacement of the talus from the posterior lip of the tibia to the nearest articular surface of the talus. It would have been interesting to have also included anterior X-P views to assess the degree of talar tilt, but it is more difficult to standardize the amount of inversion stress applied during radiography. The imaging reader had no knowledge of the patient's clinical history and physical examination—thereby making this a single-blind evaluation; addition of another reader could have added useful information on intraobserver reliability. Nevertheless, this study is valuable in that it demonstrates greater clinical accuracy, sensitivity, and specificity with US (Fig 2) and MR than with stress X-P in the evaluation of ATFL injuries. Given that MR imaging is time consuming and expensive, these findings portend the ever-increasing value of diagnostic US in the management of musculoskeletal soft tissue injuries.

C. Lebrun, MD

Bone Geometry, Strength, and Muscle Size in Runners with a History of Stress Fracture

Popp KL, Hughes JM, Smock AJ, et al (Univ of Minnesota, Minneapolis; et al)
Med Sci Sports Exerc 41:2145-2150, 2009

Purpose.—Our primary aim was to explore differences in estimates of tibial bone strength, in female runners with and without a history of stress fractures. Our secondary aim was to explore differences in bone geometry, volumetric density, and muscle size that may explain bone strength outcomes.

Methods.—A total of 39 competitive distance runners aged 18–35 yr, with (SFX, $n = 19$) or without (NSFX, $n = 20$) a history of stress fracture were recruited for this cross-sectional study. Peripheral quantitative computed tomography (XCT 3000; Orthometrix, White Plains, NY) was used to assess volumetric bone mineral density (vBMD, $mg \cdot mm^{-3}$), bone area (ToA, mm^2), and estimated compressive bone strength (bone strength index (BSI) = ToA × total volumetric density (ToD^2)) at the distal tibia (4%). Total (ToA, mm^2) and cortical (CoA, mm^2) bone area, cortical vBMD, and estimated bending strength (strength–strain index (SSIp), mm^3) were measured at the 15%, 25%, 33%, 45%, 50%, and 66% sites. Muscle cross-sectional area (MCSA) was measured at the 50% and 66% sites.

Results.—Participants in the SFX group had significantly smaller (7%–8%) CoA at the 45%, 50%, and 66% sites ($P \leq 0.05$ for all), significantly lower SSIp (9%–10%) at the 50% and 66% sites, and smaller MCSA (7%–8%) at the 66% site. The remaining bone parameters including vBMD were not significantly different between groups. After adjusting for MCSA, there were no differences between groups for any measured bone outcomes.

Conclusions.—These findings suggest that cortical bone strength, cortical area, and MCSA are all lower in runners with a history of stress fracture. However, the lower strength was appropriate for the smaller muscle size, suggesting that interventions to reduce stress fracture risk might be aimed at improving muscle size and strength.

▶ Not everyone in sports medicine will be aware of the shift in emphasis from bone density to measures of bone strength as a measure of the properties of athletes' skeletons. Bone density is traditionally measured by dual-energy x-ray absorptiometry (DXA), which provides a 2-dimensional image of the lumbar spine and proximal femur. High-school level physics and mathematics are enough to alert us that a 2-dimensional measure cannot be a true density measure, so the convention of calling DXA outcomes "density" leads to obvious challenges. Specifically, a limitation of this measure is that it does not take into account the bone size—and a larger bone, even of identical material composition, is more difficult to break than a smaller bone.

Hence the importance of this article—the authors used the more cutting edge peripheral quantitative computed tomography (pQCT) method to evaluate the distal tibia as a marker of the athelete's overall bone health. This novel method, now gaining popularity as progressively more laboratories obtain the necessary pQCT instrument, allows the calculation of bone strength. This is done by applying mathematics/engineering principles to the 3-dimensional image of bone cross-sections provided by the pQCT instrument.

Having got these important issues out of the way, what was the finding? First, the author acknowledges that this was a cross-sectional study design, so conclusions need to remain limited. Bearing this in mind, the key findings were that the athletes with the stress fractures had smaller bones, but they were smaller people with smaller muscle. The ratio of muscle to bone was normal—generally the case for bone and muscle. Thus, the take-home message for coaches, clinicians, and athletes was that strength training—aiming to increase muscle mass at key skeletal sites—might be the best preventive strategy. This is consistent with Kim Bennell's[1] important prospective stress fracture study of the mid-1990s. That may seem like a long time ago, but I argue in this case that the article has moved to a classic status. Also, it's worth checking out if you are in the business of preventing stress fractures.

K. M. Khan, MD, PhD

Reference

1. Bennell KL, Malcolm SA, Thomas SA, et al. Risk factors for stress fractures in track and field athletes: A twelve-month prospective study. *Am J Sports Med.* 1996;24:810-818.

Effect of Eccentric Exercise Program for Early Tibialis Posterior Tendinopathy

Kulig K, Lederhaus ES, Reischl S, et al (Univ of Southern California, Los Angeles)

Foot Ankle Int 30:877-885, 2009

Background.—Morphology and vascularization of painful tibialis posterior (TP) tendons before and after an intervention targeting the degenerated tendon were examined. Functional status and pain level were also assessed.

Materials and Methods.—A10-week twice daily, progressive eccentric tendon loading, calf stretching program with orthoses was implemented with ten, early stage TP tendinopathy subjects. TP tendons were imaged by grayscale and Doppler ultrasound at INITIAL and POST evaluations to assess the tendon's morphology and signs of neovascularization. The Foot Functional Index (FFI), Physical Activity Scale (PAS), 5-Minute Walk Test, and single heel raise (SHR) test were completed at INITIAL and POST evaluations. The Global Rating Scale (GRS) was completed at 6 months followup. One-way ANOVA was used to compare the FFI at INITIAL, POST, and 6-MONTH time points. Paired t-tests were used to compare means between the remaining variables. The level of significance was $p = 0.05$.

Results.—There was a significant difference in FFI total, pain, and disability at the three time-points. Post-hoc paired t-tests revealed that the FFI scores were lower for the total score and pain and disability subcategories when comparing from INITIAL to POST and INITIAL to 6-MONTH evaluations ($p < 0.05$ for all). The number of SHR increased significantly on the involved side from INITIAL to POST evaluation ($p = 0.041$). The GRS demonstrated minimum clinically important differences for improvements in symptoms at 6-MONTH. Tendon morphology and vascularization remained abnormal following the intervention.

Conclusion.—A 10-week tendon specific eccentric program resulted in improvements in symptoms and function without changes in tendon morphology or neovascularization.

▶ This study uses a pre- and post-test design on 10 individuals with tibialis posterior tendinopathy (case-series). The sample is small and there are multiple comparisons made (multiple outcomes are studied with this small sample) which make many of the conclusions tenuous. There was improvement in function, pain, and disability following a 10-week program that consisted of progressive eccentric exercise. However, the absence of a control group also precludes a definitive conclusion regarding the efficacy of such a program. One of the main objectives was to correlate improvement with change in tendon morphology and vascularization; however, there were no such changes upon ultrasound. All in all the study is not conclusive, but it does provide some preliminary support regarding the use of eccentric exercise for this problem, demonstrating that patients improved and that these exercises were not harmful. What is needed next is a clinical trial (with control[s]) to demonstrate whether in fact this intervention is more effective.

D. E. Feldman, PT, PhD

Biological Aspects and Clinical Importance of Ultrasound Therapy in Bone Healing

Erdogan Ö, Esen E (Diyarbakir Military Hosp, Turkey; Cukurova Univ, Adana, Turkey)
J Ultrasound Med 28:765-776, 2009

Objectives.—The purpose of this study was to review past and recent literature findings regarding the effects of ultrasound therapy on bone healing and its clinical efficacy in medical and dental interventions.

Methods.—A literature review was conducted on the effects of ultrasound therapy on bone healing. The studies regarding clinical applications in long bones and maxillofacial bones were evaluated separately from each other.

Results.—The effects of therapeutic ultrasound on bone healing have been studied for half a century. Numerous clinical and experimental studies have addressed this relationship, and many of them have shown positive correlations. Although several theories have been proposed to explain the mechanism of action, the exact mechanism has not been fully understood.

Conclusions.—Therapeutic ultrasound therapy in clinical settings is a noninvasive application and has no serious complications or side effects.

It may be an acceptable treatment of choice in many types of clinical procedures involving maxillofacial bones.

▶ This is a review of the benefits of therapeutic ultrasound therapy over the past century. The authors document the physical and biological effects and review the results of animal and clinical studies. The review focuses on the results of the studies and unfortunately does not assess the quality of the studies. Even in their table regarding effects of ultrasound therapy on maxillofacial bones, it appears that all studies on the subject were included and there is no judgment on the validity of the studies. I believe that this review is nevertheless useful in documenting the history of ultrasound therapy for bone healing. There is clearly the need for more research on this subject. However, there is a need for a more critical analysis of the clinical studies before being able to conclude that it is beneficial.

D. E. Feldman, PT, PhD

3 Biomechanics, Muscle Strength and Training

Intrarater and Interrater Reliability of 22 Clinical Measures Associated With Lower Quarter Malalignment

Leard JS, Crane BA, Ball KA (Univ of Hartford, CT)

J Manipulative Physiol Ther 32:270-276, 2009

Objective.—The purpose of this study was to assess the intrarater and interrater reliability of a broad range of techniques commonly used to assess the lower quarter.

Methods.—A test-retest single group design was used to investigate the intrarater and interrater reliability of 22 lower quarter evaluation measures. Two raters conducted each measure twice on a total of 18 unimpaired subjects with an average age of 23.7 years. This study was conducted in the Human Performance Research laboratory in a university setting. Intraclass correlation coefficients were used to assess reliability of continuous variables, and weighted κ was used to assess nominal or ordinal results.

Results.—Side differences were not found ($P > .05$); thus, data for right and left legs were pooled ($n = 36$) where applicable. Intraclass correlation coefficient and weighted κ results ranged from a low of 0.06 to a high of 0.99. Intrarater reliability results were generally higher than interrater reliability results.

Conclusion.—Many of the clinical measures demonstrated good overall reliability. For those tests where acceptable intrarater and interrater reliability cannot be demonstrated, additional training of raters, modification of the technique, or elimination of the technique's use should be considered.

▶ Frequently used clinical tests were assessed for reproducibility, specifically intra and interrater reliability. As expected, intrarater reliability was high for all measures. Interrater reliability was high for many measures although not for Thomas test hip flexion, frontal pelvic inclination, genu varum knee, genu varum ankle, and Q angle. For the most part, the results are reassuring. The authors propose some modification for those measures that demonstrated lower reliability. The analysis incorporated both legs from each subject, which are correlated, and this may have inflated the intraclass correlations of the single leg measures.

D. E. Feldman, PT, PhD

Torque Interaction among Adjacent Joints due to the Action of Biarticular Muscles

Nozaki D (Univ of Tokyo, Hongo, Bunkyo-ku)
Med Sci Sports Exerc 41:205-209, 2009

In our musculoskeletal system, multiple muscles are involved in the generation of torque about a joint. Hence, an infinite number of combinations of muscle activities may exist in producing a certain amount of joint torque. Many studies have assumed that the level of muscle activity level depends on torque about the joint it spans. However, this assumption does not hold true in the presence of biarticular muscles. Here we show that the muscle activity level is modulated according to a scheme called "cosine tuning" based on our experiment on the isometric force exerted by the lower limb, that is, the muscle activity about the knee and the hip joints can be represented by a linear summation of the knee and hip joint torques. This way of modulation is very simple, but it is unintuitive on the point that the activation level of the monoarticular muscles explicitly depends on the torque of the adjacent joint that they do not span. It is demonstrated that such nontrivial, cosine tuning can be mathematically explained by assuming that the muscle activity pattern is determined so as to minimize the variability of the end point force. Finally, the implications of the cosine tuning for muscle strength training and motor control are discussed.

▶ This article furthers one's understanding of how the body's neurological system controls the activation of both uniarticular and biarticular muscles during a purposeful activity. Using an elegantly simple mathematical model of a 2-joint system that contains muscles that cross either 1 or 2 of the modeled joints, the author convincingly demonstrates that each muscle's activity level is linearly dependent upon the desired torque at both joints. Further, the mathematical model explains why the neurological system attempts to minimize the sum of the squared force muscle activations that are thought to minimize tissue stress. The author also provides experimental evidence that suggests that the muscles that only cross the knee are influenced by the hip torque during a knee flexion-extension task. This finding has implications for strength training. For example, the hip joint torque must be actively monitored to allow the knee joint muscles to be activated consistently. Changes in the hip torque requirements alter the knee muscle activation patterns.

M. R. Pierrynowski, PhD

Glenohumeral Rotational Range of Motion in Collegiate Overhead-Throwing Athletes During an Athletic Season

Dwelly PM, Tripp BL, Tripp PA, et al (Univ of Arkansas, Fayetteville; Univ of Florida, Gainesville; et al)

J Athl Train 44:611-616, 2009

Context.—Repetitive throwing at high velocities leads to altered range of motion (ROM) in the dominant shoulder compared with the nondominant shoulder in overhead-throwing athletes. Loss of glenohumeral internal rotation (IR), or glenohumeral internal-rotation deficit (GIRD), is associated with shoulder injuries. Therefore, GIRD should be evaluated during the clinical examination of the thrower's shoulder.

Objective.—To assess glenohumeral ROM in competitive baseball and softball athletes at 3 intervals over the course of an athletic season in order to (1) examine changes in ROM over time and (2) monitor the prevalence of GIRD.

Design.—Observational, repeated-measures study.

Setting.—Collegiate athletic training room.

Patients or Other Participants.—Forty-eight healthy National Collegiate Athletic Association (NCAA) Division I or Division II athletes (age = 19 ± 1 years, height = 174 ± 14 cm, mass = 77.8 ± 18.1 kg; 19 softball, 29 baseball players).

Main Outcome Measure(s).—We measured glenohumeral IR, external rotation (ER), total arc (ER + IR), and GIRD at 3 times: prefall, prespring, and postspring. We calculated GIRD in 2 ways: as the difference in IR between dominant and nondominant shoulders and as the percentage of the total arc.

Results.—In the dominant shoulder, ER increased during the season ($F_{2,96} = 17.433$, $P < .001$), but IR remained the same ($F_{2,96} = 1.839$, $P = .17$). The total arc in the dominant shoulder increased between time intervals ($F_{2,96} = 14.030$, $P < .001$); the mean difference between prefall and postspring measurements was 9.694° ($P < .001$), and the mean difference between prefall and postspring measurements was 10.990° ($P < .001$). In the nondominant shoulder, ER increased over the season ($F_{2,96} = 23.395$, $P < .001$), but IR did not change over the season ($F_{2,96} = 0.087$, $P = .90$). The total arc in the nondominant shoulder increased between prefall and prespring measurements and between prefall and postspring measurements ($F_{2,96} = 18.552$, $P < .001$). No changes were noted in GIRD over time. However, more athletes with GIRD were identified with the GIRD (IR difference) calculation in prefall (n = 6) than in prespring (n = 1) and postspring (n = 4) (Cochran $Q = 5.2$, $P = .07$). In addition, more athletes with GIRD were identified with the GIRD (% total arc) calculation in postspring (n = 6) than in prefall (n = 5) or prespring (n = 4) (Cochran $Q = 2.6$, $P = .27$).

Conclusions.—Healthy NCAA Division I and Division II athletes did not display changes in glenohumeral IR over an athletic season. However, they gained in ER and total arc during the season in both shoulders. Future researchers should investigate changes over multiple seasons. The 2 methods of calculating GIRD identified different athletes as having GIRD, indicating that additional investigation is warranted to determine the clinical benefits of each method.

▶ Some glenohumeral rotational range of motion changes in athletes participating in overhead and throwing sports are postulated to be associated with pain, decreased performance, and shoulder disorders. It is therefore important that the clinician be cognizant of this possibility and understand the subtleties of these changes and how to measure them. This study is an observational, repeated measures study of 48 healthy National Collegiate Athletic Association (NCAA) Division I or Division II athletes in either softball or baseball, observed by investigators independent of the team athletic trainer, without any modification in practice, game exposures, or in stretching and warm-up routines. A mechanical inclinometer (Sears, Roebuck & Co, Hoffman Estates, IL) was used to measure glenohumeral internal rotation deficit (GIRD), and a visual inspection technique ensured that the scapula was well stabilized (Fig 1 in the original article). From prefall to postspring, external rotation (ER) and total arc of motion increased in both shoulders but internal rotation (IR) did not change. In the dominant shoulder, ER increased by about 11 degrees and this was thought to be due to the demands of throwing. The 2 calculations used to determine GIRD in the dominant shoulder—(1) GIRD (IR difference) = nondominant IR−dominant IR and (2) GIRD (% total arc) = (nondominant total arc−dominant total arc)/nondominant total arc—were shown to represent different deficits in range of motion and identified different athletes with GIRD. Further studies on this topic are warranted in other populations (eg, younger and older athletes with and without shoulder pathology and female subjects).

C. Lebrun, MD

Correlation of Throwing Mechanics With Elbow Valgus Load in Adult Baseball Pitchers

Aguinaldo AL, Chambers H (Rady Children's Hosp, San Diego, CA)

Am J Sports Med 37:2043-2048, 2009

Background.—Studies have shown that various biomechanical factors affect valgus extension overload during baseball pitching; yet, their relationships are not clearly defined, and factors such as trunk rotation and arm slot have not been investigated.

Hypothesis.—The onset of trunk rotation, with other biomechanical variables that define sequential body motion, will significantly predict elbow valgus loading.

Study Design.—Descriptive laboratory study.

Methods.—Sixty-nine adult baseball players pitched off an indoor mound during 3-dimensional motion analysis to measure whole body kinematics and kinetics at 240 Hz. Thirteen biomechanical variables were calculated and extracted for regression analysis to investigate their associations with elbow valgus load. A 2-way analysis of variance compared valgus torques between pitchers with 2 onsets of trunk rotation (before and after front-foot contact) and 2 arm slot positions (overhand and sidearm).

Results.—Six biomechanical variables had significant correlations ($P < .02$) with elbow valgus torque–with maximum shoulder external rotation, elbow flexion at peak valgus torque, and elbow valgus loading rate accounting for 68% of its variance. Reduced elbow valgus torques were associated with increased elbow flexion ($P < .01$). Players who initiated trunk rotation before front-foot contact had significantly higher elbow valgus torques than did those who rotated afterward ($P = .02$). Fourteen pitchers displayed a sidearm delivery and had significantly higher elbow valgus torques than did those with an overhand arm slot position.

Conclusion.—Valgus torque at the elbow during baseball pitching is associated with 6 biomechanical variables of sequential body motion. A condition of late trunk rotation, reduced shoulder external rotation, and increased elbow flexion appeared to be most closely related to valgus torque. Sidearm pitchers appeared to be more susceptible than overhand pitchers to reduced elbow valgus torque.

Clinical Relevance.—The biomechanical findings of this study offer scientific feedback for developing methods used to minimize the effects of valgus load on pitching-related elbow injuries.

▶ This article should be of interest to all sports medicine personnel that care for the throwing athlete – especially baseball players.

It has long been generally held that the overuse elbow injuries in baseball are the result of excessive valgus loading of the throwing elbow. This study looked at different valgus loading forces that were related to the overhand or 3 quarters throwing motion versus the sidearm motion and whether the onset of trunk rotation occurred well before the front foot was planted or after it was planted. Generally speaking, the analysis found greater valgus forces generated by the sidearm throwing motion and by those who had trunk rotation sooner rather than later. This information could be of significant value in teaching the proper mechanics to baseball players and other throwing athletes, especially those that may have incurred elbow injuries.

R. C. Cantu, MD, MA

Quantifying scapula orientation and its influence on maximal hand force capability and shoulder muscle activity

Picco BR, Fischer SL, Dickerson CR (Univ of Waterloo, Canada)

Clin Biomech 25:29-36, 2010

Background.—Non-neutral scapular orientations are often implicated as potential causes of shoulder pathologies. However, their specific influence on shoulder functional capabilities is largely unknown. This study objectively measured scapular orientation and quantified its influence on shoulder muscle activity levels and hand force capabilities during vertical and horizontal manual exertions.

Methods.—Ten healthy male university students performed 24 exertions in combinations of scapular orientation (protracted, neutral and retracted), exertion direction (up, down, medial, lateral) and intensity (maximal or 40 N). Scapular orientation was quantified using an acromion marker cluster method. An orientation by intensity repeated measures ANOVA identified differences in quantified scapular orientation. A two-way multivariate ANOVA identified the influence of scapular orientation and hand force direction on muscle activity and hand force capability.

Findings.—Participants assumed consistent retracted, neutral, and protracted scapular *orientations* during exertions, and these three orientations were different from each other ($F(2, 99) = 158.57$; P-value: 0.0001). Scapular orientation and exertion direction influenced muscle recruitment almost universally (P-value: 0.05). Scapular orientation did not influence hand force capability ($F(2, 99) = 1.34$; P-value: 0.05), but a hand force direction effect on force existed ($F(3, 99) = 144.19$; P-value: 0.0001).

Interpretation.—These findings support recommendations of health practitioners who advocate neutral scapular orientations to reduce injury risk, as a neutral orientation achieved a balanced overall muscle use pattern between retraction and protraction. Also, lowered muscle activity and higher maximal forces suggest that downward exertion forces may be preferable when possible (Fig 4).

▶ This study was motivated by the authors' assertion that knowledge of the orientation and movement of the scapula during functional tasks is critical in assessing shoulder pathologies, such as impingement, instability, and thoracic outlet syndrome. They studied a small group of healthy male university students performing a series of hand force exertions at 2 intensities and 4 directions while statically holding their scapulae in standardized protracted, neutral, and retracted positions (24 trials). Electromyography (EMG) from 7 shoulder and upper limb muscles and hand force were measured, processed, and then statistically analyzed. The authors report statistically different scapular orientations for the 3 experimentally dictated scapular positions. However, scapular position did not influence hand force in most directions (see Fig 4). Both scapular position and exertion direction influenced the EMG magnitudes of the muscle activities. Generally, lower muscle exertions were required to generate the same

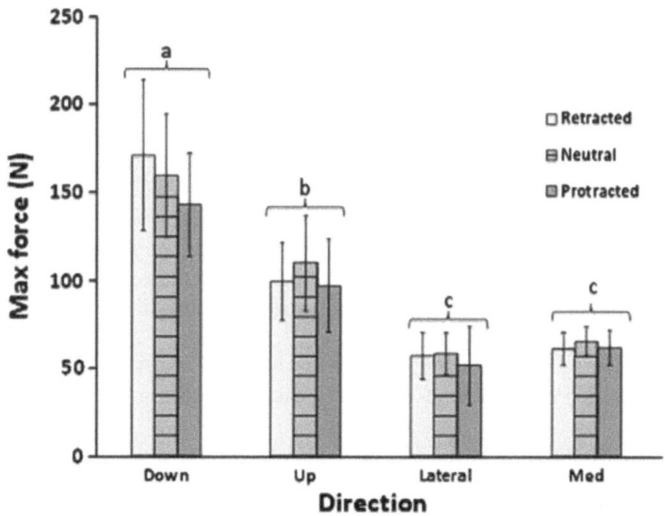

FIGURE 4.—Maximal isometric hand force capability in each direction and scapular posture combination. Groups of bars with different letters are significantly different (*P*-value: 0.05). (Reprinted from Picco BR, Fischer SL, Dickerson CR. Quantifying scapula orientation and its influence on maximal hand force capability and shoulder muscle activity. *Clin Biomech*. 2010;25:29-36, with permission from Elsevier.)

external hand force when the scapula was in the neutral position compared with non-neutral orientations. The authors conclude that health care providers must continue to recommend to their patients the adoption of neutral scapula positions during hand force exertions.

M. R. Pierrynowski, PhD

The effect of valgus bracing on the knee adduction moment during gait and running in male subjects with varus alignment

Fantini Pagani CH, Potthast W, Brüggemann G-P (German Sport Univ Cologne)

Clin Biomech 25:70-76, 2010

Background.—Increased mechanical load is one risk factor for osteoarthritis. One possible treatment for this disorder is the use of knee braces in order to redistribute joint loading, which may inhibit the progression of the disease. The hypothesis was: knee adduction moment can be reduced with the use of a dedicated knee orthosis, which applies an abduction moment at the knee.

Methods.—Sixteen healthy male subjects with varus alignment were analysed during walking and running while using an adjustable valgus orthosis. Peak knee adduction moments and knee adduction angular impulses were evaluated through inverse dynamics. Additionally, the abduction moment produced by the orthosis was measured in three different adjustments of valgus angulations (neutral, 4° and 8° valgus) using a strain gauge device.

Findings.—During walking, mean reductions of 25% and 36% in the knee adduction angular impulse were found between the conditions without orthosis and 4° and between without orthosis and 8°, respectively. For the running trials mean reductions of 18% and 23% were observed between these same conditions. The first and second peak knee adduction moments also decreased during walking with different orthosis adjustments (changes from 5% to 33%). During running, a significant reduction was observed only between the conditions without orthosis and 8° valgus adjustments (change of 11%).

Interpretation.—The orthosis tested in this study was effective in reducing the knee adduction moments during walking and running. This

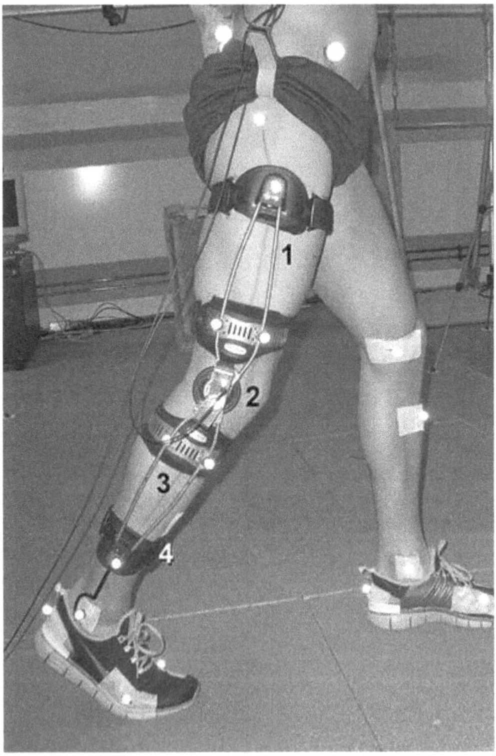

FIGURE 1.—Genu Arthro Knee Orthosis 28K20/21. 1 – Femoral Module; 2 – Orthosis' axis with the strain gauge instrumentation; 3 – Tibial Module; 4 – Straps. (Reprinted from Fantini Pagani CH, Potthast W, Brüggemann G-P. The effect of valgus bracing on the knee adduction moment during gait and running in male subjects with varus alignment. *Clin Biomech*. 2010;25:70-76, with permission from Elsevier.)

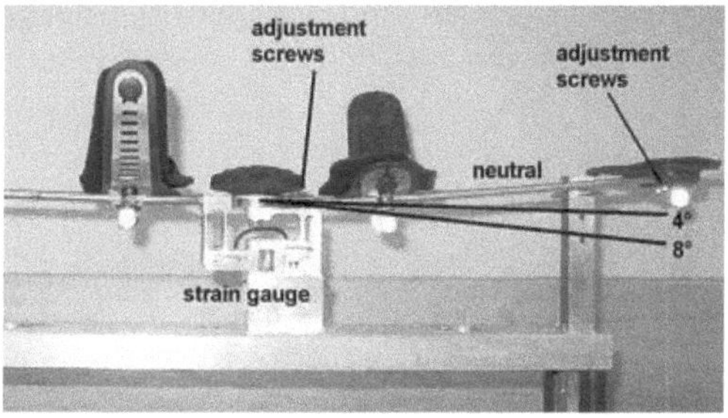

FIGURE 2.—Orthosis positioning for the valgus adjustments. The figure shows the orthosis in the neutral position. Black lines indicate the 4° and 8° valgus adjustments. (Reprinted from Fantini Pagani CH, Potthast W, Brüggemann G-P. The effect of valgus bracing on the knee adduction moment during gait and running in male subjects with varus alignment. *Clin Biomech*. 2010;25:70-76, with permission from Elsevier.)

reduction of knee adduction moments during locomotion should contribute to decelerate osteoarthritis progression.

▶ The fields of biomechanics, engineering, and medicine all converge when it comes to conservative management of osteoarthritis of the knee. Beginning as early as 1998[1] and 1999,[2] many different author groups have investigated the effects of valgus bracing in subjects with varus alignment, postulating that decreased load on the medial compartment of the knee in patients with osteoarthritis will diminish symptoms and slow the rate of progression of disease. Early studies focused more on the outcomes, such as clinical measurements, pain, and quality-of-life questionnaires, whereas more recent ones attempt to elucidate the mechanism of unloading and to somehow quantify it. Both load and loading time are known to be important variables that define the wear conditions in the knee. This study only includes young healthy male subjects with varus alignment and without significant osteoarthritis. It only examines the effects of 1 particular commercially available valgus brace (Genu Arthro Knee Orthosis 28K20/21—Fig 1). There are many more braces on the market, particularly in North America—many of them more compact in design and less cumbersome looking than this one. What makes this study unique, however, is that this orthosis was also instrumented with an external strain gauge (Fig 2). As the subjects stood, walked, or ran over a force plate, with collection of 3-dimensional kinematic data, a sophisticated software system (BodyBuilder version 3.6, VICON Motion Systems, Oxford, UK) was able to calculate simultaneous 3-dimensional external moments. Use of this information in conjunction with the measures from the strain gauge enabled the determination of net adduction moment, which may be a more sensitive marker of the load placed on the joint. It is still not possible to determine, with any degree of certainty, how this load is distributed between the knee structures (ie, the medial and lateral compartments, ligaments, and muscles) and mechanical devices such as orthosis. In any case, this orthosis was shown to support a significant portion of the total load normally supported by the knee joint and soft tissues. Ongoing research in this vein will hopefully enhance current knowledge of the conservative management of knee gonarthrosis.

C. Lebrun, MD

References

1. Hewett TE, Noyes FR, Barber-Westin SD, Heckmann TP. Decrease in knee joint pain and increase in function in patients with medial compartment arthrosis: a prospective analysis of valgus bracing. *Orthopedics.* 1998;21:131-138.
2. Kirkley A, Webster-Bogaert S, Litchfield R, et al. The effect of bracing on varus gonarthrosis. *J Bone Joint Surg Am.* 1999;81A:531-548.

The knee in full flexion: an anatomical study

Pinskerova V, Samuelson KM, Stammers J, et al (Charles Univ, Czech Republic; Intermountain Joint Replacement Centre LDS Hosp, Salt Lake City, UT; Core Trainee Surgery London Deanery, United Kingdom; et al)

J Bone Joint Surg [Br] 91-B:830-834, 2009

There has been only one limited report dating from 1941 using dissection which has described the tibiofemoral joint between 120° and 160° of flexion despite the relevance of this arc to total knee replacement. We now provide a full description having examined one living and eight cadaver knees using MRI, dissection and previously published cryosections in one knee.

In the range of flexion from 120° to 160° the flexion facet centre of the medial femoral condyle moves back 5 mm and rises up on to the posterior horn of the medial meniscus. At 160° the posterior horn is compressed in a synovial recess between the femoral cortex and the tibia. This limits flexion. The lateral femoral condyle also rolls back with the posterior horn of the lateral meniscus moving with the condyle. Both move down over the posterior tibia at 160° of flexion.

Neither the events between 120° and 160° nor the anatomy at 160° could result from a continuation of the kinematics up to 120°. Therefore hyperflexion is a separate arc. The anatomical and functional features of this arc suggest that it would be difficult to design an implant for total knee replacement giving physiological movement from 0° to 160°.

▶ Contemplate the number of times you flex your knee beyond 120° (hyperflexion) and then ponder the fact that little has been published on the arthrokinematics of the tibiofemoral motion during hyperflexion. This lack of knowledge has implications for the design of total knee prosthesis for individuals who desire to hyperflex their knee to participate in certain activities of daily living. In this study, a series of static MR images of 5 cadaveric knees and one living volunteer's knee were obtained. Although these images were not from knees performing unconstrained hyperflexion with associated physiological muscle, ligament, and bone-on-bone forces, they demonstrated that the knee in hyperflexion is not a continuation of the less than 120° kinematic motion of the knee. Hyperflexion has a unique arthrokinematic signature, and as such the authors conclude that it would be difficult to design a total knee prosthesis that has 0° to 160° range.

M. R. Pierrynowski, PhD

Static and dynamic correlates of the knee adduction moment in healthy knees ranging from normal to varus-aligned

Barrios JA, Higginson JS, Royer TD, et al (Univ of Dayton, OH; Univ of Delaware, Newark)

Clin Biomech 24:850-854, 2009

Background.—Individuals with medial knee osteoarthritis often present with varus knee alignment and ambulate with increased knee adduction moments. Understanding the factors that relate to the knee adduction moment in healthy individuals may provide insight into the development of this disease. Thus, this study aimed to examine the relationships of both static and dynamic lower extremity measures with the knee adduction moment. We hypothesized that the dynamic measures would be more closely related to this moment.

Methods.—Arch height index, hip abduction strength and two static measures of knee alignment were recorded for 37 young asymptomatic knees that varied from normal to varus-aligned. Overground gait analyses were also performed. Correlation coefficients were used to assess the relationships between the static and dynamic variables to the knee adduction moment. Hierarchical regression analyses were then conducted using the static measures, the dynamic measures, and the static and dynamic measures together.

Results.—Among the static measures, the tibial mechanical axis and the distance between the medial knee joint lines were correlated with the knee adduction moment. The best predictive static model ($R^2 = 0.53$) included only the tibial mechanical axis. Among the dynamic variables, knee adduction and rearfoot eversion angles were correlated with the knee adduction moment. Knee adduction and rearfoot eversion, together, were the best dynamic model ($R^2 = 0.53$). The static and dynamic measures together created the strongest of the three models ($R^2 = 0.59$).

Conclusions.—These results suggest that dynamic measures slightly enhance the predictive strength of static measures when explaining variation in the knee adduction moment.

▶ Identifying the factors that increase dynamic knee joint loading may help clinicians counsel and treat patients at risk of developing knee osteoarthritis. In this article, a set of static (tibial mechanical axis [TMA]; hip extension and internal rotation range of motion; hip abduction strength; distance between the medial joint lines; and arch height index) and dynamic angle outcomes measured when the knee was at peak knee adduction moment (ankle eversion; knee adduction; and hip adduction) were correlated, singly and collectively, to the knee adduction moment, which is thought to be associated with medial joint loading and subsequently medial knee osteoarthritis disease progression. This study tested 37 young asymptomatic knees and report a good ($R^2 = 0.59$) association between the combined TMA and knee adduction angle outcomes. However, this association is only modestly better than just using the TMA outcome ($R^2 = 0.53$). These findings suggest that clinicians could use the TMA to predict knee joint loading or wait until better outcomes are developed and validated.

M. R. Pierrynowski, PhD

Co-activation differences in lower limb muscles between asymptomatic controls and those with varying degrees of knee osteoarthritis during walking

Hubley-Kozey CL, Hill NA, Rutherford DJ, et al (Dalhousie Univ, Halifax, NS, Canada)

Clin Biomech 24:407-414, 2009

Background.—Increased muscle co-activation during gait has been identified as a neuromuscular alteration associated with knee osteoarthritis, however levels of co-activation among different osteoarthritis severity have not been established. The purpose of this study was to determine if differences in co-activation could be detected among asymptomatic controls, those with moderate and those with severe osteoarthritis using a co-activation index and a pattern recognition technique.

Methods.—Surface electromyograms from vastus lateralis and medialis, lateral and medial hamstring and gastrocnemius pairs were recorded from 63 asymptomatic, 59 moderate and 48 severe osteoarthritic subjects during self-selected walking. A co-activation index was calculated over the initial stance for four medial and lateral muscle pairs. The four co-activation indices were tested among groups using a one factor ANOVA ($\alpha = 0.05$). Gait waveform pattern recognition procedures were applied to yield a principal pattern, scored for each muscle site and subject. A mixed model ANOVA (group-muscle) tested for principal pattern score differences.

Findings.—A significant group effect was found ($P < 0.05$) for all four co-activation indices. Principal pattern one captured the amplitude and general shape of activity throughout the entire stance phase. ANOVA revealed a significant ($P < 0.05$) group by muscle interaction for the principal pattern scores. Significant differences were found among all three groups and between the two osteoarthritic groups for both measures.

Interpretation.—The co-activation indices and principal patterns identified that lateral site differences occurred among all three groups with medial site differences between the two osteoarthritic groups. These findings suggest that measures of muscle co-activity provide additional information related to knee osteoarthritis severity.

▶ This article proposes that the activation patterns of 6 muscles that cross the knee can be used to classify knees with various degrees of osteoarthritis (OA). Specifically, the muscle co-contraction index (CCI) and waveform analyses of the surface electromyography (EMG) collected from the medial and lateral vasti, hamstrings, and gastrocnemius muscles can clearly identify knees without and with moderate and severe OA. The methods are reported to be objective and noninvasive and, along with radiographic and patient reported signs and symptoms, can provide clinicians an enhanced tool to score knee OA severity. Clinically, this article is also important because the findings suggest that (1) patients with moderate OA and high lateral CCI and normal medial CCI could benefit using knee valgus unloader braces and lateral heel wedges, (2) patients with severe OA and generally elevated CCI could benefit using knee joint stability braces, and (3) patients with extremely high CCI are the best candidates for joint replacement.

M. R. Pierrynowski, PhD

Immediate Effects of the Suboccipital Muscle Inhibition Technique in Subjects With Short Hamstring Syndrome

Aparicio ÉQ, Quirante LB, Blanco CR, et al (Policínica FisioTex, Badajoz, Spain; et al)

J Manipulative Physiol Ther 32:262-269, 2009

Objective.—The purpose of this study is to identify the effects of the suboccipital muscle inhibition technique in patients with short hamstring syndrome by means of tests designed to evaluate the elasticity of the hamstring muscles and pressure algometry of myofascial trigger points.

Methods.—Randomized clinical trial (pre and postintervention). The study population comprised young adult students following their studies at the Physiotherapy School at the University of Extremadura (Spain) and footballers from an Extremadura Football Club with short hamstring syndrome. The sample (70 subjects = 47 male and 23 female) was randomly divided into a control group (n = 34) and an intervention group (n = 36). Mean sample age was 23.40 ± 3.82 years. The control group was subjected to a placebo technique, whereas the intervention group was subjected to the suboccipital muscle inhibition technique. Pre and postintervention evaluation was used for the assessment of hamstring elasticity, and pressure algometry was also used (myofascial trigger points). Statistical analyses were performed using the SPSS 14.5 package (SPSS Inc, Chicago, Ill), comparing the sample between groups (Kolmorogov-Smirnov test, Student t test, 2-way analysis of variance [ANOVA], the χ^2 test).

Results.—The distribution of the quantitative variables was normal, and the mean time doing physical activity per week was 2.82 ± 4.03 hours.

Two-way ANOVA afforded statistically significant results for the finger-floor test, straight leg raise test-left, straight leg raise test-right, left popliteal angle test (P values < .001), and right popliteal angle test (P =.005). For pressure algometry, only the right semimembranosus muscle afforded statistically significant differences (P =.021).

Conclusions.—According to the finger-floor distance test, the straight leg raise test, and the popliteal angle test, the suboccipital muscle inhibition technique modified the elasticity of the hamstring muscles for this group of subjects. The suboccipital muscle inhibition technique modifies the pressure algometry of the semimembranosus muscle but does not modify that of the semitendinosus muscle or biceps femoris.

▶ The suboccipital muscle inhibition technique is a manual therapy intervention that was shown to be effective in improving the elasticity of the hamstrings in the immediate term. Although this randomized clinical trial (RCT) indicates improved hamstring flexibility as shown by fingertip to floor distance, straight leg raise, and popliteal angle tests, the application was a 1-time intervention. Thus, it is not known whether there is a long-term effect, or whether a certain treatment protocol of several applications are required to achieve a longer-term effect. Nevertheless, the study is informative, indicating that this technique is effective and suggesting that further research be undertaken to determine its long-term effects.

D. E. Feldman, PT, PhD

Biomechanical variables associated with Achilles tendinopathy in runners

Azevedo LB, Lambert MI, Vaughan CL, et al (Univ of Worcester, UK; Univ of Cape Town, South Africa; et al)

Br J Sports Med 43:288-292, 2009

Objective.—The aim of this study was to investigate the kinetics, kinematics and muscle activity in runners with Achilles tendinopathy.

Design.—Case–control study.

Setting.—Biomechanics laboratory.

Participants.—21 runners free from injury and 21 runners with Achilles tendinopathy performed 10 running trials with standardised running shoes. Injured runners were diagnosed clinically according to established diagnostic criteria. Uninjured runners had been injury-free for at least 2 years.

Main Outcome Measurements.—During each trial, kinetic and lower limb kinematic data were measured using a strain gauge force plate and six infrared cameras respectively. Electromyographic (EMG) data from six muscles (tibialis anterior (TA), peroneus longus (PE), lateral gastrocnemius (LG), rectus femoris (RF), biceps femoris (BF) and gluteus medius (GM)) were measured with a telemetric EMG system.

Results.—Knee range of motion (heel strike to midstance) was significantly lower in injured runners than in uninjured runners. Similarly, preactivation (integrated EMG (IEMG) in 100 ms before heel strike) of TA was lower for injured runners than uninjured runners. RF and GM IEMG activity 100 ms after heel strike was also lower in the injured group. However, impact forces were not different between the two groups.

Conclusion.—Altered knee kinematics and reduced muscle activity are associated with Achilles tendinopathy in runners. Rehabilitation exercises or other mechanisms (e.g. footwear) that affect kinematics and muscle activity may therefore be beneficial in the treatment of runners with Achilles tendinopathy.

▶ Numerous biomechanical articles have examined the multitude of temporal-spatial, kinematic, kinetic, and electromyographic gait variables with the goal of detecting the smaller set of key outcomes that diagnose the presence or absence of some movement disorder condition. In this article, a one-stride full clinical gait analysis was performed on 42 habitual runners, approximately 40 years old, running at a self-selected speed, 5 times over force platform. All of the runners had no physical deformities, neurological disorders, and diabetes of previous lower extremity surgeries that influenced their activities. The purpose of this biomechanical article was to identify the 21 runners that had a sports physician diagnosed Achilles tendinopathy. The key finding was that the runners with Achilles tendinopathy presented with lower muscle activities in their tibialis anterior, rectus femoris, and the gluteus medius muscles just previous and just following foot floor contact. The clinical implication of this finding is that health care professionals involved with the rehabilitation of runners with Achilles tendinopathy may find muscle-strengthening exercises for these 3 muscles of some benefit for the patient.

M. R. Pierrynowski, PhD

In Vivo Kinematics of the Tibiotalar Joint After Lateral Ankle Instability

Caputo AM, Lee JY, Spritzer CE, et al (Duke Univ, Durham, NC)
Am J Sports Med 37:2241-2248, 2009

Background.—Previous studies have suggested that injury to the anterior talofibular ligament (ATFL) may be linked to altered kinematics and the development of osteoarthritis of the ankle joint. However, the effects of ATFL injury on the in vivo kinematics of the ankle joint are unclear.

Hypothesis.—Based on the orientation of the ATFL fibers, ATFL deficiency leads to increased anterior translation and increased internal rotation of the talus relative to the tibia.

Study Design.—Descriptive laboratory study.

Methods.—The ankles of 9 patients with unilateral ATFL injuries were compared as they stepped onto a level surface. Kinematic measurements were made as a function of increasing load. With use of magnetic resonance imaging and orthogonal fluoroscopy, the in vivo kinematics of the tibiotalar joint were measured in the ATFL-deficient and intact ankles of the same individuals.

Results.—A statistically significant increase in internal rotation, anterior translation, and superior translation of the talus was measured in ATFL-deficient ankles, as compared with the intact contralateral controls. For example, at 100% body weight, ATFL-deficient ankles demonstrated an increase of 0.9 ± 0.5 mm in anterior translation ($P = .008$), an increase of 5.7° ± 3.6° in internal rotation ($P = .008$), and a slight increase of 0.2 ± 0.2 mm in the superior translation ($P = .02$) relative to the intact contralateral ankles.

Conclusion.—Deficiency of the ATFL increases anterior translation, internal rotation, and superior translation of the talus.

Clinical Relevance.—Altered kinematics may contribute to the degenerative changes observed with chronic lateral ankle instability. These findings might help to explain the degenerative changes frequently observed on the medial talus in patients with chronic ATFL insufficiency and so provide a baseline for improving ankle ligament reconstructions aimed at restoring normal joint motion.

▶ Osteoarthritic degenerative changes occur in 10% to 40% of patients with lateral ankle instability. This study examined precursors of osteoarthritis changes, specifically increased ankle triplanar rotation and increased triaxial translation, in 9 patients with confirmed unilateral anterior talofibular ligament (ATFL) failure. (As a footnote, the authors state that 4 of the patients had attendant calcaneofibular ligament (CFL) failure.) Using magnetic resonance imaging and orthogonal fluoroscopy, which can measure 0.08 mm translation and 0.4° rotation changes (95% confidence interval), they found an increased internal rotation (5.7°), increased anterior translation (0.9 mm), and increased superior translation of talus (0.2 mm) comparing the patients' unstable to stable ankle when the ankles were loaded to 100% body weight. The clinical significance of these findings is that surgical procedures that aim to reduce ankle joint instability should focus on reducing internal rotation and anterior translation. If this is done, the improved stability has the potential to reduce the prevalence of osteoarthritis in patients who had lateral ankle instability.

M. R. Pierrynowski, PhD

Ankle and Subtalar Kinematics During Dorsiflexion-Plantarflexion Activities

Yamaguchi S, Sasho T, Kato H, et al (Gainesville, FL)

Foot Ankle Int 30:361-366, 2009

Background.—Understanding the effect of weightbearing on subtalar and ankle joint kinematics is critical for the diagnosis and treatment of foot disorders. However, dynamic in vivo kinematics of these joints are not well studied. The purpose of this study was to compare in vivo kinematics during nonweightbearing and weightbearing activities in healthy subjects.

Methods.—Seven healthy subjects with a mean age of 32 (range, 23 to 42) years were enrolled. Oblique lateral fluoroscopic images of nonweightbearing and weight- bearing dorsiflexion-plantarflexion activities were recorded. Three dimensional subtalar, ankle, and ankle-subtalar joint complex kinematics were determined using 3D-2D model registration techniques with 3D bone models and single-plane fluoroscopy.

Results.—During the weightbearing activity from 20 degrees dorsiflexion to 15 degrees plantarflexion, the subtalar joint was significantly more everted, dorsiflexed, and abducted, and the calcaneus showed a significantly more posterior position, than during the nonweightbearing activity. The ankle joint was significantly more plantarflexed and adducted during the weightbearing activity than the nonweightbearing activity. The ankle-subtalar joint complex was significantly more everted, and the calcaneus showed significantly greater posterior position than the nonweightbearing activity.

Conclusion.—These observations provide basic quantitative descriptions of weightbearing and nonweightbearing kinematics for healthy joints.

Clinical Relevance.—These data can serve as the basis for comparison with pathologic feet for both diagnostic and therapeutic purposes.

▶ Foot care professionals frequently examine the rear foot (talocrural and subtalar) joints using hand-applied loads to assess joint alignment and range. However, these hand-applied loads are much smaller than those experienced by the rear foot during standing and dynamic weight bearing activities such as gait and stair climbing. In this article, the investigators examined alterations in the alignment of the bones of the nonweight bearing and weight bearing rear foot using oblique lateral fluoroscopy. Subject specific digital models of the bones of the rear foot fitted to the fluoroscopic images were used to measure alignment. Although the authors used limited joint range and a specific type of foot loading (such as that during toe off during gait), and only 7 healthy young subjects, tested only once (to minimize radiation exposure), their results convincingly demonstrate marked changes in rear foot alignment and stability between the unloaded and loaded conditions. The clinical implication of this finding is that the alignment and stability of the rear foot joints must be examined when they are loaded and not hand loaded. Because foot orthoses are frequently prescribed for feet that present with a nonneutral subtalar joint static alignment while hand loaded, the assessment of the rear foot during loaded functional activities should be considered.

M. R. Pierrynowski, PhD

Augmentation of Tendon–Bone Interface Healing With Low-intensity Pulsed Ultrasound

Lu C-C, Liu Y-C, Cheng Y-M, et al (Kaohsiung Med Univ; Mackay Memorial Hosp, Taipei; et al)
Orthopedics 32:173, 2009

The capacity of low-intensity pulsed ultrasound to accelerate the integration of grafted tendon–within–bone tunnel was evaluated. The extensor digitorum longus tendons of 20 New Zealand white rabbits were transplanted into bone tunnels in both proximal tibias. One side was chosen randomly to receive low-intensity pulsed ultrasound. The other side served as control. Six rabbits each were sacrificed at 2 and 3 weeks postoperatively for biomechanical testing, and 2 rabbits each were sacrificed at 1, 3, 6, and 12 weeks postoperatively for histological study. At 2 weeks postoperatively, the mean maximal tensile strength in the ultrasound-treated group (30.676 N) was significantly stronger ($P<.05$) than the control group (17.924 N). There was no significant difference of the maximal tensile strength (33.674 vs 33.340 N; $P=.753$) between the ultrasound-treated and control groups at 3 weeks postoperatively. In the ultrasound-treated group, the histological study revealed the interface filled with denser granulation tissue and diffuse perpendicular anchored fibers in the 1- and 3-week specimens, and interface new bone formation in the 6- and 12-week specimens. The biomechanical and histological studies demonstrated that the low-intensity pulsed ultrasound enhanced the healing of grafted tendon–to–bone tunnel in the early stages. Our findings indicate that low-intensity pulsed ultrasound is a potentially promising mechanical tool to accelerate early tendon healing to bone tunnel.

▶ This animal study suggests that low-intensity pulsed ultrasound enhances tendon-bone tunnel healing. These results were demonstrated at 2 weeks post-surgery, but there were no differences at 3 weeks. The implications for this animal model were that the ultrasound accelerated healing, but at 3 weeks there was no difference between the 2 sides (ultrasounded side vs the non-ultrasounded side). The authors did not report any adverse effects from the intervention. The gains from the intervention of improvement 1 week earlier in the rabbits do not seem huge, however, it remains to be seen what the effects are in humans.

D. E. Feldman, PT, PhD

Symptomatic and Functional Responses to Concentric-Eccentric Isokinetic Versus Eccentric-Only Isotonic Exercise

Parr JJ, Yarrow JF, Garbo CM, et al (Univ of Florida, Gainesville)

J Athl Train 44:462-468, 2009

Context.—Rehabilitation protocols involving eccentric resistance exercise performed with loading more than 100% concentric 1-repetition maximum are effective in increasing muscle function in both healthy and injured populations. The mode of eccentric exercise (isokinetic versus isotonic) may be an important factor in limiting symptoms of delayed-onset muscle soreness and in improving muscle function after training.

Objective.—To compare functional and symptomatic responses after an eccentric-only (ECC) isotonic exercise protocol and after a combined concentric-eccentric (CON-ECC) isokinetic exercise protocol matched for total exercise volume.

Design.—Observational study.

Setting.—Controlled research laboratory.

Patients or Other Participants.—Twenty-four healthy, untrained, college-aged men (n = 12) and women (n = 12).

Intervention(s).—Participants were randomly assigned to the ECC isotonic or CON-ECC isokinetic exercise group and performed a single bout of resistance exercise involving the elbow flexors.

Main Outcome Measure(s).—Measurements of elbow flexion and extension, isometric strength, and muscle point tenderness were obtained before exercise (baseline) and during follow-up sessions (days 2, 4, 7, and 14). Separate 1-way analyses of variance and repeated-measures analyses of variance were used to determine outcome differences. Tukey post hoc testing was performed when indicated.

Results.—At baseline, no differences were present between groups for any measure. The ECC isotonic exercise protocol resulted in a 30% to 36% deficit in muscle strength, a 5% to 7% reduction in elbow flexion, and a 6% to 8% reduction in elbow extension at follow-up days 2 and 4 ($P < .01$). The CON-ECC isokinetic exercise protocol did not alter muscle strength or range of motion at any time when compared with baseline. Muscle point tenderness increased from baseline on days 2 and 4 in both groups ($P < .05$) but was not different between groups throughout the recovery period.

Conclusions.—Our results indicated more pronounced functional deficits occurred after a single bout of ECC isotonic exercise than with a CON-ECC isokinetic exercise protocol matched for training volume.

▶ This article compares responses after eccentric isotonic exercise and concentric-eccentric isokinetic exercise for the elbow flexors. The rationale is to try and learn more about delayed onset muscle soreness and determine which of these 2 exercise protocols have worse short-term outcomes in terms of range of motion, isometric strength, and muscle point tenderness. The intervention was a single bout of exercise. The sample size was small (12 in each group); nevertheless, the authors were able to demonstrate that those in the eccentric isotonic group as compared with those in the isokinetic group had short-term deficits with respect to range of motion (decrease on days 2 and 4 postintervention), strength (decrease on days 2 and 4 postintervention), but no differences in muscle point tenderness. The clinical implications are that perhaps isokinetic exercise programs are superior to eccentric exercise for rehabilitation purposes; however, this needs to be shown in persons who have had injuries (this study was done on healthy volunteers).

D. E. Feldman, PT, PhD

Eccentric exercises; why do they work, what are the problems and how can we improve them?

Rees JD, Wolman RL, Wilson A (Defence Med Rehabilitation Centre, Surrey, UK; The Royal Natl Orthopaedic Hosp, London, UK; The Royal Veterinary College, Hatfield, UK)

Br J Sports Med 43:242-246, 2009

Eccentric exercises (EE) have proved successful in the management of chronic tendinopathy, particularly of the Achilles and patellar tendons, where they have been shown to be effective in controlled trials. However, numerous questions regarding EE remain. The standard protocols are time-consuming and require very motivated patients. EE are effective in some tendinopathies but not others. Furthermore, the location of the lesion can have a profound effect on efficacy; for example, standard EE in insertional lesions of the Achilles are ineffective. Until recently little was known of the effect of EE on tendinopathic tendons, although a greater understanding of this process is emerging. Additionally, recent in vivo evidence directly comparing eccentric and concentric exercises provides a possible explanation for the therapeutic benefit of EE. The challenge now is to make EE more effective. Suggestions on areas of future research are made.

▶ This commentary-type article does a nice job of evaluating various elements of the evidence relating "eccentric" versus "concentric" training for tendinopathy. The authors are from a well-published group. The authors propose that the main difference between eccentric and concentric loading from the tendon's perspective is that there is a pattern of sinusoidal loading and unloading in the eccentric phase that was not present when they measured concentric exercise for Achilles tendinopathy. This is illustrated in the Fig in the original article; note that the eccentric exercise (EE) has the sinusoidal wave. The authors debunk the idea that eccentric exercise might provide more substantial loading to the tendon; that is not the case. Does this have immediate clinical applicability? Not yet, but it provides an important avenue for further research as we try to refine the exercise prescription for tendinopathy. In the meantime, it seems sensible, from a clinical study standpoint, to keep promoting focused eccentric exercise.

K. M. Khan, MD, PhD

No Impaired Hemoglobin Oxygenation in Forearm Muscles of Patients With Chronic CRPS-1

Brunnekreef JJJ, Oosterhof J, Wolff AP, et al (Radboud Univ Nijmegen Med Ctr, The Netherlands; et al)

Clin J Pain 25:513-519, 2009

Objectives.—Physiotherapy is considered an important treatment option in patients with upper limb complex regional pain syndrome type-1 (CRPS-1). In case of chronic CRPS-1, exercise therapy of the affected limb forms an important part of the physiotherapeutic program. We investigated whether muscle loading in chronic CRPS-1 patients is associated with impairments in muscle circulation of the forearm of the affected limb.

Methods.—Thirty patients with chronic CRPS-1 unilaterally affecting their upper limbs, and 30 age-matched and sex-matched control participants were included in this study. Local muscle blood flow and hemoglobin oxygenation were measured by near infrared spectroscopy within the muscles of the forearm at rest, after 1-minute isometric handgrip exercises, and after arterial occlusion. Main outcome parameters were: local muscle blood flow, O_2 consumption (mVO_2), and postischemic reoxygenation (ReOx).

Results.—We found no differences in baseline muscle blood flow, mVO_2, and ReOx between the affected CRPS-1, unaffected CRPS-1, and control arms. After exercise, mVO_2 of the affected CRPS-1 arms was not different from the clinically unaffected CRPS-1 arms. Furthermore, in comparison with the control arms, unaffected CRPS-1 arms showed no difference in mVO_2 or ReOx.

Conclusions.—Muscle loading does not seem to be related to impairments in muscle oxygen uptake in forearm muscles of upper limbs affected by chronic CRPS-1. Our results suggest that exercise therapy can be safely used in physiotherapeutic training programs for chronic CRPS-1 of the upper limb.

► Patients with complex regional pain syndrome are known to benefit from physical therapy interventions, even though the intervention often causes pain during its application. The authors of this article showed that there were no signs of muscle hypoxia in the forearm muscles of patients with complex regional pain syndrome type-1 (CRPS-1) at rest, after exercise, and after arterial occlusion. There seems to be no detrimental effects in terms of hypoxia secondary to muscle loading in these patients, even though these exercises cause pain. Thus, they conclude that loading (or exercising) does not adversely affect hemoglobin oxygenation in muscle tissues of patients with CRPS-1.

This study supports the use of physiotherapy training programs in patients with CRPS-1 affecting the upper limb. It would be interesting to replicate these results in patients with lower limb impairments who require higher loading (weight bearing exercise).

D. E. Feldman, PT, PhD

Muscle Forces or Gravity: What Predominates Mechanical Loading on Bone?

Kohrt WM, Barry DW, Schwartz RS (Univ of Colorado Denver, Aurora)
Med Sci Sports Exerc 41:2050-2055, 2009

Most mechanical forces acting on the skeleton are generated either through impact with the ground (i.e., gravitational loading) or through muscle contractions (i.e., muscle loading). If one of these conduits for activating mechanotransduction in bone is more effective than the other with respect to developing or maintaining bone strength, this would have important clinical implications for prescribing physical activity for the prevention or treatment of osteoporosis. This section of the symposium considered whether there is evidence from studies of humans that the effectiveness of physical activity to preserve bone health is dependent on whether the activities stimulate the skeleton primarily through gravitational or muscle loading. Conclusive evidence is lacking, but several lines of research suggest that physical activities that involve impact forces, and therefore generate both gravitation and muscle loading, are most likely to have beneficial effects on bone metabolism and reduce fracture risk.

▶ This discussion article opens with a statement of the clinical use of the phrases "nonweight-bearing" and "weight-bearing" to characterize the magnitude of the desired loads to be applied to lower extremity joint surfaces during locomotion activities. These phrases are most prevalent when dictating the maximal load magnitudes when prescribing crutch use. The intended goal is to upper limit constrain the lower extremity joint loads due to the application of the ground reaction force on the foot (gravitation loading) during crutch-assisted gait. However, lower extremity joint loading is influenced by gravitational loading and the locomotion muscles applying joint compressive loads (muscle loading). If clinicians want to reduce joint loading they must state that both the gravitational and muscle loadings must be reduced—a message not explicitly conveyed by the "nonweight-bearing" and "weight-bearing" instructions.

In this article, the authors extensively discuss whether it is the presence of the gravitational loading, the muscle loading, or a combination of the two that best maintains or increases bone mineral density which has been shown to lower the risk of bone fracture. The authors strongly suggest that both gravitational and muscle loadings are important. Physical activities that gravitationally and muscle load the lower extremity joints, such as walking, can significantly reduce fracture risk (see Fig 3 in the original article). This information can be used by clinicians to help convince patients who are at risk of bone fracture to maintain a physically active lifestyle.

M. R. Pierrynowski, PhD

Is explosive performance influenced by androgen concentrations in young male soccer players?

Baldari C, Di Luigi L, Emerenziani GP, et al (Univ of Rome "Foro Italico", Italy)
Br J Sports Med 43:191-194, 2009

Objective.—There is growing interest in the implementation and assessment of strength and conditioning programmes among young children. The purpose of this study was to examine the association between given anthropometric characteristics, pubertal development, salivary androgen hormones and explosive leg power in young soccer players.

Methods.—51 (age range 10–14 years) soccer players were investigated. The relations between age, pubertal developmental stages, testicular volume, weight, height, body fat, fat free mass, salivary DHEAS concentrations, salivary testosterone concentrations and lower limb explosive power were evaluated.

Results.—Standing long jump length was positively correlated ($p<0.05$) with age (11.7 (SD 1.2) years, $r=0.66$), pubertal developmental stages (mode and range: 1 (1–4), $r=0.64$), testicular volume (8.8 (5.2) ml, $r=0.58$), height (1.50 (0.10) m, $r=0.34$), weight (43.7 (9.1) kg, $r=0.34$), fat free mass (35.4 (7.2) kg, $r=0.67$), salivary DHEAS concentrations (4.4 (1.2) ng/ml, $r=0.38$) and negatively correlated with body fat (18.6 (7.0) kg; $r=-0.49$, $p<0.05$). There was no significant correlation between salivary testosterone concentrations (0.3 (0.1) ng/ml, $r=0.12$) and standing long jump.

Conclusions.—Results of the present investigation demonstrated that age, pubertal developmental stages, testicular volume, weight, height, fat free mass, and salivary DHEAS concentrations were associated with standing long jump performance. In addition, salivary testosterone concentrations were not related to explosive leg power. Results of the present investigation suggest that the teacher/coach should evaluate long jump performance relative to the subject's given biological characteristics, and not simply established standards based on chronological age.

► The message conveyed in these authors' conclusion needs to be reinforced regularly to youth coaches, parents, and sports administrators. Athletic performance in sports activities is strongly influenced by the level of sexual development, and pubertal status serves to discriminate between stages of development of athletic prowess much better than chronological age. Yes, there are certain reasons for grouping competitors by age, mainly social and psychologic, but the best means of leveling the playing field for child athletes (and perhaps reducing injury risk) is matching competitors by level of biological maturation rather than age. Just how to best do this remains problematic. At least in males, salivary testosterone values as used in this study might be worth exploring as a feasible way of maturity matching in competitive sports (particularly community football teams) in the pre or early teen years.

T. Rowland, MD

The Influence of Estrogen on Skeletal Muscle: Sex Matters

Enns DL, Tiidus PM (Wilfrid Laurier Univ, Waterloo, Ontario, Canada)

Sports Med 40:41-58, 2010

As women enter menopause, the concentration of estrogen and other female hormones declines. This hormonal decrease has been associated with a number of negative outcomes, including a greater incidence of injury as well as a delay in recovery from these injuries. Over the past two decades, our understanding of the protective effects of estrogen against various types of injury and disease states has grown immensely. In skeletal muscle, studies with animals have demonstrated that sex and estrogen may potentially influence muscle contractile properties and attenuate indices of post-exercise muscle damage, including the release of creatine kinase into the bloodstream and activity of the intramuscular lysosomal acid hydrolase, β-glucuronidase. Furthermore, numerous studies have revealed an estrogen-mediated attenuation of infiltration of inflammatory cells such as neutrophils and macrophages into the skeletal muscles of rats following exercise or injury. Estrogen has also been shown to play a significant role in stimulating muscle repair and regenerative processes, including the activation and proliferation of satellite cells. Although the mechanisms by which estrogen exerts its influence upon indices of skeletal muscle damage, inflammation and repair have not been fully elucidated, it is thought that estrogen may potentially exert its protective effects by: (i) acting as an antioxidant, thus limiting oxidative damage; (ii) acting as a membrane stabilizer by intercalating within membrane phospholipids; and (iii) binding to estrogen receptors, thus governing the regulation of a number of downstream genes and molecular targets. In contrast to animal studies, studies with humans have not as clearly delineated an effect of estrogen on muscle contractile function or on indices of post-exercise muscle damage and inflammation. These inconsistencies have been attributed to a number of factors, including age and fitness level of subjects, the type and intensity of exercise protocols, and a focus on sex differences that typically involve factors and hormones in addition to estrogen. In recent years, hormone replacement therapy (HRT) or estrogen combined with exercise have been proposed as potentially therapeutic agents for postmenopausal women, as these agents may potentially limit muscle damage and inflammation and stimulate repair in this population. While the benefits and potential health risks of long-term HRT use have been widely debated, controlled studies using short-term HRT or other estrogen agonists may provide future new and valuable insights into understanding the effects of estrogen on skeletal muscle, and greatly benefit the aging female population. Recent studies with older females have begun to demonstrate their benefits.

▶ Human activities can result in disruptions of the muscle membranes, especially if those activities are unexpected or involve lengthening (eccentric) muscular contractions. Following these, muscle injuries regeneration and repair of the skeletal muscle fibers are initiated. In this article, the authors review the role of estrogen in the muscle repair process. They report that in animal studies, estrogen and exercise limits activity-induced muscle damage and may accelerate the repair processes. However, the review of the human literature suggested that these associations are not as clear in the human studies. This article is important for clinicians advising older women who present with diminished muscle mass, muscle power, and reduced estrogen levels. The lower estrogen levels in older women may diminish their muscle repair processes and lead to decreased functional ability. The authors cautiously suggest "that hormone (estrogen) replacement therapy, combined with exercise, may be the most beneficial method for preserving muscle mass and strength in older woman."

M. R. Pierrynowski, PhD

Enhancing Muscular Qualities in Untrained Women: Linear versus Undulating Periodization

Kok L-Y, Hamer PW, Bishop DJ (The Univ of Western Australia, Perth; The Univ of Notre Dame Australia, Fremantle)

Med Sci Sports Exerc 41:1797-1807, 2009

Purpose.—This study compared linear (LP) and undulating periodization (UP) on strength changes in untrained women when total workload and average training intensity were matched by the end of training.

Methods.—Twenty females (20 ± 2 yr) were conditioned (3 wk) and assessed for one-repetition maximum squat (1RMSQ) and bench press (1RMBP) before being assigned to LP or UP training (9 wk), with training performed at 3 $d \cdot wk^{-1}$. Maximal strength, average power output during squat jumps with countermovement (SQJpwr) and bench press throws (BPTpwr), body mass, limb girth, and muscle cross-sectional area (CSA) were assessed at baseline (T1) and after every 3 wk (T2, T3, and T4) to differentiate the efficacy of LP and UP training.

Results.—Both groups improved significantly ($P < 0.05$) in 1RMSQ (LP 34.8%, UP 41.2%), 1RMBP (LP 21.8%, UP 28.3%), SQJpwr (LP 10.4%, UP 9.5%), BPTpwr (LP 11.1%, UP 13.8%), arm girth (LP 1.14%, UP 1.73%), and thigh girth (LP 1.58%, UP 1.99%), with no significant difference between them. Muscle CSA for the LP group increased significantly at T2 before maintaining similar hypertrophic responses until T4, whereas the UP group recorded significant increments

TABLE 2.—Alternation of Volume and Intensity for LP and UP Programs

Pretraining Conditioning: Weeks 1–3			T1: Division of Subjects Into Groups	Training Phase I: Weeks 4–6			Training Phase II: Weeks 7–9			Training Phase III: Weeks 10–12		
All subjects perform the same training			LP	Week 1 (H)	Week 2 (H)	Week 3 (H)	Week 1 (S)	Week 2 (S)	Week 3 (S)	Week 1 (P)	Week 2 (P)	Week 3 (P)
				$\frac{75}{10}3$	$\frac{77}{10}3$	$\frac{80}{10}3$	$\frac{85}{6}3$	$\frac{90}{6}3$	$\frac{90}{6}4$	$\frac{30}{8}3$	$\frac{40}{8}3$	$\frac{40}{8}4$
				10RM × 3	10RM × 3	10RM × 3	6RM × 3	6RM × 3	6RM × 3	$\frac{30}{8}3$	$\frac{40}{8}3$	$\frac{40}{8}3$
Week 1	Week 2	Week 3	UP	Day 1 (H)	Day 2 (S)	Day 3 (P)	Day 1 (H)	Day 2 (S)	Day 3 (P)	Day 1 (H)	Day 2 (S)	Day 3 (P)
$\frac{70}{10}2$	$\frac{70}{10}3$	$\frac{70}{12}3$		$\frac{75}{10}3$	$\frac{85}{6}3$	$\frac{30}{8}3$	$\frac{77}{10}3$	$\frac{90}{6}3$	$\frac{40}{8}3$	$\frac{80}{10}3$	$\frac{90}{6}4$	$\frac{40}{8}4$
15RM × 2	12RM × 3	10RM × 3		10RM × 3	6RM × 3	$\frac{30}{8}3$	10RM × 3	6RM × 3	$\frac{40}{8}3$	10RM × 3	6RM × 3	$\frac{40}{8}3$

$[\frac{70}{10}2]$ denotes $\left[\frac{\%\ of\ 1RM}{reception\ s}\ number\ of\ sets\right]$ for the bench press and squat exercises, and all power exercises.

\(15RM × 2) denotes the number of maximum repetitions to be performed for the required number of sets for all other exercises (except abdominal and back exercises). (H), hypertrophy training; (P), power training; (S), maximal strength training.

from T1 to T2 and T2 to T3, before stabilizing between T3 and T4. Pooled CSA increase was higher than previously found (6.8% at T2, 11.3% at T3, and 11.8% at T4).

Conclusions.—The comparison of LP and UP training with matched volume load and intensity suggests that both programs were equally adept in improving different strength qualities in active but untrained women. In addition, muscle hypertrophic responses were larger and occurred earlier than previously reported (Table 2).

▶ This is the first study to compare changes in muscle function in women in response to linear periodization (LP) and undulating periodization (UP) resistance training plans. LP refers to training that starts with high-volume and low-intensity exercises and progresses toward a low-volume high-intensity peak. This is a traditional training plan comprising, for example, 3-week training intervals within 3 months. In contrast, UP mixes training volume and intensity on a daily or weekly basis. The rationale for UP is to avoid the neural fatigue and compromised strength gains seen in response to LP. Two important aspects of this study are that training volume (repetitions × mass lifted) was matched between LP and UP and the participants were women who were not trained in resistance exercises. Both training approaches included 3 aspects of muscle quality: hypertrophy, maximal strength, and power. Hypertrophy was measured as right thigh muscle cross-sectional area using B-mode ultrasound. Maximal strength of bench press and leg press was measured using a one-repetition maximum (1-RM) test, whereas power was measured using the bench press throw and squat jump tests. These assessments were completed 5 times to establish a baseline and then after every 3 weeks of training. The training included 10 exercises completed in 3 days per week. Training intensities of 75% to 85% of the 1-RM were used for hypertrophy, 85% to 95% for maximal strength, and 30% to 40% for muscular power training (Table 2). At the end of the training, the LP and UP groups had significant increases in muscle size, strength, and power but neither strategy proved superior to the other. An interesting outcome was that upper- and lower-body strength gains continued during the final low-volume, low-intensity power training phase of LP. The participants reported that the 3 weeks of lighter intensity training provided a psychological respite from the previous phases of training. Women who completed UP also reported that the lighter training days alleviated physical and psychological stress of training from the higher intensity and volume days. Either periodization plan may prove useful to retain novice exercisers in resistance training. For example, a novice may be more motivated to complete the third exercise session within a week if she or he knows that the session would be of lighter volume (ie, undulating plan). Notably, a 3-week preconditioning phase was used to familiarize participants with the exercises before the periodization was initiated. It is not clear if either UP or LP is advantageous for sport performance, for athletes already experienced in weight training, or if carried out over a longer time frame.

C. M. Jankowski, PhD

Effect of Eccentric Exercise Program for Early Tibialis Posterior Tendinopathy

Kulig K, Lederhaus ES, Reischl S, et al (Univ of Southern California, Los Angeles)

Foot Ankle Int 30:877-885, 2009

Background.—Morphology and vascularization of painful tibialis posterior (TP) tendons before and after an intervention targeting the degenerated tendon were examined. Functional status and pain level were also assessed.

Materials and Methods.—A10-week twice daily, progressive eccentric tendon loading, calf stretching program with orthoses was implemented with ten, early stage TP tendinopathy subjects. TP tendons were imaged by grayscale and Doppler ultrasound at INITIAL and POST evaluations to assess the tendon's morphology and signs of neovascularization. The Foot Functional Index (FFI), Physical Activity Scale (PAS), 5-Minute Walk Test, and single heel raise (SHR) test were completed at INITIAL and POST evaluations. The Global Rating Scale (GRS) was completed at 6 months followup. One-way ANOVA was used to compare the FFI at INITIAL, POST, and 6-MONTH time points. Paired t-tests were used to compare means between the remaining variables. The level of significance was $p = 0.05$.

Results.—There was a significant difference in FFI total, pain, and disability at the three time-points. Post-hoc paired t-tests revealed that the FFI scores were lower for the total score and pain and disability subcategories when comparing from INITIAL to POST and INITIAL to 6-MONTH evaluations ($p < 0.05$ for all). The number of SHR increased significantly on the involved side from INITIAL to POST evaluation ($p = 0.041$). The GRS demonstrated minimum clinically important differences for improvements in symptoms at 6-MONTH. Tendon morphology and vascularization remained abnormal following the intervention.

Conclusion.—A 10-week tendon specific eccentric program resulted in improvements in symptoms and function without changes in tendon morphology or neovascularization.

▶ Our understanding of the pathogenesis, morphology, and treatment of tendon problems in various parts of the body has evolved significantly from the days when all injuries were thought to be tendonitis, with associated inflammation being the source of pain and the target of interventions. Currently much more is known about the entity of tendinosis, characterized by fibroblastic hypercellularity and neovascularization. Progress in this field has been greatly enhanced by the advent of ultrasonographic imaging (US) and usage of color Doppler mode to determine the presence or absence of neovascularization. Previous studies have demonstrated the success of eccentric loading exercise programs (various protocols, number of repetitions, and duration of treatment) for Achilles tendinosis in conjunction with a normalized tendon structure on US (thinner and less hypoechoic without neovascularization) following successful intervention.

This study was designed to relate changes in pain, disability, and function with changes in the morphology of degenerated tibialis posterior tendons in response to 2 weeks of unloading followed by a 10-week tendon-specific intervention with orthoses wear. Inclusion/exclusion criteria, correction of foot biomechanics with custom orthoses, and a 2-week program of unloading of the tendon and stretching and strengthening exercises served to standardize the subjects at baseline. The exercise protocol was administered using a commercial device called a TibPost Loader (Fig 1A, B in the original article), but practically speaking, these exercises could also be done using a simple elastic band. The condition of the participants improved over the course of the 10-week trial with regard to pain and disability as assessed by the Foot Functional Index, visual analog scales for pain after walking, and number of single heel rises and remained clinically meaningful 6 months following the intervention. Concurrent imaging of the tendon structure, morphology, and neovascularity of the tendon using color Doppler did not demonstrate any associated changes over this time. This study has been rigorously designed and well referenced. The only weakness is the low power (n = 10) and the lack of a control group. Nevertheless, it is of high quality and will be of great benefit to the reader.

C. Lebrun, MD

Skeletal Benefits After Long-Term Retirement in Former Elite Female Gymnasts

Eser P, Hill B, Ducher G, et al (Deakin Univ, Burwood, Australia)

J Bone Miner Res 24:1981-1988, 2009

Bone strength benefits after long-term retirement from elite gymnastics in terms of bone geometry and volumetric BMD were studied by comparing retired female gymnasts to moderately active age-matched women. In a cross-sectional study, 30 retired female gymnasts were compared with 30 age-matched moderately active controls. Bone geometric and densitometric parameters were measured by pQCT at the distal epiphyses and shafts of the tibia, femur, radius, and humerus. Muscle cross-sectional areas were assessed from the shaft scans. Independent *t*-tests were conducted on bone and muscle variables to detect differences between the two groups. The gymnasts had retired for a mean of 6.1 ± 0.4 yr and were engaged in ≤2 h of exercise per week since retirement. At the radial and humeral shafts, cortical cross-sectional area (CSA), total CSA, BMC, and strength strain index (SSIpol) were significantly greater (13–38%, $p \leq 0.01$) in the retired gymnasts; likewise, BMC and total CSA were significantly greater at the distal radius (22–25%, $p \leq 0.0001$). In the lower limbs, total CSA and BMC at the femur and tibia shaft were greater by 8–11%, and trabecular BMD and BMC were only greater at the tibia (7–8%). Muscle CSA at the forearm

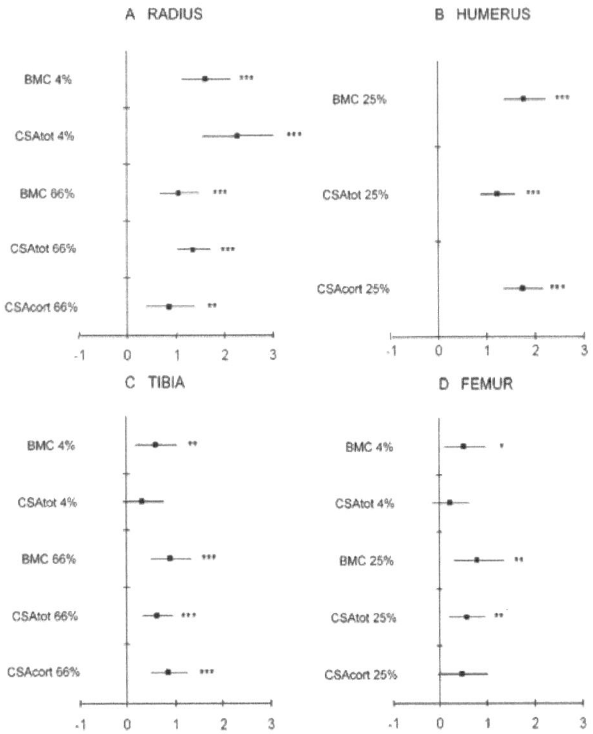

FIGURE 1.—Effect size of gymnasts over controls in SD of measured bone parameters at the (A) radius, (B) humerus, (C) tibia, and (D) femur. Shown are mean effect sizes with 95% CIs. $*p \leq 0.05$, $**p \leq 0.01$, and $***p \leq 0.0001$. (Reprinted from Eser P, Hill B, Ducher G, et al. Skeletal benefits after long-term retirement in former elite female gymnasts. *J Bone Miner Res*. 2009;24:1981-1988, with permission from the American Society for Bone and Mineral Research.)

and upper arm was greater by 15–17.6% ($p \leq 0.001$) but was not different at the upper and lower leg. Past gymnastics training is associated with greater bone mass and bone size in women 6 yr after retirement. Skeletal benefits were site specific, with greater geometric adaptations (greater bone size) in the upper compared with the lower limbs (Figs 1 and 2).

▶ Eser and colleagues conducted an elegant cross-sectional study of geometric and densitometric properties in retired, elite female gymnasts and controls of comparable age (18-36 years) and body size to better understand the prevailing effects of bone loading during gymnastics training on bone quality. An emerging technology, peripheral quantitative computed tomography (pQCT), was used to measure the geometry and bone mineral content (BMC) of the epiphyses (ends) and diaphyses (shafts) of upper (radius, ulna, and distal humerus) and lower (tibia and distal femur) long bones. This technology captures trabecular, cortical, and medullary dimensions of bone. The cross-sectional areas (CSA) of muscle and subcutaneous fat in the upper and lower limbs were also measured with pQCT. Dual energy x-ray absorptiometry

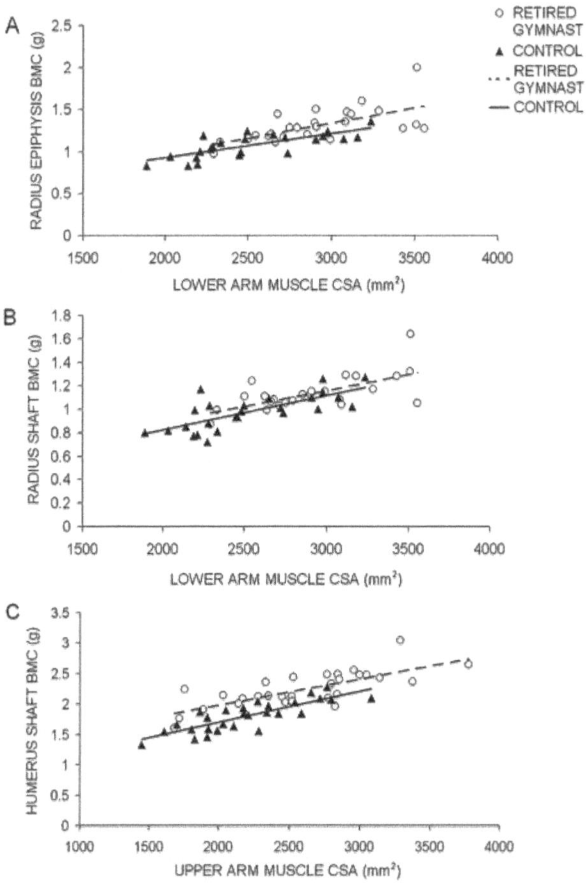

FIGURE 2.—Relationship between lower arm muscle CSA and BMC at the (A) distal radius in retired gymnasts (○) and controls (▲), as well as (B) radial shaft BMC. Relationship between upper arm muscle CSA and humeral shaft BMC is shown in C. Regression lines for the two separate groups are also shown. BMC is reported as grams per centimeter slice thickness. (Reprinted from Eser P, Hill B, Ducher G, et al. Skeletal benefits after long-term retirement in former elite female gymnasts. *J Bone Miner Res.* 2009;24:1981-1988, with permission from the American Society for Bone and Mineral Research.)

(DXA) was used to measure the total body composition. Some of the important confounding factors for bone health were addressed, including training history, retirement history of the gymnasts, menstrual history, and current physical activity (duration and intensity). The average length of the gymnasts' retirement was 6 years. The main finding was that gymnastics training was associated with site- and property-specific benefits to bone that were more pronounced in the arms (Fig 1). The CSA, BMC, and strength index of the radial distal epiphysis, radial diaphysis, and humerus diaphysis were significantly greater (20%-30%) in the gymnasts compared with controls. In the legs, gymnastics training conferred benefits (5%-20%) to BMC of the tibia epiphysis, tibia diaphysis, and femur diaphysis and the CSA of the tibia diaphysis. Total body lean mass and fat mass and lower limb muscle CSA of the gymnasts were not significantly different than controls. However, the gymnasts had significantly larger muscles in the arms. In both groups, BMC of the radius epiphysis, radius diaphysis, and humerus diaphysis were linearly related to muscle CSA (Fig 2). The adaptations in the gymnasts were the result of repetitive loading exposures to bone, particularly in the arms, over an average 10-year training career. At the highest level of training, gymnasts trained on average 23 hours per week. The recent physical activity of the gymnasts and controls was similar. In fact, the controls spent more time in moderate physical activity than the gymnasts, perhaps explaining the muted differences in the leg parameters between groups. The greater geometry and densitometry in the upper arms of the retired gymnasts may be due to the maintenance of muscle size in this region. The differences seen in bone geometry and densitometry may have been less pronounced if retirement had been longer. However, the greater prevalence of primary and secondary amenorrhea in the gymnasts may have mitigated the osteogenic adaptations during training. This study lends support to the long-term effects of mechanical loading on bone in young women.

C. M. Jankowski, PhD

Metabolomic investigation into variation of endogenous metabolites in professional athletes subject to strength-endurance training

Yan B, Jiye A, Wang G, et al (China Pharmaceutical Univ, Nanjing)

J Appl Physiol 106:531-538, 2009

Strength-endurance type of sport can lead to modification of human beings' physiological status. The present study aimed to investigate the alteration of metabolic phenotype or biochemical compositions in professional athletes induced by long-term training by means of a novel systematic tool, metabolomics. Resting venous blood samples of junior and senior male rowers were obtained before and after 1-wk and 2-wk training. Venous blood from healthy male volunteers as control was also sampled at rest. Endogenous metabolites in serum were profiled by GC/TOF-MS and multivariate statistical technique, i.e., principal component analysis (PCA), and partial least squares projection to latent structures and discriminant analysis (PLS-DA) were used to process the data. Significant metabolomic difference was observed between the professional athletes and control subjects. Long-term strength and endurance training induced distinct separation between athletes of different exercise seniority, and training stage-related trajectory of the two groups of athletes was clearly shown along with training time. However, most of these variations were not observed by common biochemical parameters, such as hemoglobin, testosterone, and creatine kinase. The identified metabolites contributing to the classification included alanine, lactate, β-D-methylglucopyranoside, pyroglutamic acid, cysteine, glutamic acid, citric acid, free fatty acids, valine, glutamine, phenylalanine, tyrosine, and so on, which were involved in glucose metabolism, oxidative stress, energy metabolism, lipid metabolism, amino acid metabolism. These findings suggest that metabolomics is a promising and potential tool to profile serum of professional athletes, make a deep insight into physiological states, and clarify the disorders induced by strength-endurance physical exercise.

► Metabolomics technology holds high promise for better understanding how the body responds to exercise and nutrition intervention.[1,2] Metabolomics involves the quantitative measurement of the global, dynamic metabolic response to biological stimuli or genetic manipulation. It is typically carried out using spectroscopic tools followed by statistical analyses and pattern recognition methods to determine the low molecular weight metabolites (typically MW < 1000) that correlate with physiological change through time. Mass spectrometry (MS) coupled to chromatographic seperations, including gas chromatography (GC) and liquid chromatography (LC), can achieve higher detection sensitivity and therefore can provide a broader range of metabolites. In this exercise-related study, the first one involving metabolomics, metabolic differences were detected between rowers and control subjects before and after intensive training. Perturbations in glucose metabolism, lipid metabolism, oxidative stress, and amino acid metabolism were measured. The authors concluded that metabolomics is a promising technique in monitoring the physiological status of athletes.

D. C. Nieman, DrPH

References

1. Kaddurah-Daouk R, Kristal BS, Weinshilboum RM. Metabolomics: a global biochemical approach to drug response and disease. *Annu Rev Pharmacol Toxicol.* 2008;48:653-683.
2. Manach C, Hubert J, Llorach R, Scalbert A. The complex links between dietary phytochemicals and human health deciphered by metabolomics. *Mol Nutr Food Res.* 2009;53:1303-1315.

Explaining the hip adduction moment variability during gait: Implications for hip abductor strengthening

Rutherford DJ, Hubley-Kozey C (Dalhousie Univ, Halifax, Canada)
Clin Biomech (Bristol, Avon) 24:267-273, 2009

Background.—There is emerging interest in hip abductor function during gait and its potential relationship to knee joint pathology. During gait, the hip abductor muscles are primarily responsible for generating moments of force to control frontal plane movement. The current study investigated the relationship between hip abductor muscle function and frontal plane hip moments of force during gait.

Methods.—Frontal plane hip moments of force and electromyographic features of gluteus medius were measured during walking in 22 healthy individuals. Hip abductor strength, subject anthropometrics and gait velocity were recorded. Multiple regression models were used to evaluate

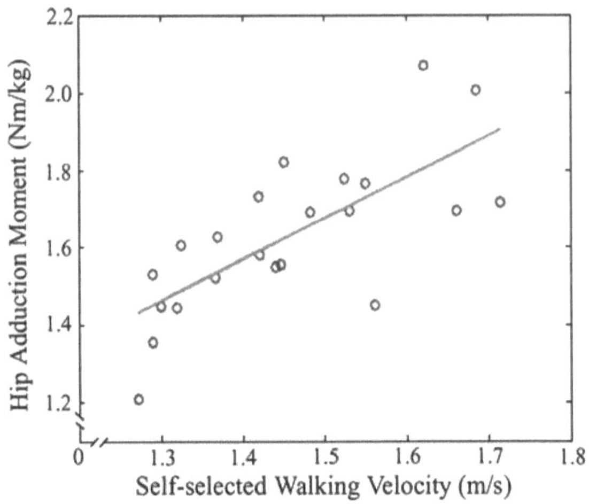

FIGURE 3.—The association between self-selected walking velocity and the peak net external hip adduction moment normalized to body mass captured during the stance phase of the gait cycle $r = 0.724$, $P = 0.000$. (Reprinted from Rutherford DJ, Hubley-Kozey C, Explaining the hip adduction moment variability during gait: implications for hip abductor strengthening. *Clin Biomech (Bristol, Avon)*. 2009;24:267-273, with permission from Elsevier Ltd.)

the relationship between the anthropometric, velocity, strength and electromyographic variables and the initial and mid-stance magnitude of the hip adduction moment.

Findings.—A positive relationship was found between the initial peak moment (Nm), and both body mass and gait speed ($R^2 = 90\%$). Body mass (positive) and hip abductor strength (negative) explained significant levels of mid-stance magnitude variability ($R^2 = 62.5\%$). Gait speed (positive) explained significant levels of variability in the normalized initial peak moment (Nm/kg) ($R^2 = 52\%$). No variables were included in the normalized mid-stance moment model ($P > 0.05$).

Interpretation.—Body mass was the key factor associated with high hip adduction moments during initial and mid-stance of the gait cycle. Increased gait velocity was associated with higher initial peaks and higher muscle strength was associated with lower mid-stance magnitude of the external hip adductor moment during walking. These findings suggest that in a healthy adult population, hip abductor strength and activation were not directly related to the hip adduction moment magnitude during gait (Fig 3).

▶ This study examined how a subject's walking speed and their weight influences the magnitude of the hip extensor moment during gait. This question is clinically important because weak hip abductors can cause excessive frontal plane motion which influences medial knee joint loading which has been associated with the progression and severity of knee osteoarthritis. Twenty-two healthy subjects were assessed in a clinical gait laboratory (measures the temporal-spatial, kinematic, kinetic, and electromyographic gait outcomes) and positive associations between the hip abduction moment during middle stance and walking speed and subject weight were reported (Fig 3 for the moment-speed relationship). However, the subject's isometric hip adduction strength was not associated with the hip adduction moment during gait. The authors suggest that the lack of association is because the hip abductors are never maximally recruited during gait, therefore are active below capacity. The authors further suggest that if one wants to increase the hip abduction moment during gait to potentially reduce the severity and progression of knee osteoarthritis, having the subject increase their weight or walk faster, not strengthen the hip abductors, would achieve this goal.

M. R. Pierrynowski, PhD

Physical examination of the foot and ankle by orthopaedic and accident and emergency clinicians

Roche A, Hunter L, Pocock N, et al (The Royal Liverpool and Broadgreen Univ Hosps Trust, Prescot, UK)

Injury 40:136-138, 2009

Our aim was to test the knowledge of clinicians in the Orthopaedic clinic and in the Emergency department of the surface anatomical landmarks that should be examined routinely in the assessment of foot and ankle injuries. A survey of 109 clinicians was conducted. Each participant was asked to palpate six important surface landmarks. Two participants failed to identify even a single landmark. Of 109 assessed only 27% correctly identified all six landmarks. The mean number of landmarks correctly identified by each clinician was 4.1 with a standard deviation of 1.5 and range of 0–6. The knowledge of surface anatomy overall by junior Orthopaedic and Emergency clinicians was found to be very poor. Clinicians are becoming more reliant on potentially unnecessary and expensive imaging investigations. They have neglected the basic art of physical examination based on a sound knowledge of human anatomy. At present, the authors believe that the anatomical teaching that should begin in undergraduate medicine is inadequate.

▶ The use of the Ottawa ankle rules (OAR) has been shown to have near 100% sensitivity to detect a foot or ankle fracture in those individuals presenting to emergency departments following an ankle sprain. The correct use of the OAR has significantly reduced the need to image and read a radiograph of the foot and ankle. To use the OAR, a health care professional must have a good knowledge of the surface anatomy of the foot and ankle. Specifically, the clinician must be able to confidently locate 6 surface anatomy landmarks: the medial malleolus, lateral malleolus, head of the fibula, the navicular, the base of the fifth metatarsal, and the anterior talo-fibular ligament. In this article, the ability of 109 emergency nurse practitioners (senior students and those with specialty training) to identify the 6 foot and ankle landmarks was reported. Although 98% of the clinicians correctly identified the lateral malleolus, only

45% and 50% could locate the anterior talofibular ligament and the navicular. The authors of this study suggest that the anatomical training health care professionals receive during their problem-based learning education is grossly inadequate.

M. R. Pierrynowski, PhD

4 Physical Activity, Cardio-respiratory Physiology and Immune Function

Increasing Our Understanding of Reactivity to Pedometers in Adults

Clemes SA, Parker RAA (Loughborough Univ, Leicestershire, UK)

Med Sci Sports Exerc 41:674-680, 2009

Purpose.—To investigate the presence of reactivity, if any, to wearing sealed and unsealed pedometers, with and without step count recording.

Methods.—On the first visit to the laboratory, 63 participants (41 females and 22 males; age = 23.6 ± 9.6 yr, body mass index = 22.7 ± 3.0 kg·m^{-2}), blinded to the study aim, were provided with a sealed pedometer (New Lifestyles NL-1000) and informed that it was a "body posture monitor" (covert monitoring). Participants wore the pedometer throughout waking hours for 1 wk. On return to the laboratory, stored step counts were downloaded, and participants were informed that the device was a pedometer. Participants wore the pedometer under three more conditions—sealed, unsealed, and unsealed plus logging daily steps in an activity diary—each having a duration of 1 wk. The order of participation in each condition (sealed/unsealed/diary) was balanced across participants. Mean daily step counts recorded during the four conditions were compared using a repeated-measures ANOVA.

Results.—There was a significant overall effect of condition ($P < 0.001$; covert monitoring = 8362 ± 2600 steps per day; sealed condition = 8832 ± 2845 steps per day; unsealed condition = 9176 ± 3299 steps per day; diary condition = 9635 ± 2709 steps per day), with *post hoc* analyses revealing that mean step counts were significantly higher in the diary condition than those reported during both the covert and sealed conditions (both $P < 0.003$). No significant gender effects were observed ($P = 0.33$).

Conclusion.—The greatest increase in step counts occurred in the diary condition, suggesting that reactivity to pedometers is greatest when participants are requested to wear an unsealed pedometer and record

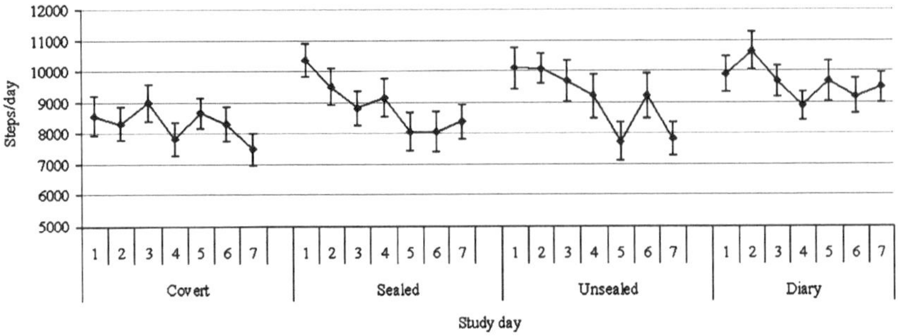

FIGURE 1.—Mean daily step counts recorded during each study day within each condition along with SE bars. (Reprinted from Clemes SA, Parker RAA, Increasing our understanding of reactivity to pedometers in adults. *Med Sci Sports Exerc.* 2009;41:674-680.)

their step counts. This has validity implications for short-term pedometer studies investigating habitual free-living activity that require participants to provide a daily log of their step counts (Fig 1).

▶ The accurate assessment of human movement is essential to progress in understanding relationships between health and physical activity. There has been a tendency to regard pedometer and accelerometer estimates of daily step counts as objective and accurate, but if the device is worn for only a few days and subjects can view their count, this can lead to a substantial increase over normal habitual activity (the problem of reactivity).[1] Some observers were reassured by the similarity of data whether the pedometer was visible or sealed; however, in either case, subjects were aware that they were participating in a study of their physical activity, and this likely augmented their active behavior.[2] In fact, one study found that the normal step count was boosted by almost 20% relative to covert monitoring.[3] This study shows the effect was greatest when the subjects were not only wearing a pedometer, but also completing a diary (Fig 1). We became aware of reactivity to keeping a diary many years ago.[4] However, the data also show a significant effect even when a diary is not being kept. This effect declines with time (Fig 1), and the remedy is thus to wear the instrument for longer than a few days. Our recent studies in Japan have underlined that many accelerometer studies are too short to collect representative data on an individual's behavior.[5]

R. J. Shephard, MD (Lond), PhD, DPE

References

1. Measurement issues in the assessment of physical activity in children. *Res Q Exerc Sport.* 2000;71:S59-S73.
2. Eastep E, Beveridge S, Eisenman P, Ransdell L, Shultz B. Does augmented feedback from pedometers increase adults' walking behavior? *Percept Mot Skills.* 2004;99:392-402.
3. Clemes SA, Matchett N, Wane SL. Reactivity: an issue for short-term pedometer studies? *Br J Sports Med.* 2008;42:68-70.

4. Shephard RJ, ed.. Endurance Fitness. 2nd ed. Toronto: University of Toronto Press; 1977:200.
5. Aoyagi Y, Shephard RJ. Steps per day: the road to senior health? *Sports Med.* 2009;39:423-438.

Effectiveness of the 2006 Commonwealth Games 10,000 Steps Walking Challenge

Harvey JT, Eime RM, Payne WR (Univ of Ballarat, Victoria, Australia)
Med Sci Sports Exerc 41:1673-1680, 2009

Introduction.—There is little evidence supporting sustainability of public health interventions based upon the 10,000 steps concept conducted in "real-world" settings. This study investigated the effectiveness of the 10,000 Steps Walking Challenge, initiated in conjunction with the 2006 Commonwealth Games in Melbourne, Australia, in March 2006.

Methods.—This study analyzed characteristics of registrants ($n = 1836$), pedometer counts logged onto a Web site between February 2006 and February 2007 ($n = 18,032$ entries by 914 participants), and two surveys of participants in June 2006 ($n = 128$) and December 2006 ($n = 62$).

Results.—The program reached its target population of females aged 30–49 yr (40.2% of participants), a group known to have low activity levels, which also has potential to influence the behavior of family, friends, and workmates. Compliance was poor; only 49.8% of registrants ever logged steps, and of these, only 45.5% continued beyond the period of the challenge and 16.6% for more than 1 month. Mean (9527 ± 297, 95% confidence interval) and median (9638) recorded steps per day came close to the target of 10,000 steps; 80.1% of participants reached 10,000 steps at least once and 21.9% did so every time they logged steps. For survey respondents who provided complete data ($n = 53$), the mean estimated daily steps increased significantly ($P < 0.001$) from 6401 ± 884 steps before the program to 9921 ± 1039 steps at the first survey and then fell back significantly ($P = 0.026$) to 8727 ± 1284 steps at the second survey but remained significantly higher than the baseline figure ($P < 0.001$).

Conclusion.—The program had immediate effectiveness and was sustainable for a small proportion of participants, but effectiveness was limited by problems with long-term motivation and compliance/adherence (Fig 3).

► It has often been argued that the enormous expense associated with the hosting of the Olympic and Commonwealth Games is warranted because this incites a substantial increase in the physical activity of the general population. However, there is a dearth of published evidence to support such claims. Moreover, most of the available studies of compliance with home or work-site exercise programs have been based on individuals who themselves had decided that they wished to become more active, and (unlike the "real" world) the subjects

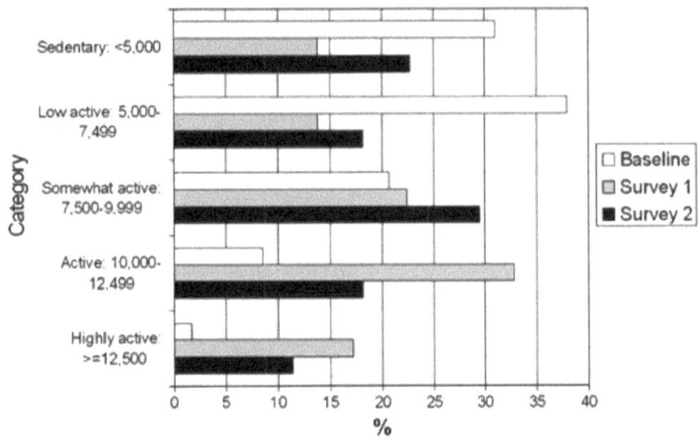

FIGURE 3.—Activity categories. (Reprinted from Harvey JT, Eime RM, Payne WR. Effectiveness of the 2006 commonwealth games 10,000 steps walking challenge. *Med Sci Sports Exerc.* 2009;41: 1673-1680, with permission from the American College of Sports Medicine.)

concerned have had access to specialized resources of personnel and facilities.[1] The trial reported in this article began with the services of an experienced marketing company, extensive newspaper publicity, and the boost associated with the hosting of the 2006 Commonwealth Games; there were also prizes for compliance in the initial 12 days of the challenge, and there was finally the continuing practical stimulus of using a pedometer to log the number of steps taken. Registration was at a booth in the Commonwealth Games precinct, further biassing data in terms of an interested sample; despite the large numbers attending the Commonwealth Games, only 1836 subjects registered for the challenge. Given all the favorable features of the intervention, the overall response rate and compliance must be very discouraging to all who are hoping to embark on the mass promotion of physical activity; less than a half of the initial registrants even began the trial, and less than 16% were still recording data 1 month later. Even in the best 5% of participants, a mere 53 individuals, the daily step count never reached the desired value of 10 000 steps/day, and activity was waning at the time of the second survey (after 9 months). Nevertheless, at the 9-month mark, some 27% of continuing participants claimed to be walking nearly every day, and many of this group had not been doing so before the intervention (Table 3 in the original article). Although not meeting the intended 10 000 steps/day target, their volume of physical activity was likely sufficient to have some health benefit. Several practical lessons can be drawn from this study. Firstly, any motivational effect of a massive sports event is very small. Secondly, social marketing does not seem a very effective means of promoting physical activity; success may be greater with one on one advice from a physician or exercise scientist. Finally, there is a need to test whether mass campaigns could be made more effective if the power of electronic technology was exploited to provide periodic reinforcement of the desired physical activity.

R. J. Shephard, MD (Lond), PhD, DPE

Reference

1. Glasgow R, Lichtenstein E, Marcus A. Why don't we see more translation of health promotion research to practice? Rethinking the efficacy-to-effectiveness transition. *Am J Public Health*. 2003;93:1261-1267.

Congestion Road Tax and Physical Activity

Bergman P, Grjibovski AM, Hagströmer M, et al (Karolinska Inst, Huddinge, Sweden; Univ of Tromsø, Norway)
Am J Prev Med 38:171-177, 2010

Background.—Large-scale policy and environmental changes, such as congestion road taxes, may be a way to promote active transportation.

Purpose.—This study aimed to examine the potential effect of a congestion road tax on physical activity.

Methods.—Baseline data were collected during October-November 2003, follow-up data in May 2006, and analysis was performed in September 2008. The short self-administered version of the International Physical Activity Questionnaire was used to assess physical activity. Data from those with access to motorized vehicles in the Stockholm region ($n = 165$), where the tax was in place, were compared with those from the Göteborg/Malmö regions ($n = 138$). Within each region before and during the road tax implementation, the data were analyzed for differences in time spent at different intensity levels of physical activity, in addition to sitting, as well as for changes in reported time in overall (weighted) physical activity.

Results.—There were no significant differences in the magnitude of the changes of the intensity levels of physical activity, weighted overall physical activity, or sitting, between Stockholm and Göteborg/Malmö. Among those exposed to the congestion road tax and with access to motorized vehicles, an increase in moderate physical activity ($p = 0.036$); overall physical activity ($p = 0.015$); and a reduction in time spent sitting ($p = 0.009$) was observed. No differences were observed among those unexposed.

Conclusions.—The results from this study on the influence of a congestion road tax on levels of physical activity, though inconclusive, suggest that policy changes such as a congestion road tax might promote improvements in physical activity levels in individuals with motorized vehicles (Fig 3).

► This is a rather nice set of observations examining the possibility of an increase in physical activity from legislative action designed to control urban pollution and vehicle congestion. The hope is that the introduction of a congestion tax will increase some combination of public and active transportation, and some studies have suggested that active transportation can make a positive contribution to an individual's health.[1,2] The tax studied in this report was quite modest, equivalent to United States $1.5 to 2.5, increasing during rush

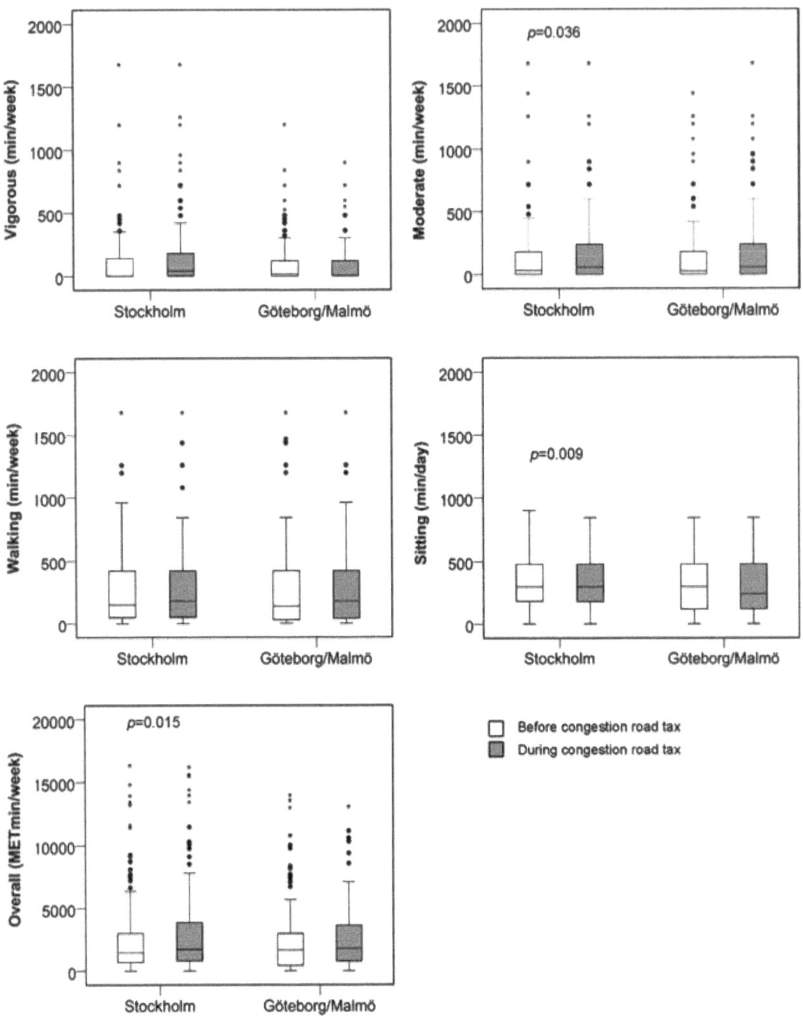

FIGURE 3.—Box-plots showing the physical activity from baseline to follow-up in Stockholm and Göteborg/Malmö. Filled circles indicate an outlier (1.5–3 times the interquartile range) and asterisks an extreme value (>3 times the interquartile range). (Reprinted from Bergman P, Grjibovski AM, Hagströmer M, et al. Congestion road tax and physical activity. *Am J Prev Med.* 2010;38:171-177.)

hours. It was applied to all vehicles entering Stockholm for a trial period during 2006. Traffic into Göteborg/Malmö, Sweden's second and third cities, was not regulated in this way, and the citizens from these regions thus provided a source of control data. Physical activity was assessed by a short international physical activity questionnaire. Traffic into Stockholm was reduced by some 25% during the trial, there was no increase of car-pooling or working at home, and the use of public transportation increased by only 6%, suggesting that there had been some increase in active transportation among the residents of the Stockholm area. However, the changes shown by the physical activity questionnaire were not particularly impressive (Fig 3). Moreover, these changes were seen in both Stockholm and the control cities, suggesting that seasonal factors may have been an issue. If opportunity arises, it would be interesting to carry out a similar trial, but with objective electronic monitoring of daily activity patterns over an entire year.

R. J. Shephard, MD (Lond), PhD, DPE

References

1. Andersen LB, Schnohr P, Schroll M, Hopkins LN. All-causemortality associated with physical activity during leisure time, work, sports, and cycling to work. *Arch Intern Med.* 2000;160:1621-1628.
2. Besser LM, Dannenberg AL. Walking to public transit:steps to help meet physical activity recommendations. *Am J Prev Med.* 2005;29:273-280.

A 5-yr Change in Norwegian 9-yr-Olds' Objectively Assessed Physical Activity Level

Kolle E, Steene-Johannessen J, Klasson-Heggebø L, et al (Norwegian School of Sport Sciences, Oslo, Norway)
Med Sci Sports Exerc 41:1368-1373, 2009

Purpose.—To describe changes in objectively assessed physical activity by socioeconomic status (SES) between 1999–2000 and 2005 in 9-yr-old children living in Oslo, Norway.

Methods.—Two cross-sectional studies were conducted in 1999–2000 and 2005. The participation rate was 70.9% in 1999–2000 and 91.4% in 2005. Participants were identified by SES based on whether the school they attended was in an area designated as high, middle, or low mean income. Physical activity was assessed objectively by accelerometers. A total of 718 children (1999–2000, $n = 340$; 2005, $n = 378$) provided valid physical activity assessments that met all inclusion criteria. General linear models were used to assess the changes in physical activity between 1999–2000 and 2005.

Results.—A significant increase in mean physical activity level and physical activity during weekends was observed between the two study periods ($P = 0.02$ and <0.001, respectively), with the patterns being similar for girls and boys. Interactions were found between change in physical activity and SES. Although the mean physical activity level and moderate-to-vigorous physical activity (MVPA) among children from low-SES groups showed no change over time, an increase was seen among children from middle-SES groups. Moreover, in high-SES groups, an increase was observed for mean physical activity level (girls only) between study periods, whereas no change was seen for MVPA participation.

Conclusions.—Nine-year-old children living in Oslo, Norway, have increased both their mean and weekend physical activity level between 1999–2000 and 2005. However, because these opportunities are not equal across SES groups, interventions are required to focus on the needs of children from low-SES groups.

▶ This study reminds us that identification of high-risk groups for sedentary behavior is important when designing strategies for improving physical activity in youth. In this case, changes in activity over time were related to socioeconomic status (SES) with improvements observed in high- but not low-SES groups. Importantly, these investigators used objective measures of activity (accelerometers) rather than relying on diary or questionnaire methods, which has been a weakness in similar studies in the past. It is interesting in this study that similar patterns were observed for males and females because other reports have indicated that girls rather than boys may be at greater risk for developing poor activity habits over time. Also, unexpected in this study is the finding that activity levels of both males and females increased as these youth passed into the teenage years. Other studies have indicated that this is a particularly common time for habits of physical activity in young people to decrease rather than increase. Perhaps there is something going on regarding the promotion of physical activity in children and adolescents in Norwegian culture that we should learn more about.

T. Rowland, MD

The Role of Free-Living Daily Walking in Human Weight Gain and Obesity

Levine JA, McCrady SK, Lanningham-Foster LM, et al (Mayo Clinic, Rochester, MN)

Diabetes 57:548-554, 2008

Objective.—Diminished daily physical activity explains, in part, why obesity and diabetes have become worldwide epidemics. In particular, chair use has replaced ambulation, so that obese individuals tend to sit for ~2.5 h/day more than lean counterparts. Here, we address the hypotheses that free-living daily walking distance is decreased in obesity compared with lean subjects and that experimental weight gain precipitates decreased daily walking.

Research Design and Methods.—During weight-maintenance feeding, we measured free-living walking using a validated system that captures locomotion and body movement for 10 days in 22 healthy lean and obese sedentary individuals. These measurements were then repeated after the lean and obese subjects were overfed by 1,000 kcal/day for 8 weeks.

Results.—We found that free-living walking comprises many (~47) short-duration (<15 min), low-velocity (~1 mph) walking bouts. Lean subjects walked 3.5 miles/day more than obese subjects ($n = 10$, 10,3 ± 2.5 vs. $n = 12$, 6.7 ± 1,8 miles/day; $P = 0.0009$). With overfeeding, walking distance decreased by 1.5 miles/day compared with baseline values (−1.5 ± 1.7 miles/day; $P = 0.0005$). The decrease in walking

TABLE 2.—Free-living walking characteristics for obese ($n = 12$) and lean ($n = 10$) subjects and the total group ($n = 22$)

	Walking Bouts (*n*/day)	Time Engaged in Walking (Minutes/Day)	Average Distance of a Walking Bout (Miles)	Free-Living Walking Velocity (mph)
Baseline				
Lean	46 ± 8	448 ± 111	0.22 ± 0.04	1.19 ± 0.21
Obese	47 ± 5	339 ± 74*	0.14 ± 0.04†	1.10 ± 0.20
Total	47 ± 6	389 ± 106	0.18 ± 0.06	1.14 ± 0.20
Overfed				
Lean	48 ± 11	459 ± 119	0.19 ± 0.06‡	1.09 ± 0.28
Obese	47 ± 9	334 ± 79*	0.11 ± 0.03§¶	0.96 ± 0.15‖
Total	47 ± 10	391 ± 116	0.15 ± 0.06**	1.02 ± 0.20**
Change with overfeeding				
Lean	1.6 ± 5	11 ± 43	−0.03 ± 0.04	−0.10 ± 0.14
Obese	−0.3 ± 7	−5 ± 51	−0.03 ± 0.05	−0.14 ± 0.15
Total	0.6 ± 6	2 ± 47	−0.03 ± 0.04	−0.12 ± 0.14

Data are means ± SD. Data were gathered every 0.5 s for 10 days continuously during weight-maintenance feeding and after 8 weeks of overfeeding by 1,000 kcal/day using validated posture and motion sensors worn under clothing (7). Statistical differences are indicated: obese subjects compared with lean.

*$P = 0.01$.

†$P = 0.002$.

§$P = 0.001$; overfed compared with baseline.

‡$P = 0.05$.

¶$P = 0.005$.

‖$P = 0.01$.

**$P < 0.001$.

that accompanied overfeeding occurred to a similar degree in the lean (−1.4 ± 1.9 miles/day; $P = 0.04$) and obese (−1.6 ± 1.7 miles/day; $P = 0.008$) subjects.

Conclusions.—Walking is decreased in obesity and declines with weight gain. This may represent a continuum whereby progressive increases in weight are associated with progressive decreases in walking distance. By identifying walking as pivotal in weight gain and obesity, we hope to add credence to an argument for an ambulatory future (Table 2).

▶ Although many nutritionists have pointed to changes in our diet that have contributed to the current epidemic of obesity, it is likely that a more important factor has been a progressive decrease in the habitual physical activity of the general population,[1,2] caused by both automation at work and in the home, and increased concentration of the population in high-rise towers that do not encourage any incidental physical activity. Some of the physical activity that distinguishes the lean from the obese is deliberate walking for health, but much comprises very short bursts of walking. This article confirms an earlier report that lean people are out of their chairs for a much longer part of the day than those who are obese; they thus accumulate an extra 5.6 km of walking per day, or perhaps 90 minutes of mostly casual activity. The method of determining these differences in physical activity (twin tri-axial accelerometers) was relatively precise, although obesity was judged simply on the body mass index, and the sample size was relatively small. During this casual physical activity the rate of metabolism is at least doubled so that there is a potential to burn at least an extra 600 kJ of energy per day, equivalent to some 20 g of fat; repeated throughout the year, with the same food intake as an obese person this could lead to a 6 kg loss of body fat in a lean subject. The other interesting aspect of this study is that when a substantial increase of food intake (4 MJ/day of excess food) was provided, this reduced the incidental activity in both lean and obese individuals (Table 2). The practical lesson seems that it is important to encourage patients to get out of their chairs in addition to fostering their participation in deliberate sustained bouts of such activities as walking to work in order to reduce the prevalence of obesity.

R. J. Shephard, MD (Lond), PhD, DPE

References

1. Prentice AM, Jebb SA. Obesity in Britain: gluttony or sloth? *Br Med J*. 1995;311: 437-439.
2. Hill JO, Wyatt HR, Reed GW, Peters JC. Obesity and the environment: where do we go from here? *Science*. 2003;299:853-855.

Physiological Demands of the Firefighter Candidate Physical Ability Test

Williams-Bell FM, Villar R, Sharratt MT, et al (Univ of Waterloo, Ontario, Canada)

Med Sci Sports Exerc 41:653-662, 2009

Purpose.—The Candidate Physical Ability Test (CPAT) is used by fire departments across North America to screen for minimal physical capabilities in potential candidates, but its physiological demands are unknown.

Methods and Results.—We examined oxygen uptake and carbon dioxide output ($\dot{V}O_2$, $\dot{V}CO_2$) and heart rate (HR) responses with the portable system in 57 subjects (23 females) who were familiarized before completing the CPAT in times similar to those of actual candidates. Two men and nine women failed to complete the circuit because of fatigue. Thirty-two men (91%) and four women (15%) completed the circuit under the criterion time (10 min 20 s) with mean completion times for men (8 min 32 s ± 51 s) and women (11 min 16 s ± 1 min 28 s, $P < 0.05$). For all finishers, $\dot{V}O_2$ during the test was 38.5 and 36.6 $mL \cdot kg^{-1} \cdot min^{-1}$, corresponding to 73% and 71% of $\dot{V}O_{2max}$ for men and women, and HR was 90% and 91% of maximum ($P > 0.05$). RER averaged 1.02 for men and 0.97 for women suggesting elevated anaerobic metabolism. Women had a drop in RER after the second event, and they were significantly slower at each event after the step mill than the men. Prediction of circuit completion time by backward stepwise regression yielded models with absolute $\dot{V}O_{2max}$ alone or relative $\dot{V}O_{2max}$ plus body mass and handgrip strength accounting for more than 67% of the variance but with large errors of estimation exceeding 75 s.

TABLE 2.—Group Means for Predicted 1-RM Muscular Strength Measurements (Handgrip, Bench Press, Shoulder Press, Biceps Curls, and Leg Press), Muscular Endurance to Fatigue (Bench Press and Leg Press), and Wingate Performance for those who Completed Irrespective of Time (a) and those who did not Complete (b) the CPAT.

	Predicted 1-RM					Muscular Endurance		Wingate Test	
	Handgrip (kg)	Bench Press (kg)	Shoulder Press (kg)	Biceps Curls (kg)	Leg Press (kg)	Leg Press (reps)	Bench Press (reps)	Peak Power (W)	Fatigue Index
(a) Completed									
Men ($n = 32$)	56.2 ± 8.1*	82.7 ± 23.0*	51.7 ± 15.9*	36.8 ± 7.2*	340.9 ± 89.1*	41.7 ± 29.2*	35.1 ± 14.0*	633.8 ± 160.5*	43.9 ± 11.8
Women ($n = 14$)	34.5 ± 3.6	42.5 ± 10.2	26.7 ± 4.2	20.2 ± 3.4	204.1 ± 70.2	20.1 ± 15.9	13.2 ± 9.5	412.9 ± 92.9	41.1 ± 9.1
(b) Did not complete									
Men ($n = 2$)	44.4 ± 19.2	44.6 ± 25.7	30.0 ± 7.1	27.1 ± 7.4	245.5 ± 38.6	17.5 ± 9.2	14.0 ± 4.2	413.1 ± 184.8	41.0 ± 4.9
Women ($n = 9$)	30.9 ± 4.1†	34.5 ± 6.6†	21.0 ± 4.7†	17.9 ± 2.9	129.8 ± 24.8†	4.9 ± 7.2†	6.2 ± 5.0	323.7 ± 76.6†	47.5 ± 7.9

*Significant difference between men and women who "completed" ($P < 0.05$).
†Significant difference between women who "completed" and "did not complete" ($P < 0.05$).

Conclusion.—The CPAT challenged both the aerobic and anaerobic energy supply systems, and the average $\dot{V}O_2$ and HR were similar to reported values during firefighting simulations with incumbent firefighters (Table 2).

▶ Many countries now have legislation requiring equal opportunity of employment for women and the elderly; however, in physically demanding occupations such as police and firefighters, candidates must generally meet some objective criterion of fitness – a "bonafide occupational requirement"; this must be a figure that can be defended before an equal employment opportunity tribunal. In the case of firefighters the test choice has usually been that of the "content" approach (evaluating performance on a circuit comprising likely elements in firefighting)[1-3] rather than a "construct" approach (looking at individual components of fitness such as the maximal oxygen intake). There has been much discussion of the necessary maximal oxygen intake, with different authors proposing lower limits that have ranged from 33.5 mL/kg·min to 4 L/min (50 mL/kg·min in an 80 kg man). The present data show that those unable to complete the most commonly accepted field test for firefighters not only have a low maximal oxygen intake, but also poor scores on tests of muscular strength, muscular endurance, and anaerobic power (Table 2), all typical requirements of firefighting. The oxygen consumption during the test was 38.5 mL/kg·min in men and 36.7 mL/kg·min in women, suggesting that some investigators may have underestimated the aerobic demands of firefighting. The weakness in all of this objective assessment is that unions usually resist the annual testing of older individuals who have already been hired as firefighters. Probably some workers manage to retain their job by moving more slowly and sharing heavy work with a colleague, although this probably reduces their efficacy as firefighters.

R. J. Shephard, MD (Lond), PhD, DPE

References

1. Davis PO, Dotson CO, Santa Maria DL. Relationship between simulated fire fighting tasks and physical performance measures. *Med Sci Sports Exerc.* 1982; 14:65-71.
2. Gledhill N, Jamnik VK. Development and validation of a fitness screening protocol for fighter applicants. *Can J Sport Sci.* 1992;17:199-206.
3. International Association of Fire Chiefs (IAFC). The IAFF/IAFC fire service joint labor management candidate physical ability test program summary, http://www.iaff.org/safe/content/wellness/peer.htm. Accessed August 29 2009.

Physical Activity and Health Outcomes Three Months After Completing a Physical Activity Behavior Change Intervention: Persistent and Delayed Effects

Rogers LQ, Hopkins-Price P, Vicari S, et al (SIU School of Medicine, Springfield, IL)

Cancer Epidemiol Biomarkers Prev 18:1410-1418, 2009

Purpose.—We previously reported the effectiveness of a 12-week physical activity behavior change intervention for breast cancer survivors postintervention with this report, aiming to determine delayed and/or persistent effects 3 months after intervention completion.

Methods.—Forty-one sedentary women with stage I, II, or IIIA breast cancer currently receiving hormonal therapy were randomly assigned to receive the 12-week Better Exercise Adherence after Treatment for Cancer intervention or usual care. Assessments occurred at baseline, postintervention, and 3 months postintervention.

Results.—Weekly minutes of greater than or equal to moderate intensity physical activity measured by accelerometer showed a significant group by time interaction ($F = 3.51$; $P = 0.035$; between group difference in the mean change from baseline to 3 months postintervention, 100.1 minute, $P = 0.012$). Significant group by time interactions also showed sustained improvements from baseline to 3 months postintervention in strength ($F = 3.82$; $P = 0.027$; between group difference, 11.2 kg; $P = 0.026$), waist-to-hip ratio ($F = 3.36$; $P = 0.041$; between group difference, −0.04; $P = 0.094$), and social well-being ($F = 4.22$; $P = 0.023$; between group difference, 3.9; $P = 0.039$). A delayed reduction in lower extremity dysfunction 3 months postintervention was noted ($F = 3.24$; $P = 0.045$; between group difference in the mean change from postintervention to

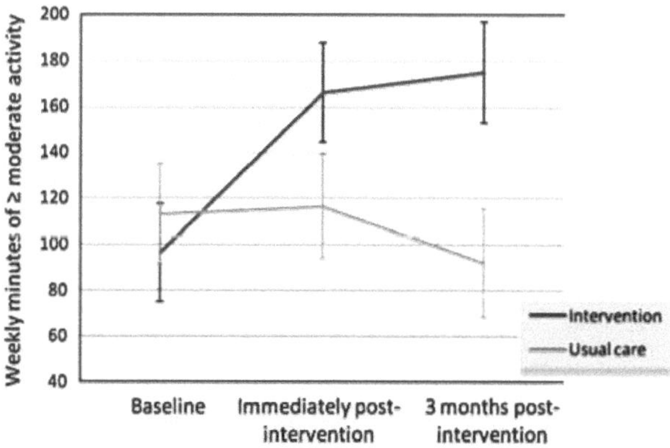

FIGURE 1.—The effects of the BEAT Cancer physical activity behavior change intervention on back/leg extensor muscle strength immediately postintervention and 3 months postintervention (least square means ± SE). (Reprinted from Rogers LQ, Hopkins-Price P, Vicari S, et al. Physical activity and health outcomes three months after completing a physical activity behavior change intervention: persistent and delayed effects. *Cancer Epidemiol Biomarkers Prev.* 2009;18:1410-1418.)

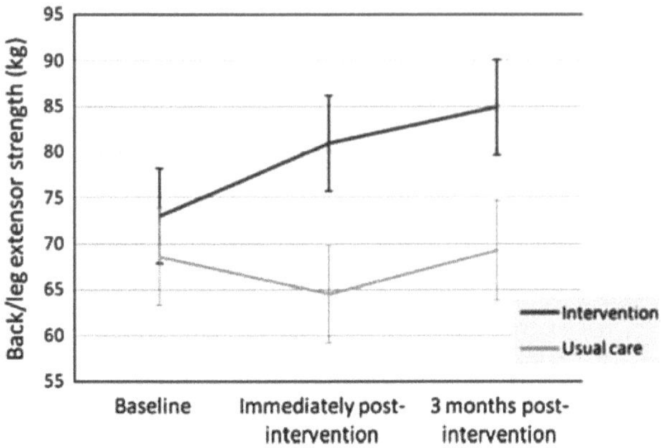

FIGURE 2.—The effects of the BEAT Cancer physical activity behavior change intervention on weekly minutes of moderate plus vigorous physical activity immediately postintervention and 3 mo postintervention (least square means ± SE). Physical activity assessed with accelerometer. (Reprinted from Rogers LQ, Hopkins-Price P, Vicari S, et al. Physical activity and health outcomes three months after completing a physical activity behavior change intervention: persistent and delayed effects. *Cancer Epidemiol Biomarkers Prev.* 2009;18:1410-1418.)

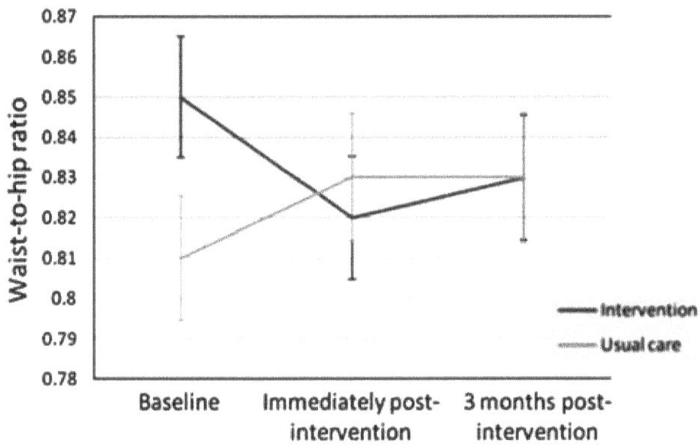

FIGURE 3.—The effects of the BEAT Cancer physical activity behavior change intervention on waist-to-hip ratio immediately postintervention and 3 mo postintervention (least square means ± SE). (Reprinted from Rogers LQ, Hopkins-Price P, Vicari S, et al. Physical activity and health outcomes three months after completing a physical activity behavior change intervention: persistent and delayed effects. *Cancer Epidemiol Biomarkers Prev.* 2009;18:1410-1418.)

3 months follow-up; $P = -7.6$; $P = 0.015$). No group by time effect was noted for fitness, body mass index, percent fat, bone density, total quality of life (Functional Assessment of Cancer Therapy-General), fatigue, endocrine symptoms, cognitive function, or sleep.

Conclusions.—The intervention resulted in sustained improvements in physical activity, strength, central adiposity, and social well-being with

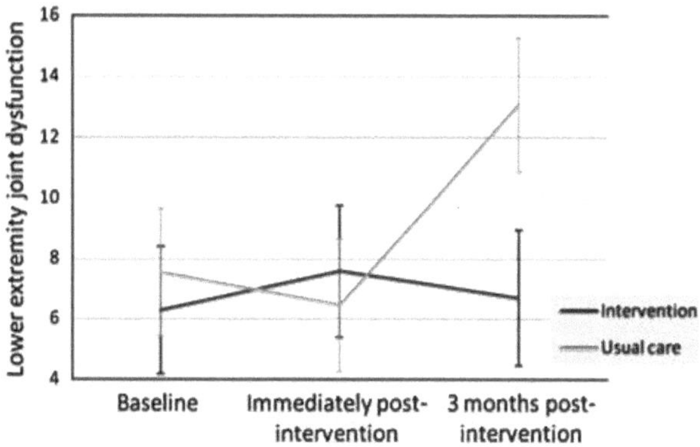

FIGURE 4.—The effects of the BEAT Cancer physical activity behavior change intervention on lower extremity joint dysfunction immediately postintervention and 3 mo postintervention (least square means ± SE). (Reprinted from Rogers LQ, Hopkins-Price P, Vicari S, et al. Physical activity and health outcomes three months after completing a physical activity behavior change intervention: persistent and delayed effects. *Cancer Epidemiol Biomarkers Prev.* 2009;18:1410-1418.)

lower extremity function benefits appearing 3 months after intervention completion. Testing translation in a multisite study is warranted (Figs 1-4).

▶ This study provides evidence that women with breast cancer experience sustained improvements in physical activity and function 3 months after completion of an exercise intervention. Women with stages I to IIIa breast cancer treated with antihormone therapies were enrolled in a randomized controlled study of a 12-week exercise and lifestyle intervention.[1] This intervention successfully improved objective measures of moderate intensity, physical activity (via accelerometer counts), muscle strength, and waist-to-hip ratio in exercisers compared with controls. These changes were sustained over an additional 3 months of follow-up without any further contact with the study team (Figs 1-3). Perhaps the most interesting finding was that lower extremity function exhibited a delayed improvement in the exercisers (Fig 4). Joint pain and total Western Ontario and McMaster Universities Osteoarthritis (WOMAC) Index also improved during follow-up in the exercisers compared with controls. Arthralgia is a common side effect of antihormone therapy. It appears that although an increase in physical activity may initially exacerbate arthralgia and lower extremity function in breast cancer survivors, these effects do not become worse with maintained activity. To the contrary, joint pain and leg function may become worse if women remain physically inactive following breast cancer treatment.

C. M. Jankowski, PhD

Reference

1. Rogers LQ, Hopkins-Price P, Vicari S, et al. A randomized trial to increase physical activity in breast cancer survivors. *Med Sci Sports Exerc.* 2009;41:935-946.

Physical Activity, Mortality, and Cardiovascular Disease: Is Domestic Physical Activity Beneficial? The Scottish Health Survey—1995, 1998, and 2003

Stamatakis E, Hamer M, Lawlor DA (Univ College London, UK; Univ of Bristol, UK)

Am J Epidemiol 169:1191-1200, 2009

Intense domestic physical activity (IDPA) is promoted by preventive health campaigns, but this recommendation is not supported by evidence. The authors used data from the 1995, 1998, and 2003 Scottish Health Survey samples and the associated mortality and hospital episode records to determine the independent effects of IDPA on cardiovascular disease (CVD) events and all-cause mortality. The sample comprised 13,726 (6,102 men) CVD-free respondents (≥35 years). Multivariable survival analysis assessed the relation between IDPA and the risk for CVD (fatal/nonfatal combined) or all-cause mortality. During 8.4 (standard deviation, 3.4) years of follow-up, there were 1,103 deaths (573 among men) and 890 CVD events (521 among men). Participation in IDPA was associated with lower all-cause mortality (men: relative risk = 0.68, 95% confidence interval: 0.50, 0.91; women: relative risk = 0.70, 95% confidence interval: 0.52, 0.93). In both sexes, IDPA was unrelated to the risk for CVD. Total physical activity (including IDPA) was unrelated to fatal/nonfatal CVD, but when domestic activity was excluded from the calculations there was an association (men: relative risk = 0.76, 95% confidence interval: 0.58, 0.98; women: relative risk = 0.68, 95% confidence interval: 0.50, 0.93). These results indicate that IDPA may not offer protection against CVD, but it may protect against all-cause mortality. CVD preventive efforts may need to focus on moderate-to-vigorous-intensity physical activities other than those performed in and around the household (Table 2).

▶ Population surveys of physical activity commonly include domestic physical activity as one response item on questionnaires. When interest in the energy cost of various types of physical activity was first aroused by Durnin and his colleagues in Glasfow (in the 1950s), items on an inventory might well include such things as the scrubbing of floors; in the 1950s, the scrubbing of stone tenement floors was undoubtedly quite hard work, and it is interesting that this historical activity remained one of the questions asked in the present Scottish surveys. However, labor-saving appliances have now removed most of the drudgery from housework in developed societies, probably including Scotland, and it may not be too surprising that the 1995-2003 data from Scotland showed no association between domestic activity and cardiovascular mortality in an 8.4-year follow-up. Indeed, the inclusion of domestic activity in the overall activity total seemed enough to mask associations with the remainder of an individual's physical activity. There are several caveats to the

TABLE 2.—Cox Regression Models for Physical Activity Levels and All-Cause Mortality Among Men Aged 35 or More Years, 1995, 1998, and 2003 Scottish Health Survey Samples[a]

	No. of Cases (N=499)	Total (N=5,896)	Age Adjusted Hazard Ratio	Age Adjusted 95% Confidence Interval	Model 1[b] Hazard Ratio	Model 1[b] 95% Confidence Interval	Model 2[c] Hazard Ratio	Model 2[c] 95% Confidence Interval
Domestic activity sessions (median)[d]								
None (0)	363	3,362	1.00		1.00		1.00	
Medium[e] (1.0)	53	1,219	0.47	0.35, 0.62	0.53	0.40, 0.71	0.68	0.50, 0.91
High[f] (2.5)	83	1,315	0.64	0.50, 0.81	0.71	0.56, 0.91	0.89	0.69, 1.14
P_{trend}				<0.001		<0.001		0.034
Walking activity sessions (median)[d]								
None (0)	294	3,157	1.00		1.00		1.00	
Medium[e] (2.0)	87	1,206	0.87	0.68, 1.10	0.91	0.72, 1.16	1.10	0.86, 1.14
High[f] (7.0)	118	1,533	0.79	0.64, 0.98	0.77	0.62, 0.95	0.91	0.73, 1.13
P_{trend}				0.088		0.058		0.394
Sports activity sessions (median)[d]								
None (0)	458	4,502	1.00		1.00		1.00	
Medium[e] (1.0)	19	689	0.43	0.27, 0.69	0.51	0.32, 0.80	0.69	0.42, 1.08
High[f] (2.8)	22	705	0.50	0.32, 0.76	0.53	0.34, 0.82	0.73	0.47, 1.13
P_{trend}				<0.001		<0.001		0.117
Total activity sessions (median)[d,g]								
Low (3.0)	203	1,692	1.00		1.00		1.00	
Medium (4.8)	178	2,047	0.76	0.62, 0.93	0.80	0.65, 0.97	0.97	0.79, 1.19
High (7.0)	118	2,157	0.60	0.47, 0.75	0.65	0.52, 0.82	0.92	0.72, 1.17
P_{trend}				<0.001		0.001		0.800
Total activity sessions excluding domestic (median)[d,g]								
Low (1.0)	258	2,230	1.00		1.00		1.00	
Medium (3.0)	165	1,567	0.90	0.74, 1.09	0.88	0.72, 1.07	1.03	0.85, 1.26
High (4.3)	76	2,099	0.49	0.38, 0.63	0.54	0.42, 0.70	0.76	0.58, 0.98
P_{trend}				<0.001		<0.001		0.078

[a]Excludes deaths during the first year of follow-up and cancer registrations and cardiovascular disease events prior to the baseline measurement.
[b]Model 1 includes additional adjustment for social economic group and marital status.
[c]Model 2 incorporates model 1 with additional adjustment for body mass index category, longstanding illness, self-rated health, family disease history, smoking, and other types of physical activities.
[d]The values in parentheses correspond to the median number of sessions per category.
[e]The medium category is defined as below the sex-specific median.
[f]The high category is defined as above the sex-specific median.
[g]The categories for total physical activity correspond to sex-specific tertiles.

author's conclusions. The sample excluded all those who reported hospital admissions for cardiovascular disease from 1981 to study entry, so it is unlikely that the analysis was complicated because some of the population with cardiac disease had subsequently avoided exercise. However, the age ranges of the samples were 35 to 64 in the 1995 survey, 35 to 74 in 1998, and 35+ in 2003; this is important, because a domestic activity demanding 3 metabolic equivalents of energy expenditure is a mere bagatelle for a 35-year-old, but it can represent a substantial fraction of maximal aerobic power in a retiree. There were also unfortunate changes in the questionnaire format between the 3 surveys, necessitating some approximations of the data, and do-it-yourself activities and heavy gardening were lumped in with housework. Perhaps most importantly, involvement in domestic work was rated simply on the number of occasions performed per week rather than on any more sophisticated appraisal of the volume and intensity of activity. Finally, although no association was found between this weak measure and cardiovascular mortality, it did have a significant influence on all-cause mortality (Table 2), perhaps by influencing the accumulation of body fat.

R. J. Shephard, MD (Lond), PhD, DPE

Total mortality after changes in leisure time physical activity in 50 year old men: 35 year follow-up of population based cohort

Byberg L, Melhus H, Gedeborg R, et al (Uppsala Univ, Sweden; et al)

Br J Sports Med 43:482, 2009

Objective.—To examine how change in level of physical activity after middle age influences mortality and to compare it with the effect of smoking cessation.

Design.—Population based cohort study with follow-up over 35 years.

Setting.—Municipality of Uppsala, Sweden.

Participants.—2205 men aged 50 in 1970-3 who were reexamined at ages 60, 70, 77, and 82 years.

Main Outcome Measure.—Total (all cause) mortality.

Results.—The absolute mortality rate was 27.1, 23.6, and 18.4 per 1000 person years in the groups with low, medium, and high physical activity, respectively. The relative rate reduction attributable to high physical activity was 32% for low and 22% for medium physical activity. Men who increased their physical activity level between the ages of 50 and 60 continued to have a higher mortality rate during the first five years of follow-up (adjusted hazard ratio 2.64, 95% confidence interval 1.32 to 5.27, compared with unchanged high physical activity). After 10 years of follow-up their increased physical activity was associated with reduced mortality to the level of men with unchanged high physical activity (1.10, 0.87 to 1.38). The reduction in mortality associated with increased physical activity (0.51, 0.26 to 0.97, compared with unchanged low physical activity) was similar to that associated with smoking cessation (0.64, 0.53 to 0.78, compared with continued smoking).

Conclusions.—Increased physical activity in middle age is eventually followed by a reduction in mortality to the same level as seen among men with constantly high physical activity. This reduction is comparable with that associated with smoking cessation (Fig 2).

▶ Many of the studies lauding physical activity have been based simply on cross-sectional comparisons between active and inactive groups. This study is particularly welcome because it looks at the response to a change in behavior initiated at a relatively late age (50 years), and is based on an entire community

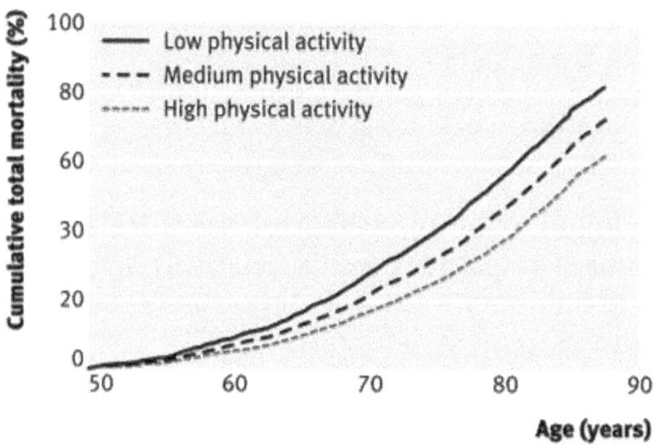

Age	50	60	70	77	82	End of study
Men at risk	2205	1904	1406	1123	933	876

FIGURE 2.—Cumulative mortality from age 50 (Cox regression) according to leisure time physical activity level and total mortality. At end of follow-up, estimated proportions of deaths were 81.4 (95% confidence interval 80.8 to 82.0) for low physical activity, 72.0 (71.5 to 72.5) for medium, and 61.8 (61.4 to 62.2) for high. (Reprinted from Byberg L, Melhus H, Gedeborg R, et al. Total mortality after changes in leisure time physical activity in 50 year old men: 35 year follow-up of population based cohort. *Br J Sports Med.* 2009;43:482, with permission from the BMJ Publishing Group.)

(the men of Uppsala of an appropriate age) rather than high-risk volunteers. It also has complete information on mortality. About 11% of men increased their reported physical activity over the survey, but a challenging 38% said that they had reduced their activity. The study offers a very long follow-up, allowing the authors to determine how long after beginning exercise benefit first appears; in this age group the lag period was 5 years. Ultimately (after 10 years), subjects who became vigorously active reached the same life expectancy as those who had been consistently active from a young age. The data show no evidence that physical activity became disadvantageous even in the ninth decade of life (Fig 2). The type of physical activity conferring substantial benefit was active recreation or heavy gardening for more than 3 hours per week, or hard training, or competitive sport. Interestingly, benefits were on a par with what would have been achieved by quitting smoking at this age. The absence of benefit in the first 5 years is an important pointer to the fact that those who adopted a high level of physical activity were not a "health conscious" group with other favorable health behaviors.

R. J. Shephard, MD (Lond), PhD, DPE

Impact of Worksite Wellness Intervention on Cardiac Risk Factors and One-Year Health Care Costs

Milani RV, Lavie CJ (Ochsner Health System, New Orleans, LA)

Am J Cardiol 104:1389-1392, 2009

Cardiac rehabilitation and exercise training (CRET) provides health risk intervention in cardiac patients over a relatively short time frame. Worksite health programs offer a unique opportunity for health intervention, but these programs remain underused due to concerns over recouping the costs. We evaluated the clinical efficacy and cost-effectiveness of a 6-month worksite health intervention using staff from CRET. Employees (n = 308) and spouses (n = 31) of a single employer were randomized to active intervention (n = 185) consisting of worksite health education, nutritional counseling, smoking cessation counseling, physical activity promotion, selected physician referral, and other health counseling versus usual care (n = 154). Health risk status was assessed at baseline and after the 6-month intervention program, and total medical claim costs were obtained in all participants during the year before and the year after intervention. Significant improvements were demonstrated in quality-of-life scores (+10%, p = 0.001), behavioral symptoms (depression −33%, anxiety −32%, somatization −33%, and hostility −47%, all p values <0.001), body fat (−9%, p = 0.001), high-density lipoprotein cholesterol (+13%, p = 0.0001), diastolic blood pressure (−2%, p = 0.01), health habits (−60%, p = 0.0001), and total health risk (−25%, p = 0.0001). Of employees categorized as high risk at baseline, 57% were converted to low-risk status. Average employee annual claim costs decreased 48% (p = 0.002) for the 12 months after the intervention, whereas control employees' costs remained unchanged (−16%, p = NS), thus creating a sixfold return on investment. In conclusion, worksite health intervention using CRET staff decreased total health risk and markedly decreased medical claim costs within 12 months (Table 2).

▶ There have been many reports on the outcomes of work-site wellness programs, but relatively few have looked at the impact on medical expenses. Our own quasi-experimental study some 25 years ago showed that the introduction of an exercise-centered work-site program did lead to small reductions in both medical consultations and the use of hospital services.[1] This study (in keeping with the general direction of work-site programs) offered a comprehensive approach to health with a relatively light exercise component (referral to off-site fitness centers, with no information on attendance). The main change in health status seems to have been in the affective domain (Table 2), and although cardiac risk factors changed in the right direction, gains in these variables were relatively small. It may well be that costs have decreased for the experimental group mainly because demand for medical services has been decreased by an improvement of mood state, and necessary interventions have been provided in a more efficient manner than the usual United States medical system. A comparison between Canada and the United States shows

TABLE 2.—Change in Health Parameters in Active Participants After Worksite Health Intervention (n = 185)

Variable	Baseline	After Intervention	Change	p Value
Anxiety (U)	3.7 ± 4.2	2.5 ± 3.6	−32%	0.0001
Depression (U)	2.4 ± 3.7	1.6 ± 3.1	−33%	0.0002
Somatization (U)	5.2 ± 4.1	3.5 ± 3.3	−33%	0.0001
Hostility (U)	3.6 ± 4.0	1.9 ± 2.8	−47%	0.0001
Quality of life (U)	117 ± 12	128 ± 14	10%	0.001
CAGE (U)	0.17 ± 1.1	0.09 ± 0.08	−47%	NS
Body mass index (kg/m^2)	28.5 ± 5.7	28.3	−1%	0.08
Fat (%)	26.7	24.4	−9%	0.001
Smoker (%)	17%	15%	−12%	NS
Sedentary (%)	79%	72%	−9%	0.14
Total cholesterol (mg/dl)	190	184	−3%	NS
HDL cholesterol (mg/dl)	47	53	13%	0.0001
TC/HDL (U)	4.2	3.6	−14%	0.0001
Systolic blood pressure (mm Hg)	124	122	−2%	0.08
Diastolic blood pressure (mm Hg)	81	79	−2%	0.01
Health habits (U)	2.0	0.8	−60%	0.0001
Total health risk score (U)	7.2 ± 5.1	5.4 ± 4.0	−25%	0.0001

Abbreviations as in Table 1.

that more effective health care can be provided at a half of the cost simply by crossing the 49th parallel!

R. J. Shephard, MD (Lond), PhD, DPE

Reference

1. Shephard RJ, Corey P, Renzland P, Cox M. The influence of an industrial fitness programme upon medical care costs. *Can J Publ Health.* 1982;73:259-263.

Evidence for a Greater Elevation in Vascular Shear Stress after Morning Exercise

Jones H, Green DJ, George KP, et al (Liverpool John Moores Univ, UK)
Med Sci Sports Exerc 41:1188-1193, 2009

Introduction.—The vascular endothelium plays an important role in the maintenance of vascular health and the modulation of vascular tone and blood pressure. Recently, it has been demonstrated that blood pressure reactivity to physical activity is greater in the morning, and possibly, diurnal variation in vascular function may also be evident. The aim of this study was to assess vascular responses after exercise at different times of day.

Methods.—After 45 min of supine rest, 12 male normotensives completed a 30-min bout of cycling at 70% peak oxygen uptake beginning on separate days at 0800 and 1600 h. Edge detection and wall tracking of high-resolution arterial B-mode ultrasound images combined with synchronized Doppler waveform analysis were used to measure brachial and femoral conduit artery diameter and to calculate blood flow and shear rate. Measurements were recorded before and 20 min after exercise.

Results.—At 5 min after exercise, the mean ± SE brachial shear rate was 72 ± 21 arbitrary unit (AU) higher in the morning compared with the afternoon ($P = 0.05$), but this was not compensated for by enlargement of arterial diameter ($P = 0.59$). No diurnal variation was observed in the femoral artery measurements.

Conclusion.—Diurnal difference in conduit artery regulatory control manifests as an elevated intravascular shear stress after morning exercise. Potentially, higher postexercise shear rate in the morning in at-risk

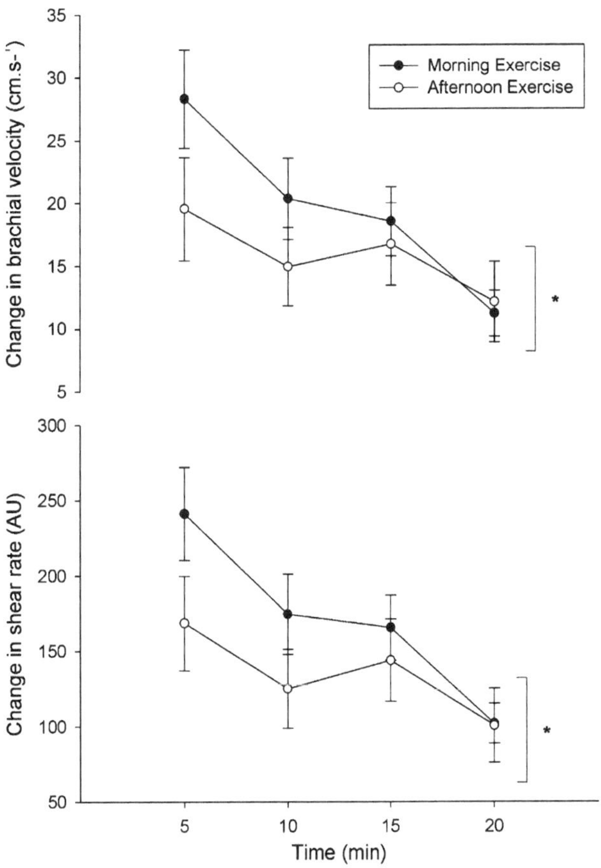

FIGURE 1.—Change from preceding baseline in mean postexercise brachial velocity (*top*) and shear rate (*bottom*) between times of day. *Significant interaction between time of day and postexercise time ($P < 0.05$). (Reprinted from Jones H, Green DJ, George KP, et al. Evidence for a greater elevation in vascular shear stress after morning exercise. *Med Sci Sports Exerc.* 2009;41:1188-1193.)

individuals could contribute to the elevated cardiovascular risk evident in the postwaking hours (Fig 1).

▶ Attempts to pin-point factors precipitating myocardial infarction have been met with little success, but there have been interesting reports that the immediate risk of infarction is greatest shortly after getting out of bed;[1-3] this has led humorists to suggest that lying in bed for most of the morning was an easy shortcut to a long life. The mechanism underlying early morning risk is as yet unclear, but suggestions include diurnal variations in blood pressure, sympathetic nerve activity, activity patterns, vascular resistance, and vascular function. Plainly, the issue is of some concern to those who take their exercise early in the morning, whether to void heat or ozone exposure. Exercise appears to induce a greater rise of blood pressure early in the morning, and it may be that endothelium-dependent vasodilatation is for some reason reduced at this time of day.[4] The present small-scale study of young, healthy, and active men used sophisticated modern techniques to compare brachial and femoral arterial diameters in the morning and the afternoon both at rest and following cycle ergometer exercise at 70% of maximal oxygen intake; the brachial (but not the femoral) artery showed evidence of narrowing in the morning (Fig 1), with a resultant increase in shear stress and the risk of rupturing atherosclerotic plaques. It was argued that in the femoral circulation, any such diurnal effect was masked by the local metabolic demands of exercise. Further evaluation of these findings could usefully focus on NO generation and responses after administration of sympatholytic drugs. It will also be necessary to assess the magnitude of effects in an older population that is more prone to coronary disease.

R. J. Shephard, MD (Lond), PhD, DPE

References

1. Kario K, Pickering TG, Umeda Y, et al. Morning surge in BP as a predictor of silent and clinical cerebrovascular disease in elderly hypertensives: a prospective study. *Circulation.* 2003;107:1401-1406.
2. Muller JE. Circadian variation in cardiovascular events. *Am J Hypertens.* 1999;12: 35S-42S.
3. Willich SN, Linderer T, Wegscheider K, Leizorovicz A, Alamercery I, Schröder R. Increased morning incidence of myocardial infarction in the ISAM Study: absence with prior beta-adrenergic blockade. ISAM Study Group. *Circulation.* 1989;80: 853-858.
4. Otto ME, Svatikova A, de Mattos Barretto RB, et al. Early morning attenuation of endothelial function in healthy humans. *Circulation.* 2004;109:2507-2510.

Sitting Time and Mortality from All Causes, Cardiovascular Disease, and Cancer

Katzmarzyk PT, Church TS, Craig CL, et al (Pennington Biomedical Res Ctr, Baton Rouge, LA; Canadian Fitness and Lifestyle Res Inst, Ontario, Canada)

Med Sci Sports Exerc 41:998-1005, 2009

Purpose.—Although moderate-to-vigorous physical activity is related to premature mortality, the relationship between sedentary behaviors and mortality has not been fully explored and may represent a different paradigm than that associated with lack of exercise. We prospectively examined sitting time and mortality in a representative sample of 17,013 Canadians 18–90 yr of age.

Methods.—Evaluation of daily sitting time (almost none of the time, one fourth of the time, half of the time, three fourths of the time, almost all of the time), leisure time physical activity, smoking status, and alcohol consumption was conducted at baseline. Participants were followed prospectively for an average of 12.0 yr for the ascertainment of mortality status.

Results.—There were 1832 deaths (759 of cardiovascular disease (CVD) and 547 of cancer) during 204,732 person-yr of follow-up. After adjustment for potential confounders, there was a progressively higher risk of mortality across higher levels of sitting time from all causes (hazard ratios (HR): 1.00, 1.00, 1.11, 1.36, 1.54; P for trend <0.0001) and CVD (HR: 1.00, 1.01, 1.22, 1.47, 1.54; P for trend <0.0001) but not cancer. Similar results were obtained when stratified by sex, age, smoking status, and body mass index. Age-adjusted all-cause mortality rates per 10,000 person-yr of follow-up were 87, 86, 105, 130, and 161 (P for trend <0.0001) in physically inactive participants and 75, 69, 76, 98, 105 (P for trend $= 0.008$) in active participants across sitting time categories.

Conclusions.—These data demonstrate a dose–response association between sitting time and mortality from all causes and CVD, independent of leisure time physical activity. In addition to the promotion of moderate-to-vigorous physical activity and a healthy weight, physicians should discourage sitting for extended periods.

▶ Our modern lifestyle has been castigated for the progressive elimination of deliberate physical activity, ranging from compulsory physical education classes to opportunities for walking or cycling to school or work. However, a second major change over the last 20 years has been the growing sedentary of the population, as people spend ever longer hours watching television, working on their computers, or playing video games. Some authors have recently suggested that the current poor health of developed nations may reflect sedentary as much as a reduction in physical activity.[1-4] This article is based on a large and representative prospective study of the Canadian population, and it demonstrates a progressive increase in overall mortality most marked in those who spend 3 quarters to almost all of their time sitting (Fig 1); moreover, this risk appears to be an independent variable, exerting its effects after allowance for reported

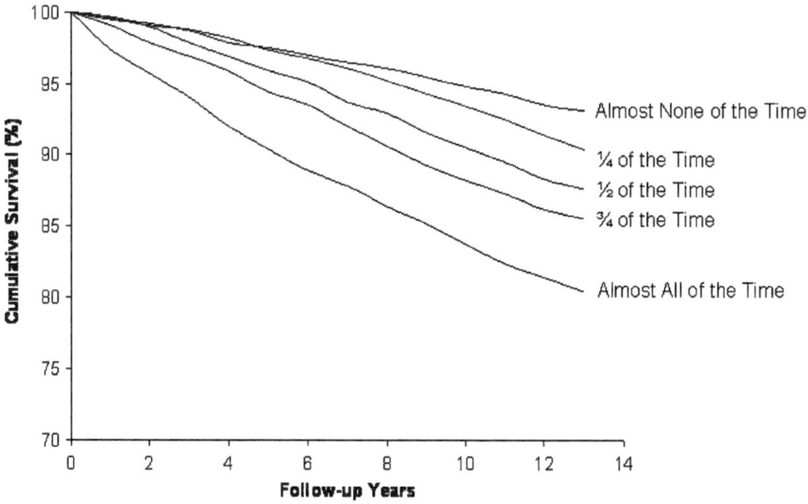

FIGURE 1.—Kaplan–Meier survival curve for all-cause mortality across categories of daily sitting time in 17,013 men and women 18–90 yr of age, in the Canada Fitness Survey, 1981–1993. Log-rank $\chi^2 = 174.4$, $df = 4$, $P < 0.0001$. The sample sizes across the categories were 3022 (17.8%), 6652 (39.1%), 4379 (25.7%), 2138 (12.6%), and 822 (4.8%), for the categories of almost none of the time, one fourth of the time, half of the time, three fourths of the time, and almost all of the time, respectively. (Reprinted from Katzmarzyk PT, Church TS, Craig CL, et al. Sitting time and mortality from all causes, cardiovascular disease, and cancer. *Med Sci Sports Exerc.* 2009;41:998-1005.)

leisure activity. One weakness in the study is that it was not possible to make a very thorough allowance for ill health on entry to the trial. Nevertheless, the issue is important, because a high proportion of the North American population have a sedentary profile that puts them in a high-risk category,[5] and further observations on this topic are urgently needed. It seems likely that policy guidelines for our populations should set maximum screen viewing times and minima of deliberate physical activity.

R. J. Shephard, MD (Lond), PhD, DPE

References

1. Hamilton MT, Hamilton DG, Zderic TW. Exercise physiology versus inactivity physiology: an essential concept for understanding lipoprotein lipase regulation. *Exerc Sport Sci Rev.* 2004;32:161-166.
2. Hamilton MT, Hamilton DG, Zderic TW. Role of low energy expenditure and sitting in obesity, metabolic syndrome, type 2 diabetes, and cardiovascular disease. *Diabetes.* 2007;56:2655-2667.
3. Healy GN, Wijndaele K, Dunstan DW, et al. Objectively measured sedentary time, physical activity, and metabolic risk: the Australian Diabetes, Obesity and Lifestyle Study (AusDiab). *Diabetes Care.* 2008;31:369-371.
4. Spanier PA, Marshall SJ, Faulkner GE. Tackling the obesity pandemic: a call for sedentary behaviour research. *Can J Public Health.* 2006;97:255-257.
5. Matthews CE, Chen KY, Freedson PS, et al. Amount of time spent in sedentary behaviors in the United States, 2003-2004. *Am J Epidemiol.* 2008;167:875-881.

Ability of Physical Activity to Predict Cardiovascular Disease Beyond Commonly Evaluated Cardiometabolic Risk Factors

McGuire KA, Janssen I, Ross R (Queen's Univ School of Kinesiology and Health Studies, Ontario, Canada)

Am J Cardiol 104:1522-1526, 2009

It is well-established that increasing physical activity (PA) is important for the prevention and management of cardiovascular disease (CVD). Although it has been demonstrated that PA predicts CVD independent of commonly measured cardiometabolic risk factors in women, it is unclear whether this association is true in men. The study participants consisted of 5,882 adults (age ≥18 years) from the 1999 to 2004 United States National Health and Nutrition Examination Survey. Blood pressure, triglycerides, low-density lipoprotein cholesterol, high-density lipoprotein cholesterol, glucose, and waist circumference were categorized using standard clinical thresholds. The participants were divided into the following groups according to the volume of their moderate-to-vigorous intensity PA: active (≥150 min/wk), somewhat active (30 to 149 min/wk), and inactive (<30 min/wk). Logistic regression analyses were used to calculate the odds ratios for CVD according to PA. After controlling for the basic confounders (age, gender, race, smoking), inactive participants were 52% (95% confidence interval 16% to 98%) more likely than the active participants to have CVD. Additional adjustment for cardiometabolic risk factors did not change the odds ratio for CVD in the inactive group. To further delineate the effects of PA on CVD, the participants were cross-classified according to their PA level and their number of cardiometabolic risk factors. Both PA and cardiometabolic risk factors were independent predictors of CVD (P_{trend} <0.0001). The results were not modified by gender. In conclusion, PA was associated with CVD, independent of the common cardiometabolic risk factors, in men and women. The association between PA and CVD risk was not mediated by the measured cardiometabolic risk factors (Table 2).

▶ Although the benefits of physical activity in preventing cardiovascular disease are well established, the biological basis of this advantage is less clearly understood. Regular physical activity corrects a number of important cardiovascular risk factors, but as the present substantial epidemiological trial demonstrates, benefit remains unattenuated after statistical adjustment for the influence of traditional risk factors (Table 2). The authors of the present report suggest that benefit may reflect such factors as direct influences of physical activity on the vascular wall, improved glucose transport, enhanced antioxidant function, and decreased cytokine production by adipose tissue. However, they fail to comment on one more likely candidate—the influence of regular physical activity on the individual's level of fitness—the sedentary and unfit individual must attend to any sudden emergency at a higher fraction of his or her maximal cardiovascular and/or muscular performance, with a correspondingly greater disturbance of body function in terms of the immediate rise of blood pressure

TABLE 2.—Odds Ratio (OR) for Cardiovascular Disease (CVD) According to Physical Activity (PA) Level

Covariates Included in Regression Model	PA Group Active (≥150 min/wk)	Somewhat Active (30–149 min/wk)	Inactive (<30 min/wk)
Age, gender, race, smoking	1.00	1.24 (0.92–1.68)	1.52 (1.18–1.97)†
Age, gender, race, smoking, cardiometabolic risk factors*	1.00	1.17 (0.85–1.59)	1.50 (1.15–1.95)†
Age, gender, race, smoking, cardiometabolic risk factors,* waist circumference	1.00	1.15 (0.84–1.57)	1.52 (1.16–1.98)†

Data are presented as odds ratios (95% confidence intervals).
*Cardiometabolic risk factors included blood pressure, low-density lipoprotein cholesterol, high-density lipoprotein cholesterol, triglyceride, and fasting glucose risk factor categories.
†Significantly greater than active group ($p < 0.05$).

and the secretion of catecholamines, and this in turn seems likely to enhance the risk of a cardiovascular catastrophe. Irrespective of causation, the present findings underscore the importance of a clear physical activity history when identifying those at an increased risk of cardiovascular disease.

R. J. Shephard, MD (Lond), PhD, DPE

Active Commuting and Cardiovascular Disease Risk: The CARDIA Study

Gordon-Larsen P, Boone-Heinonen J, Sidney S, et al (Univ of North Carolina at Chapel Hill; Division of Res, Kaiser Permanente, Oakland, CA; et al)
Arch Intern Med 169:1216-1223, 2009

Background.—There is little research on the association of lifestyle exercise, such as active commuting (walking or biking to work), with obesity, fitness, and cardiovascular disease (CVD) risk factors.

Methods.—This cross-sectional study included 2364 participants enrolled in the Coronary Artery Risk Development in Young Adults (CARDIA) study who worked outside the home during year 20 of the study (2005-2006). Associations between walking or biking to work (self-reported time, distance, and mode of commuting) with body weight (measured height and weight); obesity (body mass index [BMI], calculated as weight in kilograms divided by height in meters squared, ≥30); fitness (symptom-limited exercise stress testing); objective moderate-vigorous physical activity (accelerometry); CVD risk factors (blood pressure [oscillometric systolic and diastolic]); and serum measures (fasting measures of lipid, glucose, and insulin levels) were separately assessed by sex-stratified multivariable linear (or logistic) regression modeling.

Results.—A total of 16.7% of participants used any means of active commuting to work. Controlling for age, race, income, education, smoking, examination center, and physical activity index excluding

TABLE 5.—Association Between Active Commuting and CVD Risk Biomarkers at Examination Year 20 (2005-2006) of the CARDIA Study[a]

Variable	Model (Effect Measure)	No.	Mean/% (SE)	Model 1, Measure of Effect (95% CI)	P Value	Model 2, Measure of Effect (95% CI)	P Value
				Men			
HDL-C level[b]	$(HDL\text{-}C_{active})/(HDL\text{-}C_{nonactive})$	883	47.8 (14.2)	**1.05 (1.00 to 1.10)**	.04	1.03 (0.99 to 1.08)	.18
LDL-C level[b]	$(LDL\text{-}C_{active})/(LDL\text{-}C_{nonactive})$	862	116.9 (31.7)	0.99 (0.94 to 1.04)	.60	0.99 (0.93 to 1.04)	.58
Trig level[b]	$(trig_{active})/(trig_{nonactive})$	883	127.0 (97.5)	**0.88 (0.80 to 0.98)**	.01	**0.88 (0.80 to 0.98)**	.02
DBP level[c,d]	$(DBP_{active}) - (DBP_{nonactive})$	913	71.6 (9.2)	**−1.54 (−3.07 to −0.01)**	.05	**−1.67 (−3.20 to −0.15)**	.03
SBP level[c,d]	$(SBP_{active}) - (SBP_{nonactive})$	913	116.9 (11.3)	−1.39 (−3.29 to 0.52)[d]	.15	−1.60 (−3.51 to 0.32)[d]	.10
FG level[e]	$(FG_{active})/(FG_{nonactive})$	965	99.9 (17.4)	0.98 (0.96 to 1.00)	.12	0.98 (0.96 to 1.01)	.16
FI level[e]	$(FI_{active})/(FI_{nonactive})$	964	14.5 (9.4)	**0.84 (0.77 to 0.92)**	<.001	0.86 (0.78 to 0.93)	<.001
				Women			
HDL-C level[b]	$(HDL\text{-}C_{active})/(HDL\text{-}C_{nonactive})$	1120	60.1 (16.0)	1.02 (0.98 to 1.06)	.41	1.01 (0.97 to 1.06)	.53
LDL-C level[b]	$(LDL\text{-}C_{active})/(LDL\text{-}C_{nonactive})$	1117	108.5 (29.2)	1.01 (0.96 to 1.06)	.68	1.01 (0.97 to 1.06)	.59
Trig level[b]	$(trig_{active})/(trig_{nonactive})$	1120	90.9 (60.1)	1.02 (0.95 to 1.11)	.55	1.04 (0.96 to 1.12)	.39
DBP level[c,d]	$(DBP_{active}) - (DBP_{nonactive})$	1076	69.8 (10.7)	−0.18 (−1.84 to 1.47)	.83	−0.15 (−1.81 to 1.51)	.86
SBP level[c,d]	$(SBP_{active}) - (SBP_{nonactive})$	1076	111.4 (13.7)	0.93 (−1.20 to 3.07)	.39	0.74 (−1.39 to 2.87)[e]	.50
FG level[e]	$(FG_{active})/(FG_{nonactive})$	1143	94.2 (16.1)	1.00 (0.98 to 1.02)	.85	1.00 (0.98 to 1.02)	.99
FI level[e]	$(FI_{active})/(FI_{nonactive})$	1143	13.4 (8.3)	1.00 (0.92 to 1.08)	.93	1.00 (0.93 to 1.09)	.93

Abbreviations: BP, blood pressure; CARDIA, Coronary Artery Risk Development in Young Adults; CI, confidence interval; CVD, cardiovascular disease; DBP, diastolic blood pressure; FG, fasting glucose; FI, fasting insulin; HDL-C, high-density lipoprotein cholesterol; LDL-C, low-density lipoprotein cholesterol; SBP, systolic blood pressure; trig, triglycerides.

[a]Active commuting was defined as any walking or biking during the trip from home to work. Model 1 was adjusted for age, race, income, education, and examination center. Model 2 was adjusted for smoking, alcohol consumption, physical activity index excluding walking (self-report), and model 1 variables. Bold font indicates significant association ($P < 05$).

[b]Ratios obtained by exponentiation of coefficients from linear regression of natural log-transformed lipid measure on active commuting and control variables. Excludes individuals reporting cholesterol-lowering medications or who fasted less than 8 hours prior to blood draw.

[c]Differences obtained from linear regression of BP measure on active commuting and control variables. Excludes individuals reporting BP-lowering medications.

[d]When limiting to participants who reside within 2 miles of their work location, estimated associations were similar across sexes and outcomes, with the exception of SBP; men, model 1: $(SBP_{active})-(SBP_{nonactive}) = 3.92$ (95% CI, −0.74 to 8.59), model 2: $(SBP_{active})-(SBP_{nonactive}) = 4.40$ (95% CI, −0.24 to 9.04); women, significant interaction with physical activity, high physical activity: $(SBP_{active})-(SBP_{nonactive}) = 2.39$ (95% CI, −0.50 to 5.29), low physical activity: $(SBP_{active})-(SBP_{nonactive}) = -1.17$ (95% CI, −4.26 to 1.92).

[e]Ratios obtained by exponentiation of coefficients from linear regression of natural log-transformed fasting insulin and glucose measures on active commuting and control variables. Excludes individuals reporting diabetes medications or who fasted less than 8 hours prior to blood draw.

walking, men with any active commuting (vs none) had reduced likelihood of obesity (odds ratio [OR], 0.50; 95% confidence interval [CI], 0.33-0.76), reduced CVD risk: ratio of geometric mean triglyceride levels $(trig_{active})/(trig_{nonactive}) = 0.88$ (95% CI, 0.80 to 0.98); ratio of geometric mean fasting insulin $(FI_{active})/(FI_{nonactive}) = 0.86$ (95% CI, 0.78 to 0.93); difference in mean diastolic blood pressure (millimeters of mercury) $(DBP_{active})-(DBP_{nonactive}) = -1.67$ (95% CI, −3.20 to −0.15); and higher fitness: mean difference in treadmill test duration (in seconds) in men $(TT_{active}) - (TT_{nonactive}) = 50.0$ (95% CI, 31.45 to 68.59) and women $(TT_{active})-(TT_{nonactive}) = 28.77$ (95% CI, 11.61 to 45.92).

Conclusions.—Active commuting was positively associated with fitness in men and women and inversely associated with BMI, obesity, triglyceride levels, blood pressure, and insulin level in men. Active commuting should be investigated as a modality for maintaining or improving health (Table 5).

▶ Active commuting has frequently been suggested as a means of enhancing population health,[1] and doctors are often asked about such activity. Active commuting certainly has a number of potential attractions. In particular, most people attend their work on most days of the week, so necessary exercise is not easily forgotten. Walking also seems the most popular type of voluntary activity for many people, and with the choice of active commuting, there is no need for the exerciser to purchase expensive memberships or equipment, and no need for governments to build expensive arenas or swimming pools. There may be some initial costs to a municipality in terms of constructing walkways or cycle paths, but in the long-term costs for new highways and mass transit could decrease. Employers could encourage active commuting by installing showers, changing facilities, and cycle lockers. The critical question is whether the intensity and volume of exercise are sufficient to have a health benefit, and on this issue the opinion has been divided. Earlier reviews of the literature[1,2] suggested that cycling generally was at an appropriate intensity to enhance cardiovascular health, but walking might not provide an adequate stimulus, except in an older person or a hilly area. This article presents long-term data from the Cardia study, a 20-year follow-up of a substantial group of (initially) young adults in various parts of the United States. This is helpful information because many of the previous investigations of active commuting have been from Scandinavia. This study also included accelerometer measures of leisure activity, thus allowing for substantial correlations between active commuting and a more general interest in physical activity. As in most North American reports, few people were prepared to accept the risk of cycling to work on busy highways, but there were a substantial 16% of walkers (probably reflecting a health-conscious segment of the population). After allowing for other risk factors, health benefit was seen in male walkers but not in women (model 2 of Fig 5 in the original article); the male advantage seemed related to longer and faster commutes. However, even in the men, effects were entirely attributable to a lowering of body mass index in the walkers, confirming that their intensity of effort was insufficient for direct cardiac benefit. The inevitable limitation of the study is self-selection—the most health conscious individuals are those likely to engage in active commuting, and their lower body mass index could arise from dietary prudence rather than exercise.

R. J. Shephard, MD (Lond), PhD, DPE

References

1. Shephard RJ. Is active commuting the answer to population health? *Sports Med.* 2008;38:751-758.
2. Hamer M, Chida Y. Active commuting and cardiovascular risk: a meta-analytic review. *Prev Med.* 2008;46:9-13.

Exercise on prescription for women aged 40-74 recruited through primary care: two year randomised controlled trial

Lawton BA, Rose SB, Elley CR, et al (Univ of Otago, Wellington, New Zealand; Univ of Auckland, New Zealand; et al)

BMJ 337:a2509, 2008

Objective.—To assess the effectiveness of a primary care based programme of exercise on prescription among relatively inactive women over a two year period.

Design.—Randomised controlled trial.

Setting.—17 primary care practices in Wellington, New Zealand.

Participants.—1089 women aged 40-74 not undertaking 30 minutes of moderate intensity physical activity on at least five days of the week.

Intervention.—Brief physical activity intervention led by nurse with six month follow-up visit and monthly telephone support over nine months.

Main Outcome Measure.—Physical activity assessed at baseline and 12 and 24 months. Secondary outcomes were quality of life (SF-36), weight, waist circumference, blood pressure, concentrations of fasting serum lipids, glycated haemoglobin (HbA_{1c}), glucose, insulin, and physical fitness.

Results.—Mean age was 58.9 (SD 7) years. Trial retention rates were 93% and 89% at 12 and 24 months, respectively. At baseline, 10% of intervention participants and 11% of control participants were achieving 150 minutes of at least moderate intensity physical activity a week. At 12 months rates increased to 43% and 30% and at 24 months to 39.3% and 32.8% ($P<0.001$), respectively. SF-36 physical functioning ($P=0.03$) and mental health ($P<0.05$) scores improved more in intervention compared with control participants, but role physical scores were significantly lower ($P<0.01$). There were no significant differences in clinical outcomes. More falls ($P<0.001$) and injuries ($P=0.03$) were recorded in the intervention group.

Conclusions.—This programme of exercise on prescription increased physical activity and quality of life over two years, although falls and injuries also increased. This finding supports the use of exercise on

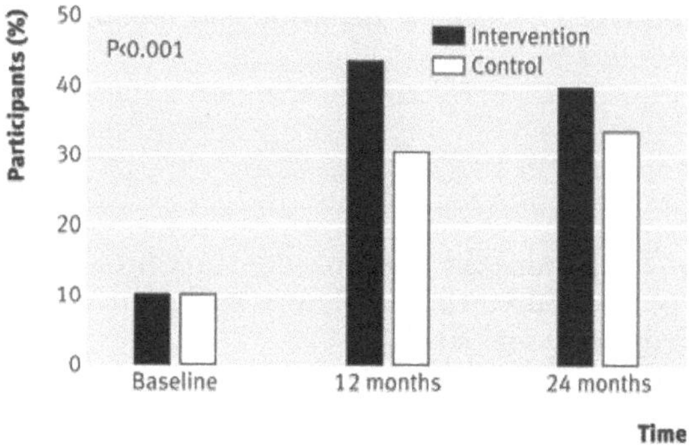

FIGURE 2.—Proportion of participants achieving at least 150 minutes of moderate intensity physical activity at baseline and 12 and 24 months. (Reprinted from Lawton BA, Rose SB, Elley CR, et al. Exercise on prescription for women aged 40-74 recruited through primary care: two year randomised controlled trial. *BMJ*. 2008;337:a2509, with permission from the BMJ Publishing Group.)

prescription programmes as part of population strategies to reduce physical inactivity (Fig 2).

▶ Exercise on prescription refers to written advice to patients from a health care professional to increase daily physical activity. In this randomized controlled trial, Lawton and colleagues tested the effectiveness and sustainability of an exercise on prescription program in sedentary women aged 40 to 70 years. This study was conducted in New Zealand, where exercise on prescription ("green prescription") is becoming a part of routine health care. The primary outcome was the proportion of women who achieved the goal of 150 min of exercise weekly. Exercise was assessed by a self-reported questionnaire, the New Zealand Physical Activity Questionnaire (NZPAQ). After baseline assessment of physical activity, quality of life, and clinical outcomes, women were randomly assigned to a telephone-based behavioral intervention group or usual care (control). The intervention group received an exercise prescription and brief counseling from a nurse who then provided telephone support for 9 months with a clinic visit at 6 months. Controls did not receive an exercise prescription or support. Follow-up clinic visits occurred at 12 and 24 months after randomization. At baseline, only 10% of women met the exercise goal. The proportion of women meeting the goal increased significantly in both groups over 1 year and was sustained over the second year (Fig 2). However, the intervention group had a greater proportion of women achieving the exercise goals (~40%) than controls (~30%). The intervention group also had more falls and injuries than the control groups at follow-up. The increase in physical activity in the control group was unexpected and could be partly attributed to the halo effect of participating in a physical activity study. Only 2% of women in the control group reported receiving an exercise prescription from other sources. A cost analysis of the study is planned. Future interventions may need to place more emphasis on fall and injury prevention, particularly in older women.

C. M. Jankowski, PhD

Associations Between Sedentary Behavior and Blood Pressure in Young Children

Martinez-Gomez D, Tucker J, Heelan KA, et al (Iowa State Univ, Ames; Univ of Nebraska at Kearney; et al)

Arch Pediatr Adolesc Med 163:724-730, 2009

Objective.—To examine the effect of sedentary behavior on blood pressure (BP) in young children using different indicators of sedentariness.

Design.—Cross-sectional study.

Setting.—A rural Midwestern US community.

Participants.—Children aged 3 to 8 years (N = 111).

Intervention.—Adiposity was assessed using dual energy x-ray absorptiometry. Objective measurements of sedentary activity were obtained from the accelerometers that participants wore continuously for 7 days. Measurements of television (TV) viewing, computer, and screen time (TV + computer) were obtained via parent report.

Main Outcome Measures.—Systolic and diastolic BP.

Results.—The sample spent a mean of 5 hours per day in sedentary activities, of which 1.5 hours were screen time. Accelerometer-determined sedentary activity was not significantly related to systolic BP or diastolic BP after controlling for age, sex, height, and percentage of body fat. However, TV viewing and screentime, but not computer use, were positively associated with both systolic BP and diastolic BP after adjusting for potential confounders. Participants in the lowest tertile of TV and screen time had significantly lower levels of systolic and diastolic BP than participants in the upper tertile.

Conclusions.—Sedentary behaviors, particularly TV viewing and screen time, were associated with BP in children, independent of body composition. Other factors that occur during excessive screen time (eg, food consumption) should also be considered in the context of sedentary behavior and BP development in children.

▶ In the past several years growing attention has been paid to sedentary behaviors in youth as a health risk factor. In fact, sedentary time may not indicate the level of a child's regular physical activity, and sedentary behaviors may track (ie, remain consistent) more than activity as a child grows. This report reflects this new focus and provides data that imply a relationship of sedentary time and blood pressure in youth. Importantly, this association was seen with screen time but not total nonactive time. The issue is not a simple one, because "sedentary time" includes time spent in what we would consider valuable endeavors—doing homework, reading, art, listening, playing music, etc. Even screen time, of course, can be included in this good sedentary time. It was a bit eye-opening to find in this study that the subjects averaged 5 hours of sedentary time per day.

T. Rowland, MD

Frontal and motor cortex oxygenation during maximal exercise in normoxia and hypoxia

Subudhi AW, Miramon BR, Granger ME, et al (Univ of Colorado Altitude Res Ctr)

J Appl Physiol 106:1153-1158, 2009

Reductions in prefrontal oxygenation near maximal exertion may limit exercise performance by impairing executive functions that influence the decision to stop exercising; however, whether deoxygenation also occurs in motor regions that more directly affect central motor drive is unknown. Multichannel near-infrared spectroscopy was used to compare changes in prefrontal, premotor, and motor cortices during exhaustive exercise. Twenty-three subjects performed two sequential, incremental cycle tests (25 W/min ramp) during acute hypoxia [79 Torr inspired PO_2 (PI_{O_2})] and normoxia (117 Torr PI_{O_2}) in an environmental chamber. Test order was balanced, and subjects were blinded to chamber pressure. In normoxia, bilateral prefrontal oxygenation was maintained during low- and moderate-intensity exercise but dropped 9.0 ± 10.7% (mean ± SD, $P < 0.05$) before exhaustion (maximal power = 305 ± 52 W). The pattern and magnitude of deoxygenation were similar in prefrontal, premotor, and motor regions ($R^2 > 0.94$). In hypoxia, prefrontal oxygenation was reduced 11.1 ± 14.3% at rest ($P < 0.01$) and fell another 26.5 ± 19.5% ($P < 0.01$) at exhaustion (maximal power = 256 ± 38 W, $P < 0.01$). Correlations between regions were high ($R^2 > 0.61$), but deoxygenation was greater in prefrontal than premotor and motor regions ($P < 0.05$). Prefrontal, premotor, and motor cortex deoxygenation during high-intensity exercise may contribute to an integrative decision to stop

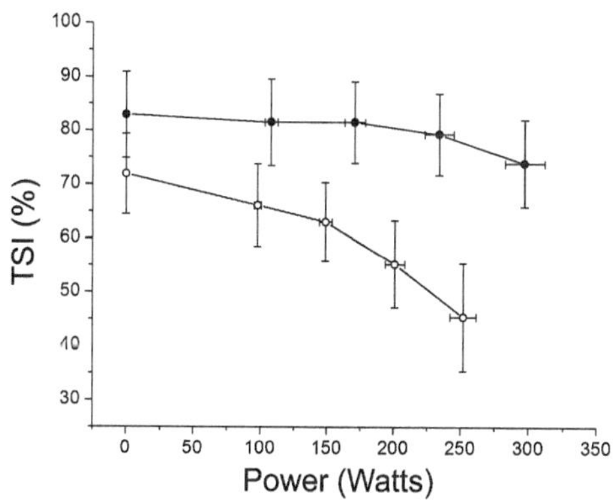

FIGURE 1.—Cerebral tissue saturation index (TSI) during exercise ($n = 12$). Data points correspond to rest and 25, 50, 75, and 100% maximal power output (W_{max}) in normoxia (Norm, ●) and hypoxia (Hypox, ○). Cerebral TSI is maintained in Norm until 75% W_{max} and declines thereafter ($P < 0.05$). In Hypox, resting TSI is reduced ($P < 0.05$) and continues to fall as exercise intensity increases ($P < 0.01$). (Reprinted from Subudhi AW, Miramon BR, Granger ME, et al. Frontal and motor cortex oxygenation during maximal exercise in normoxia and hypoxia. *J Appl Physiol.* 2009;106:1153-1158, with permission from the American Physiological Society.)

exercise. The accelerated rate of cortical deoxygenation in hypoxia may hasten this effect (Fig 1).

▶ Scientific advances in near-infrared spectroscopy (NIRS) now allows non-invasive, continuous monitoring of brain oxygenation. In previous studies, NIRS measurements during exercise were limited to the prefrontal cortex.[1] Prefrontal oxygenation is maintained or increased slightly during light- to moderate-intensity exercise but decreases near maximal exercise intensity.[2] Data from this study are the first to show that deoxygenation also occurs in pre-motor and motor regions during high-intensity aerobic exercise, raising the possibility that deoxygenation in motor areas may directly impair motor neuron excitability. Thus deoxygenation in premotor and motor cortices may contribute to fatigue and/or decisions to stop exercising. As shown in Fig 1, acute hypoxia exacerbates exercise-induced cortical deoxygenation and appears to decrease the ability to exercise at a high power output.

D. C. Nieman, DrPH

References

1. Perrey S. Non-invasive NIR spectroscopy of human brain function during exercise. *Methods*. 2008;45:289-299.
2. Bhambhani Y, Malik R, Mookerjee S. Cerebral oxygenation declines at exercise intensities above the respiratory compensation threshold. *Respir Physiol Neurobiol*. 2007;156:196-202.

Frontal and motor cortex oxygenation during maximal exercise in normoxia and hypoxia

Subudhi AW, Miramon BR, Granger ME, et al (Univ of Colorado Altitude Res Ctr)

J Appl Physiol 106:1153-1158, 2009

Reductions in prefrontal oxygenation near maximal exertion may limit exercise performance by impairing executive functions that influence the decision to stop exercising; however, whether deoxygenation also occurs in motor regions that more directly affect central motor drive is unknown. Multichannel near-infrared spectroscopy was used to compare changes in prefrontal, premotor, and motor cortices during exhaustive exercise. Twenty-three subjects performed two sequential, incremental cycle tests (25 W/min ramp) during acute hypoxia [79 Torr inspired PO_2 (Pi_{O_2})] and normoxia (117 Torr Pi_{O_2}) in an environmental chamber. Test order was balanced, and subjects were blinded to chamber pressure. In normoxia, bilateral prefrontal oxygenation was maintained during low- and moderate-intensity exercise but dropped 9.0 ± 10.7% (mean ± SD, $P < 0.05$) before exhaustion (maximal power = 305 ± 52 W). The pattern and magnitude of deoxygenation were similar in prefrontal, premotor, and motor regions ($R^2 > 0.94$). In hypoxia, prefrontal oxygenation was reduced 11.1 ± 14.3% at rest ($P < 0.01$) and fell another 26.5 ± 19.5%

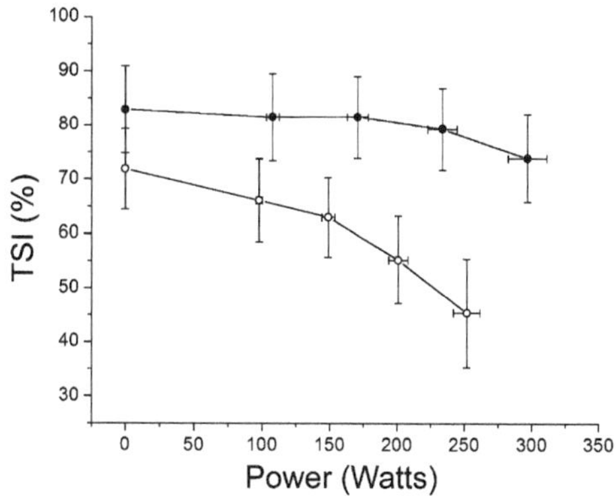

FIGURE 1.—Cerebral tissue saturation index (TSI) during exercise ($n = 12$). Data points correspond to rest and 25, 50, 75, and 100% maximal power output (W_{max}) in normoxia (Norm, ●) and hypoxia (Hypox, ○). Cerebral TSI is maintained in Norm until 75% W_{max} and declines thereafter ($P < 0.05$). In Hypox, resting TSI is reduced ($P < 0.05$) and continues to fall as exercise intensity increases ($P < 0.01$). (Reprinted with permission from Subudhi AW, Miramon BR, Granger ME, et al. Frontal and motor cortex oxygenation during maximal exercise in normoxia and hypoxia. *J Appl Physiol.* 2009;106:1153-1158.)

($P < 0.01$) at exhaustion (maximal power = 256 ± 38 W, $P < 0.01$). Correlations between regions were high ($R^2 > 0.61$), but deoxygenation was greater in prefrontal than premotor and motor regions ($P < 0.05$). Prefrontal, premotor, and motor cortex deoxygenation during high-intensity exercise may contribute to an integrative decision to stop exercise. The accelerated rate of cortical deoxygenation in hypoxia may hasten this effect (Fig 1).

▶ I have long argued that if a maximal oxygen intake test is well performed, the subject begins to show signs of cerebral hypoxia and/or hypoglycemia as an oxygen plateau is approached. This is a logical corollary if the oxygen demand of the muscles is still increasing but the cardiac output has reached a plateau value. My evidence in support of cerebral oxygen lack was primarily clinical observation of the subject; often there was a progressive loss of coordination, and 1 postdoctoral fellow who was well aware that I did not speak Spanish made the irrational decision of speaking several sentences to me in Spanish at the point when I decided to halt his test. This near infrared spectroscopy study did not carry subjects to a very convincing maximal oxygen intake (maximal heart rate of 178 beats/min in subjects of average age 29 years), but nevertheless their data supports my contention, showing a 10% decrease in tissue oxygenation at the maximum effort that was achieved (Fig 1); moreover, this drop was exacerbated when the subjects were breathing low oxygen mixtures. The issue of exercise-induced cerebral hypoxia is important to rejection of the much-touted central governor hypothesis.[1] If there were a feed-forward mechanism limiting muscle activation, and thus a person's maximal effort, we would not see a plateauing of cardiac output or a reduction in oxygen supply to the brain. The hypoxia seems particularly marked in the prefrontal cortex, and the authors of this article question how far the drop in tissue oxygenation may be a factor that leads to fatigue or a conscious restriction of effort.[2] Our clinical observation of decreasing coordination would certainly support the idea of progressive fatigue, but anyone who has experienced acute hypoxia will confirm that far from leading to rational and careful protective decision making, cerebral hypoxia encourages reckless continuation of activity.

R. J. Shephard, MD (Lond), PhD, DPE

References

1. Shephard RJ. Is it time to retire the central Governor? *Sports Med.* 2009; In press.
2. Ramnani N, Owen AM. Anterior prefrontal cortex: insights into function from anatomy and neuroimaging. *Nat Rev Neurosci.* 2004;5:184-194.

Effect of Prolonged Walking on Cardiac Troponin Levels

Eijsvogels T, George K, Shave R, et al (Radboud Univ Nijmegen Med Centre, The Netherlands; Liverpool John Moore's Univ; Brunel Univ, Uxbridge, Middlesex, UK; et al)
Am J Cardiol 105:267-272, 2010

Increased cardiac troponin I (cTnI), a marker for cardiac damage, has been reported after strenuous exercise in young subjects. However, little is known about changes in cTnI after moderate-intensity exercise in a heterogenous population or which factors may contribute to this change in cTnI levels. We examined cTnI levels before and immediately after each day of a 4-day long-distance walking event (30 to 50 km/day) in a heterogenous group (67 men, 42 women), across a broad age range (21 to 82 years), with known cardiovascular pathology or risk factors present in many subjects ($n = 24$). Walking was performed at a self-selected pace. Cardiac TnI was assessed using a standard system (Immulite) with high values (≥0.20 μg/L) cross-checked using a high-sensitive cTnI assay (Centaur). Mean cTnI levels increased significantly from 0.04 to 0.07 μg/L on day 1, with no further increase thereafter ($p < 0.001$, analysis of variance). Backward linear regression found a weak, but significant, association of age ($p < 0.001$), walking speed ($p = 0.02$), and cardiovascular pathology ($p = 0.03$) with postexercise cTnI level (combined $r^2 = 0.11$, $p < 0.001$). In 6 participants (6%), cTnI was increased above the clinical cut-off value for myocardial infarction on ≥1 day. These participants supported the regression analysis, because they were older, walked at higher relative exercise intensity, and reported a high prevalence of cardiovascular pathology. In conclusion, prolonged, moderate-intensity exercise may result in an increase in cTnI levels in a broad spectrum of

TABLE 3.—Details about Participants (n = 6) with a Positive, Clinically Relevant, Highly Sensitive Cardiac Troponin I Test Result (99th percentile 0.20 μg/L)

Subject (day)	cTnI (μg/L)	Age (years)/Sex	BMI (kg/m^2)	Distance (km)	Fitness (sport hors/week)	Speed (km/hour)	Exercise (percent HRmax)	CBT (°C)	Pathology
1 (4)	0.25	57/F	25.9	50	5	4.0	63	—	hypertension
2 (1)	0.30	53/F	30.9	50	4	5.4	78	38.6	none
3 (3)	0.20	82/M	24.7	30	0	3.7	56	37.9	none
4 (1)	1.17	79/M	26.2	30	4	3.1	59	37.9	hypertension, COPD
5 (1)	0.26	74/M	21.5	30	1	4.7	64	37.9	atherosclerosis
6 (1)	0.65	75/F	26.9	30	2	4.1	61	38.1	hypertension
6 (2)	0.74					4.1	56	38.2	
6 (3)	0.79					4.6	57	38.2	
6 (4)	0.44					4.6	55	37.9	
Average (n = 6)		70/3 M:3 F	26.0		2.7	4.3	61	38.1	78%
Average (n = 109)		57/67 M:42 F	25.2		3.3	4.5	58	38.2	22%

CBT = core body temperature; COPD = chronic obstructive pulmonary disease; HRmax = maximum heart rate.

subjects, especially in older subjects with pre-existing cardiovascular disease or risk factors (Table 3).

▶ There have been quite a number of reports of increases in cardiac troponin persisting for 1 to 3 days following marathon and ultramarathon runs and long-distance cycling events.[1-3] Although this article purports to describe exercise of more moderate intensity (a mass walking event with some 40 000 participants), and the walking speed was moderate (4.5 km/h), the distance walked was not trivial (30-50 km in different subjects, repeated on each of 4 days), particularly as this volume of exercise was performed by a randomly chosen sample of subjects covering a wide range of ages and fitness levels, and about a fifth of those who were studied had some previous cardiac pathology. The weather was relatively cool, and peak core temperatures were a little over 38°C. Six of the 109 test subjects showed an elevated cardiac troponin level (Table 3). Age, speed of walking, and previous cardiovascular disease were all pointers to this outcome. Increases in troponin level exceeded the cut-off for diagnosis of acute myocardial infraction in the 6 subjects, although they reported no symptoms suggesting cardiac damage. It is possible that exercise-induced oxidative stress in the cardiac muscle may have contributed to the troponin release.[4]

R. J. Shephard, MD (Lond), PhD, DPE

References

1. Whyte G, Stephens N, Senior R, et al. Treat the patient not the blood test: the implications of an increase in cardiac troponin after prolonged endurance exercise. *Br J Sports Med.* 2007;41:613-615.
2. Koller A. Exercise-induced increases in cardiac troponins and pro-thrombotic markers. *Med Sci Sports Exerc.* 2003;35:444-448.
3. Neumayr G, Pfister R, Mitterbauer G, Eibl G, Hoertnagl H. Effect of competitive marathon cycling on plasma N-terminal pro-brain natriuretic peptide and cardiac troponin T in healthy recreational cyclists. *Am J Cardiol.* 2005;96:732-735.
4. Goette A, Bukowska A, Dobrev D, et al. Acute atrial tachyarrhythmia induces angiotensin II type 1 receptor-mediated oxidative stress and microvascular flow abnormalities in the ventricles. *Eur Heart J.* 2009;30:1411-1420.

No Indications of Persistent Oxidative Stress in Response to an Ironman Triathlon

Neubauer O, König D, Kern N, et al (Univ of Vienna, AUSTRIA; Freiburg Univ Hosp, GERMANY)
Med Sci Sports Exerc 40:2119-2128, 2008

Introduction.—Training for and competing in ultraendurance exercise events is associated with an improvement in endogenous antioxidant defenses as well as increased oxidative stress. However, consequences on health are currently unclear.

Purpose.—We aimed to examine the impact of training- and acute exercise-induced changes in the antioxidant capacity on the oxidant/antioxidant balance after an ironman triathlon and whether there are indications for sustained oxidative damage.

Methods.—Blood samples were taken from 42 well-trained male triathletes 2 d before an ironman triathlon, then immediately postrace, 1, 5, and 19 d later. Blood was analyzed for conjugated dienes (CD), malondialdehyde (MDA), oxidized low-density lipoprotein (oxLDL), oxLDL:LDL ratio, advanced oxidation protein products (AOPP), AOPP:total protein (TP) ratio, Trolox equivalent antioxidant capacity (TEAC), uric acid (UA) in plasma, and activities of superoxide dismutase (SOD), glutathione peroxidase (GSH-Px), and catalase (CAT) in erythrocytes.

Results.—Immediately postrace, there were significant increases in CD, AOPP, TEAC, UA (for all $P < 0.001$), and AOPP:TP ($P < 0.01$). MDA rose significantly ($P < 0.01$) 1 d postrace, whereas CD ($P < 0.01$), AOPP ($P = 0.01$), AOPP:TP ($P < 0.05$), and TEAC ($P < 0.001$) remained elevated. OxLDL:LDL trended to increase, whereas oxLDL significantly ($P < 0.01$) decreased 1 d postrace. Except for GSH-Px ($P = 0.08$), activities of SOD ($P < 0.001$) and CAT ($P < 0.05$) significantly decreased postrace. All oxidative stress markers had returned to prerace values 5 d postrace. Furthermore, several relationships between training status and oxidative stress markers, TEAC, and antioxidant enzyme activities were noted.

Conclusions.—This study indicates that despite a temporary increase in most (but not all) oxidative stress markers, there is no persistent oxidative stress in response to an ironman triathlon, probably due to training- and exercise-induced protective alterations in the antioxidant defense system.

▶ Competing in an Ironman race increases oxidative stress, but the effect is transient. Thus it appears that exercise training-induced improvements in the antioxidant defense system of athletes counteract oxidative damage, even after extremely demanding exercise. Even though these data imply that acute ultraendurance exercise does not cause long-lasting alterations in systemic oxidative stress, there is still concern that competing in a high number of ultramarathon races may eventually break down the body's ability to cope with the repeated physiologic insults leading to increased disease.[1] Long-term studies of ultramarathon runners are needed to determine if cancer risk is elevated in old age.

D. C. Nieman, DrPH

Reference

1. Knez WL, Coombes JS, Jenkins DG. Ultra-endurance exercise and oxidative damage: implications for cardiovascular health. *Sports Med.* 2006;36:429-441.

Left ventricular wall segment motion after ultra-endurance exercise in humans assessed by myocardial speckle tracking

George K, Shave R, Oxborough D, et al (Liverpool John Moores Univ, UK; Brunel Univ, UK; Univ of Leeds, UK; et al)

Eur J Echocardiogr 10:238-243, 2009

Aims.—Assessment of the left ventricular responses to prolonged exercise has been limited by technology available to assess cardiac tissue movement. Recently developed strain and strain rate imaging provide the unique opportunity to assess tissue deformation in all planes of motion.

Methods and Results.—Nineteen runners (mean ± SD age; 41 ± 9 years) were assessed prior to and within 60 min (34 ± 10 min) of race finish (Comrades Marathon, 89 km). Standard echocardiography assessed ejection fraction and the ratio of early to atrial (*E/A*) peak transmitral blood flow velocities. Myocardial speckle tracking determined segmental strain as well as systolic and diastolic strain rates in radial, circumferential, and longitudinal planes. Cardiac troponin T (cTnT) assessed cardiomyocyte insult. Ejection fraction (71 ± 5 to 64 ± 6%) and *E/A* (1.47 ± 0.35 to 1.25 ± 0.30) were reduced ($P < 0.05$). Peak strain and peak systolic and diastolic strain rates were altered post-race in circumferential (e.g. peak strain reduced from 21.3 ± 2.4 to 17.3 ± 3.2%, $P < 0.05$) and radial planes. Some individual heterogeneity was observed between segments and planes of motion. A post-race elevation in cTnT (range 0.013-0.272 μg/L) in 5/12 runners did not differentiate changes in LV function.

Conclusion.—Completion of the Comrades Marathon resulted in a depression in ejection fraction, *E/A*, as well as radial and circumferential strain and strain rates. Group data, however, masked some heterogeneity in cardiac function (Table 1).

▶ Several previous reports have suggested that there is a transient depression of left ventricular function immediately following participation in an endurance or ultra-endurance competition.[1-3] Myocardial speckle tracking is a new and improved technology, but the data tell essentially the same story, with a 10% depression of resting ejection fraction and disturbance of other parameters of both systolic and diastolic performance 1 hour after running the Comrades Marathon (Table 1). Some previous authors have attributed such observations to temporary disturbances of cardiac preloading, after loading, or resting heart rate, but available evidence from this study argues against such explanations. Another possibility is a progressive β-desensitization over the course of the race, although it would be difficult to explain changes of diastolic function on this basis.[4] The final, and perhaps the most important possibility, is some transient damage to the cardiac muscle[5]; this study found elevated cardiac troponin levels in 5 of the runners, but unlike the earlier study from Rifai et al[5] the levels of cardiac troponin did not appear to be correlated with changes in myocardial performance. As a result of elimination, this left the possibility that there was a transient, nonpathological leakage of cardiac troponin mediated by reactive oxygen species,[6] and that the depression of left ventricular function

TABLE 1.—Global Indices of LV Systolic and Diastolic Function Pre- and Post-Race

Parameter	Pre-Race	Post-Race	*P*-value
Systolic			
Fractional area change (%)	59 ± 7	53 ± 7	0.004
Ejection fraction (%)	71 ± 5	64 ± 6	0.001
End-systolic pressure:volume	4.2 ± 1.3	3.3 ± 1.0	0.001
Diastolic			
Peak *E* velocity (cm s^{-1})	88 ± 14	71 ± 16	<0.001
Peak *A* velocity (cm s^{-1})	63 ± 15	58 ± 13	0.298
E/A	1.47 ± 0.35	1.25 ± 0.30	0.016
E deceleration time (ms)	203 ± 33	239 ± 48	0.002

E, early; A, atrial.

reflected local ischemia or some other undetermined transient metabolic abnormality.

R. J. Shephard, MD (Lond), PhD, DPE

References

1. Ashley EA, Kardos A, Jack ES, et al. Angiotensin-converting enzyme genotype predicts cardiac and autonomic responses to prolonged exercise. *J Am Coll Cardiol.* 2006;48:523-531.
2. Middleton N, Shave R, George KP, et al. Exercise-induced cardiac fatigue a meta-analysis. *Med Sci Sports Exerc.* 2006;38:681-687.
3. Neilan TG, Jannuzzi JL, Lee-Lewandrowski E, et al. Myocardial injury and ventricular dysfunction related to training levels among non-elite participants in the Boston Marathon. *Circulation.* 2006;114:2325-2333.
4. Hart ECJ, Dawson EA, Rasmussen P, et al. b-adrenergic receptor desensitisation in man: insight into post-exercise attenuation of cardiac function. *J Physiol.* 2006; 577:717-725.
5. Rifai N, Douglas PS, O'Toole M, Rimm E, Ginsburg GS. Cardiac troponin T and I, electrocardiographic wall motion analyses and ejection fractions in athletes participating in the Hawaii ironman triathlon. *Am J Cardiol.* 1999;83:1085-1089.
6. Neumayr G, Pfister R, Mitterbauer G, et al. Effect of the "Race Across The Alps" in elite cyclists on plasma cardiac troponins I and T. *Am J Cardiol.* 2002;89: 484-486.

Myocardial Late Gadolinium Enhancement: Prevalence, Pattern, and Prognostic Relevance in Marathon Runners

Breuckmann F, Möhlenkamp S, Nassenstein K, et al (West German Heart Ctr Essen; Dept of Diagnostic and Interventional Radiology and Neuroradiology; et al)

Radiology 251:50-57, 2009

Purpose.—To prospectively analyze the myocardial distribution of late gadolinium enhancement (LGE) with delayed-enhancement cardiac magnetic resonance (MR) imaging, to compare the prevalence of this distribution in nonprofessional male marathon runners with that in asymptomatic control subjects, and to examine the prognostic role of LGE.

Materials and Methods.—Institutional review board and ethics committee approval were obtained for this study, and all subjects provided written informed consent. Two-dimensional inversion-recovery segmented k-space gradient-echo MR sequences were performed after administration of a gadolinium-containing contrast agent in 102 ostensibly healthy male runners aged 50–72 years who had completed at least five marathons during the past 3 years and in 102 age-matched control subjects. Predominantly subendocardial regions of LGE typical of myocardial infarction (hereafter, coronary artery disease [CAD] pattern) were distinguished from a predominantly midmyocardial patchy pattern of LGE (hereafter, non–CAD pattern). Marathon runners with LGE underwent repeat cardiac MR imaging and additional adenosine perfusion imaging. Runners were followed up for a mean of 21 months ± 3 (standard deviation) after initial presentation. The χ^2, Fisher exact, and McNemar exact tests were used for comparisons. Event-free survival rates were estimated with the Kaplan-Meier method, and overall group differences were evaluated with log-rank statistics.

Results.—Of the 102 runners, five had a CAD pattern of LGE, and seven had a non–CAD pattern of LGE. The CAD pattern of LGE was located in the territory of the left anterior descending coronary artery more frequently than was the non–CAD pattern ($P = .0027$, Fisher exact test). The prevalence of LGE in runners was higher than that in age-matched control subjects (12% vs 4%; $P = .077$, McNemar exact test). The event-free survival rate was lower in runners with myocardial LGE than in those without myocardial LGE ($P < .0001$, log-rank test).

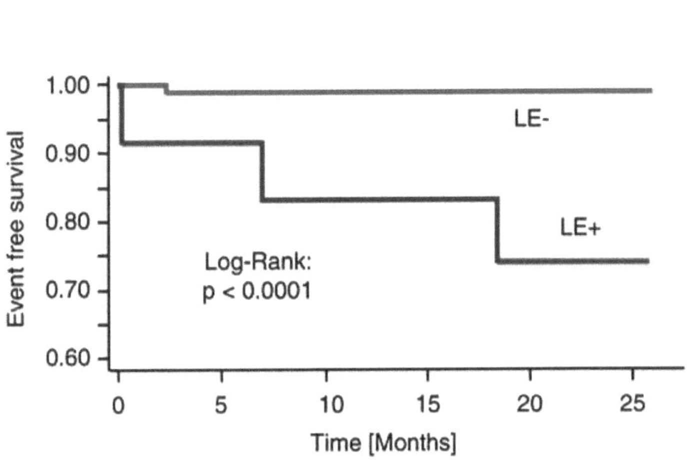

FIGURE 4.—Graph shows the rate of coronary event-free survival according to the presence of LGE. One runner without LGE (*LE*−) (1%) and three runners with LGE (*LE*+) (25%) required revascularization during follow-up. All runners who had a coronary event had a CAD pattern of LGE typical of subclinical myocardial infarction. (Reprinted from Breuckmann F, Möhlenkamp S, Nassenstein K, et al. Myocardial late gadolinium enhancement: prevalence, pattern, and prognostic relevance in marathon runners. *Radiology*. 2009;251:50-57, with permission from the RSNA.)

Conclusion.—Ostensibly healthy marathon runners have an unexpectedly high rate of myocardial LGE, and this may have diagnostic and prognostic relevance (Fig 4).

▶ Sports physicians have long recognized the paradox that regular moderate physical activity enhances survival, but vigorous exercise is associated with an increased risk of cardiac death.[1] This study compared a substantial sample of older marathon runners with age-matched controls, using a gadolinium contrast agent and magnetic resonance imaging. Late gadolinium enhancement was distinguished by site; subendocardial enhancement was thought typical of myocardial lesions. The prevalence of this sign was greater in the runners than in the controls (as many as 12% of runners had abnormal records), and the abnormality was associated with poor survival prospects (Fig 4); possibly, runners showing this phenomenon should moderate their running.

R. J. Shephard, MD (Lond), PhD, DPE

Reference

1. Shephard RJ. Sudden death- a significant hazard of exercise? *Br J Sports Med.* 1974;8:101-110.

Relation of Biomarkers and Cardiac Magnetic Resonance Imaging After Marathon Running

Mousavi N, Czarnecki A, Kumar K, et al (Univ of Manitoba, Winnipeg, Canada; et al)
Am J Cardiol 103:1467-1472, 2009

Although previous studies including endurance athletes after marathon running have demonstrated biochemical evidence of cardiac injury and have correlated these findings with echocardiographic evidence of cardiac dysfunction, particularly of the right ventricle, a study of marathon athletes incorporating biomarkers, echocardiography, and cardiac magnetic resonance (CMR) imaging has not been performed to date. The aim of this study was to demonstrate the cardiac changes associated with participation in a marathon using serial cardiac biomarkers, echocardiography, and CMR imaging. Fourteen participants (mean age 33 ± 6 years, 8 men) completed the full marathon. Myoglobin, creatine kinase, and troponin T were elevated in all athletes after the race. There was a strong linear correlation between right ventricular (RV) fractional area change as assessed by echocardiography and the RV ejection fraction as assessed by CMR imaging ($r = 0.96$) after the marathon. RV function, using echocardiography, transiently decreased from before to after the race (RV fractional area change 43 ± 4% vs 33 ± 5%, $p < 0.05$). There were also postrace changes in left ventricular and RV diastolic filling. Although RV systolic changes were transient, left ventricular and RV diastolic abnormalities persisted up to 1 week after the marathon. No evidence of delayed

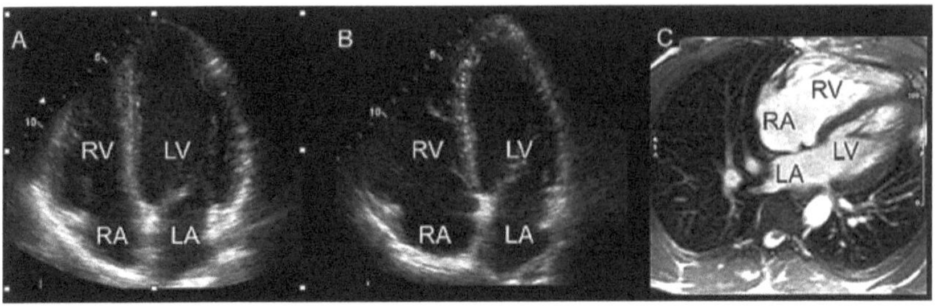

FIGURE 1.—Baseline and postmarathon transthoracic echocardiographic image in the apical 4-chamber view in a participant with a cTnT level that increased from <0.01 to 0.54 μg/L. *(A)* Baseline transthoracic echocardiographic image demonstrating normal right ventricular structure and function. *(B)* Postmarathon evidence of mild right ventricular dilatation (right ventricular end-diastolic diameter 38 mm) and a decrease in right ventricular fractional area change of 35%. *(C)* Postmarathon cine CMR image in the horizontal long-axis view confirming a decrease in the right ventricular ejection fraction of 44%. LA = left atrium; LV = left ventricle; RA = right atrium; RV = right ventricle. (Reprinted from Mousavi N, Czarnecki A, Kumar K, et al. Relation of biomarkers and cardiac magnetic resonance imaging after marathon running. *Am J Cardiol.* 2009;103:1467-1472, with permission from Elsevier Inc.)

enhancement of the left ventricular myocardium was found on CMR imaging, suggesting that the increase in cardiac biomarkers after the marathon may not have be due to myocardial necrosis. In conclusion, RV systolic dysfunction transiently occurs after a marathon and has been validated for the first time by CMR imaging. The increase in cardiac troponin after marathon running is likely due to the cytosolic release of the biomarker, not to the true breakdown of the myocyte, as confirmed by delayed enhancement CMR imaging (Fig 1).

▶ Several studies have shown leakage of cardiac troponin and transient depression of myocardial stroke volume following participation in marathon and ultramarathon endurance races,[1-5] but it is less clear whether these changes have pathological significance. One previous report suggested that frequent repetition of such changes could induce myocardial fibrosis. The present study used cardiac magnetic resonance imaging to confirm the changes previously shown by echocardiography (Fig 1). There was a striking decrease in right ventricular systolic function (probably 30-40%, although accurate quantification is difficult); this change was attributed to transient pulmonary hypertension. Some of the changes in cardiac function persisted for as long as one week following race participation. The present report argues, on the basis of the absence of any delay in enhancement of the gadolinium left ventricular myocardial image 3 days after the event, that the troponin reaches the plasma by leakage rather than a breakdown of the myocyte, as would occur with a - pathological lesion. The sensitivity of the method is such that it should detect 1 g of myocardial damage, although it cannot rule out the presence of smaller lesions. If a person raced repeatedly it remains difficult to exclude the possibility that smaller lesions could eventually progress to significant myocardial fibrosis.

R. J. Shephard, MD (Lond), PhD, DPE

References

1. Neilan TG, Januzzi JL, Lee-Lewandrowski E, et al. Myocardial injury and ventricular dysfunction related to training levels among non-elite participants in the Boston marathon. *Circulation.* 2006;114:2325-2333.
2. Neumayr G, Pfister R, Mitterbauer G, Eibl G, Hoetnagl H. Effect of competitive marathon cycling on plasma N-terminal pro-brain natriuretic peptide and cardiac troponin T in healthy recreational cyclists. *Am J Cardiol.* 2005;96:732-735.
3. Scharhag J, Herrmann M, Urhausen A, Haschke M, Herrmann W, Kindermann W. Independent elevations of N-terminal pro-brain natriuretic peptide and cardiac troponins in endurance athletes after prolonged strenuous exercise. *Am Heart J.* 2005;150:1128-1134.
4. Shave RE, Dawson E, Whyte G, et al. Evidence of exercise-induced cardiac dysfunction and elevated cTnT in separate cohorts competing in an ultra-endurance mountain marathon race. *Int J Sports Med.* 2002;23:489-494.
5. Shave R, George KP, Atkinson G, et al. Exercise-induced cardiac troponin T release: a meta-analysis. *Med Sci Sports Exerc.* 2007;39:2099-2106.

Mental fatigue impairs physical performance in humans

Marcora SM, Staiano W, Manning V (Bangor Univ, Wales, UK)
J Appl Physiol 106:857-864, 2009

Mental fatigue is a psychobiological state caused by prolonged periods of demanding cognitive activity. Although the impact of mental fatigue on cognitive and skilled performance is well known, its effect on physical performance has not been thoroughly investigated. In this randomized crossover study, 16 subjects cycled to exhaustion at 80% of their peak power output after 90 min of a demanding cognitive task (mental fatigue) or 90 min of watching emotionally neutral documentaries (control). After experimental treatment, a mood questionnaire revealed a state of mental fatigue ($P = 0.005$) that significantly reduced time to exhaustion (640 ± 316 s) compared with the control condition (754 ± 339 s) ($P = 0.003$). This negative effect was not mediated by cardiorespiratory and musculoenergetic factors as physiological responses to intense exercise remained largely unaffected. Self-reported success and intrinsic motivation related to the physical task were also unaffected by prior cognitive activity. However, mentally fatigued subjects rated perception of effort during exercise to be significantly higher compared with the control condition ($P = 0.007$). As ratings of perceived exertion increased similarly over time in both conditions ($P < 0.001$), mentally fatigued subjects reached their maximal level of perceived exertion and disengaged from the physical task earlier than in the control condition. In conclusion, our study provides experimental evidence that mental fatigue limits exercise tolerance in humans through higher perception of effort rather than cardiorespiratory and musculoenergetic mechanisms. Future research in this

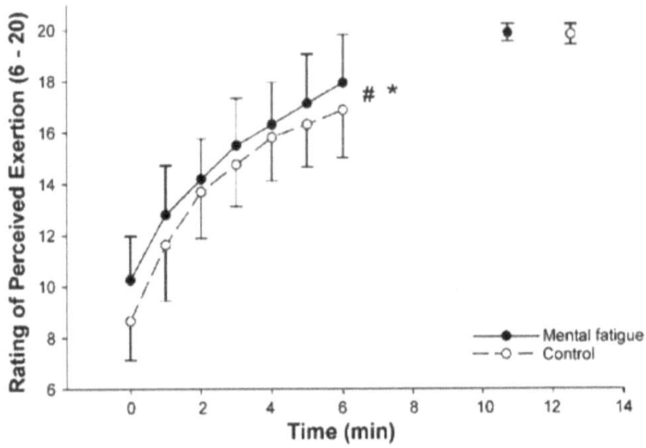

FIGURE 3.—Effect of mental fatigue on perception of effort during high-intensity cycling exercise. # Significant main effect of time ($P < 0.05$). *Significant main effect of condition ($P < 0.05$). Data are presented as means ± SD. *Minute 0* represents end of warm-up. (Reprinted from Marcora SM, Staiano W, Manning V. Mental fatigue impairs physical performance in humans. *J Appl Physiol.* 2009;106:857-864, with permission from the American Physiological Society.)

area should investigate the common neurocognitive resources shared by physical and mental activity (Fig 3).

▶ This intriguing study supports the belief that exercise performance is limited by mental fatigue and the perception of effort rather than cardiorespiratory and muscle energy factors (Fig 3). The authors propose several potential mechanisms. For example, mental fatigue before exercise may affect central processing of the sensory inputs generating perception of effort during exercise. Mental fatigue may also directly affect the anterior cingulate cortex (ACC), a cortical area in which motor control, homeostatic drive, emotion, and cognition converge. The ACC is affected by mental fatigue and is related to perception of effort during exercise[1]; and in animal studies, ACC lesions alter effort-based decision making.[2] Overall, this study provides strong evidence that brain function can limit short-term endurance performance, and future studies will determine if these results apply to long duration exercise conditions.

D. C. Nieman, DrPH

References

1. Williamson JW, Fadel PJ, Mitchell JH. New insights into central cardiovascular control during exercise in humans: a central command update. *Exp Physiol.* 2006;91:51-58.
2. Walton ME, Kennerley SW, Bannerman DM, Phillips PE, Rushworth MF. Weighing up the benefits of work: behavioral and neural analyses of effort-related decision making. *Neural Netw.* 2006;19:1302-1314.

Attentional processes and blood lactate levels

Coco M, Di Corrado D, Calogero RA, et al (Univ of Catania, Italy)
Brain Res 1302:205-211, 2009

The accumulation of lactate in the blood after a high-intensity exercise is associated to an increase of lactate extractions by the brain. However, no information has been provided about the influences of blood lactate on cognitive performances and, in particular, on attention. The present

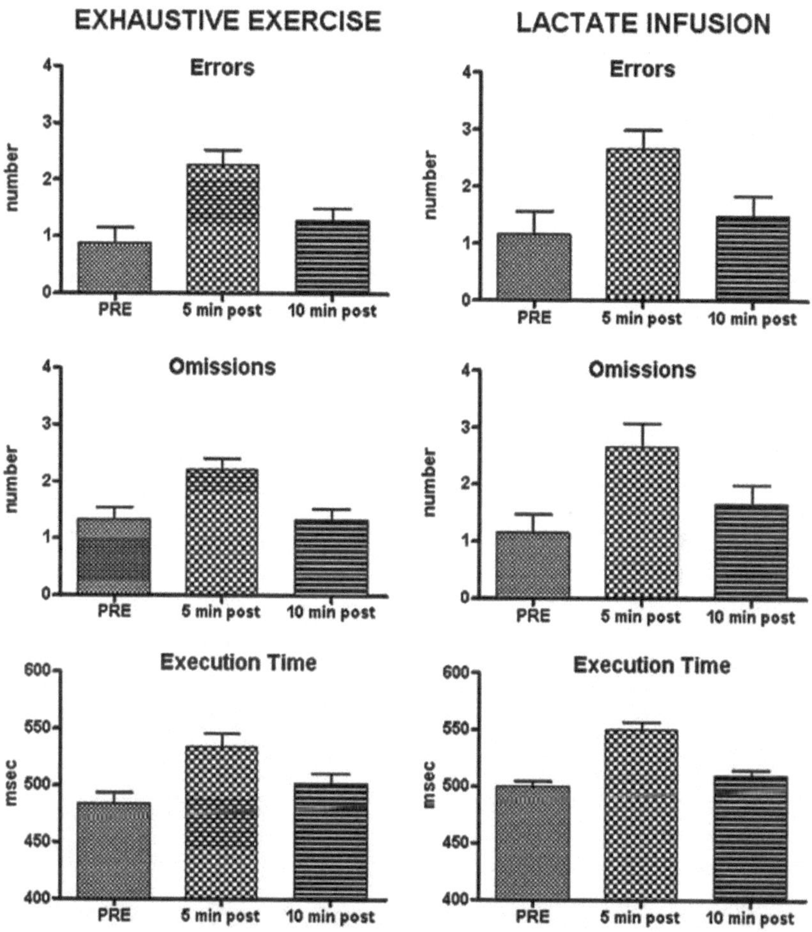

FIGURE 2.—Relationships between level of blood lactate and the three different parameters expressing selective attention, i.e. number of errors, number of omissions and duration of the performance (execution time). Graphics on the left illustrate data (± standard deviation) obtained in the 17 subjects before the exercise (PRE), as well as 5 min and 10 min after its end, whereas graphics on the right show data (± standard deviation) measured in 6 subjects before the lactate infusion (PRE), as well as 5 min and 10 min after its end. (Reprinted from Coco M, Di Corrado D, Calogero RA, et al. Attentional processes and blood lactate levels. *Brain Res.* 2009;1302:205-211, with permission from Elsevier.)

study was carried out to examine the association of high blood lactate levels, induced with a maximal cycling, with two different attentional tasks. The study was carried out on 17 male sprinters who performed exhaustive exercise. Before the exercise, as well as 5 and 10 min after the exhaustion, blood lactate was measured and intensity as well as selectivity of attention of each subject were evaluated. Same measurements were performed on 6 out of 17 subjects who accepted to receive an intravenous infusion of a lactate solution. In both experimental conditions, an inverse relation between scores in both aspects of attention and blood lactate levels was observed (Fig 2).

▶ Attention is a key component of performance in many types of competitive sport, and it is well recognized that either a fall of arterial oxygen concentration or a depletion of glucose, the main metabolic fuel of the brain, can have an adverse effect on attention. Less is known about the effects of an increase in blood lactate concentrations, although in vitro experiments have shown that elevated lactate concentrations can suppress neuronal firing and inhibit glucose metabolism in hippocampal slice cultures.[1] The decrease of cerebral performance seen with bouts of maximal exercise (Fig 2) might be attributable to factors other than lactate accumulation, such as a transient oxygen lack or the release of various hormones and cytokines, but the causal role of lactate is supported by the fact that very similar effects on cerebral performance are seen with the experimental infusion of equivalent concentrations of lactate. From a practical point of view, it seems possible that in some types of sport attention might be helped by the appropriately timed ingestion of sodium bicarbonate to counter a build-up of lactate.

R. J. Shephard, MD (Lond), PhD, DPE

Reference

1. Gilbert E, Tang JM, Ludvig N, et al. Elevated lactate suppresses neuronal firing in vivo and inhibits glucose metabolism in hippocampal slice cultures. *Brain Res.* 2006;1117:213-223.

Athletic Participation in Severe Hemophilia: Bleeding and Joint Outcomes in Children on Prophylaxis

Ross C, Goldenberg NA, Hund D, et al (Univ of Colorado Denver and Children's Hosp, Aurora)

Pediatrics 124:1267-1272, 2009

Objectives.—We sought to determine joint outcomes relative to impact level of athletic participation among school-aged children who had hemophilia and were taking prophylactic factor replacement, as well as to investigate prognostic factors for joint outcomes.

Methods.—School-aged boys with severe hemophilia A or B at a single center were included in the study. Clinical data on baseline joint status,

BMI, hemophilia treatment, bleeding episodes, joint assessments, athletic participation, and injuries were retrospectively reviewed. Data on athletic participation were supplemented, when incomplete in the medical record, via structured telephone interview.

Results.—Among 37 children with severe hemophilia A or B receiving factor prophylaxis, 73% participated in high-impact activities, whereas 27% participated in exclusively low-impact activities. The frequency of joint hemorrhages and new injuries did not appreciably differ between high- and low-impact athletics. In most instances, children developed <1 bleed or injury per season. A new target joint developed in 1 (3%) child. Sixteen percent of children met established BMI criteria for overweight, and 3% were obese. In logistic regression analyses with adjustment for prophylaxis frequency, level of athletic participation was not a significant prognostic factor for joint hemorrhage.

Conclusions.—In the setting of regular prophylaxis and adult coaching and supervision, significant bleeding complications were uncommon and level of impact of athletic participation was not a prognostic factor for joint outcomes. Athletic participation with appropriate supervision and precautions should be encouraged in children with hemophilia receiving prophylaxis, given potential health benefits in an increasingly overweight pediatric population.

▶ I have to admit to being rather surprised (yet pleased) with the findings in this report. Not long ago, worries over risk of serious bleeds (intracranial and articular) led to great concern regarding any form of vigorous physical activity, not to mention contact sports, in young patients with coagulation disorders. Times have changed. This study provides evidence that contemporary factor prophylaxis and appropriate coaching supervision permits these youth, even youth with severe hemophilia, to participate in athletics with minimal risk. The general message, too, is that we should be continuing to attempt to maximize exercise habits in young persons with chronic illnesses of all forms to the limits of either their abilities or disease risks. That such youngsters frequently develop sedentary lifestyles independent of the dictates of their disease is a recurring story.

T. Rowland, MD

5 Metabolism and Obesity, Nutrition and Doping

Cardiometabolic Abnormalities in Current National Football League Players

Selden MA, Helzberg JH, Waeckerle JF, et al (Univ of Missouri-Kansas City School of Medicine; et al)

Am J Cardiol 103:969-971, 2009

Media reports suggested an increased prevalence of cardiovascular disease and premature death in former National Football League (NFL) players. The prevalence of cardiometabolic syndrome was determined in current active NFL players. The presence of cardiometabolic syndrome was defined as ≥3 of (1) blood pressure ≥130/85 mm Hg, (2) fasting glucose ≥100 mg/dl, (3) triglycerides ≥150 mg/dl, (4) waist circumference ≥100 cm, and (5) high-density lipoprotein cholesterol ≤40 mg/dl. Sixty-nine of 91 players (76%) from 1 NFL team were studied before the 2008 preseason training camp. Cardiometabolic syndrome markers, body mass index (BMI), waist-height ratio, and triglycerides/high-density lipoprotein cholesterol ratio were compared between 69 players and an age-and gender-matched reference population from NHANES (1999 to 2002) and by player position of linemen versus nonlinemen. Blood pressure ≥130/85 mm Hg, glucose ≥100 mg/dl, and BMI ≥30 kg/m^2 were significantly more prevalent in the 69 players than the NHANES cohort (28% vs 17%, $p = 0.032$; 19% vs 7%, $p = 0.002$; and 51% vs 21%, $p < 0.001$, respectively), although cardiometabolic syndrome prevalence was similar in both groups. However, cardiometabolic syndrome prevalence, BMI >30 kg/m^2, and waist-height ratio >0.5 were significantly more common in the linemen versus the nonlinemen subgroup (22% vs 0%, $p = 0.004$; 100% vs 32%, $p < 0.001$, and 95% vs 36%, $p < 0.001$ respectively). In conclusion, cardiometabolic syndrome and its individual components were noted in current NFL players, particularly linemen.

▶ It has been recognized for many years that by middle age, major league football players and collegiate letter winners often become inactive, in part because of their inherent body build, and in part because of continued overeating and inactivity. Such individuals then become obese, and they commonly have

TABLE 1.—The Team Compared with the National Health and Nutrition Examination Survey (NHANES) Population

	Team	NHANES	p Value
Blood pressure ≥130/85 mm Hg	19 (28%)	17%	0.032
Glucose ≥100 mg/dl	13 (19%)	7%	0.002
Triglycerides ≥150 mg/dl	8 (12%)	24%	0.041
HDL cholesterol ≤40 mg/dl	6 (10%)	34%	<0.001
Triglycerides/HDL cholesterol ratio >3.5	7 (12%)	22%	0.085
Waist circumference ≥100 cm	26 (38%)	26%	0.057
Waist-height ratio >0.5	36 (52%)	55%	0.726
Cardiometabolic syndrome	4 (6%)	10%	0.355

a poorer health experience than the general population.[1-3] Premature deaths are particularly common in former athletes who have become obese, and cardiovascular disease is often the cause of their demise. However, it remains an open question as to whether football players already show an increased prevalence of obesity and the metabolic syndrome and thus a high cardiovascular risk while they are still active in their sport. The issue is of particular concern because linesmen are becoming ever heavier to an average of 113 kg in 2006. This study made a cross-sectional comparison between 69 National Football League (NFL) players and age- and sex-matched data from the United States National Health and Nutrition Examination Survey (NHANES) national reference population (Table 1). The football players fared more poorly than their peers in terms of both resting blood pressure and body mass index. The latter is plainly a fallible index of obesity in muscular individuals, although in the case of the linesmen some support for an accumulation of body fat was found in higher waist circumferences and waist circumference/height ratios than in the NHANES sample. Nevertheless, the author's conclusion of an increased cardiovascular risk must be accepted with caution because they had relatively high-density lipoprotein (HDL) cholesterol levels. There seems a need to repeat these studies with more direct measurements of body fat content either by underwater weighing or by skinfold measurements.

R. J. Shephard, MD (Lond), PhD, DPE

References

1. Miller MA, Croft LB, Belanger AR, et al. Prevalence of metabolic syndrome in retired National Football League players. *Am J Cardiol.* 2008;101:1281-1284.
2. Croft LB, Belanger A, Miller MA, Roberts A, Goldman ME. Comparison of National Football League linemen versus nonlinemen of left ventricular mass and left atrial size. *Am J Cardiol.* 2008;102:343-347.
3. Nicholas SJ, Nicholas JA, Nicholas C, Diecchio JR, McHugh MP. The health status of retired American football players. *Am J Sports Med.* 2007;35:1674-1679.

Cardiometabolic Abnormalities in Current National Football League Players

Selden MA, Helzberg JH, Waeckerle JF, et al (Univ of Missouri-Kansas City School of Medicine; et al)

Am J Cardiol 103:969-971, 2009

Media reports suggested an increased prevalence of cardiovascular disease and premature death in former National Football League (NFL) players. The prevalence of cardiometabolic syndrome was determined in current active NFL players. The presence of cardiometabolic syndrome was defined as ≥3 of (1) blood pressure ≥130/85 mm Hg, (2) fasting glucose ≥100 mg/dl, (3) triglycerides ≥150 mg/dl, (4) waist circumference ≥100 cm, and (5) high-density lipoprotein cholesterol ≤40 mg/dl. Sixty-nine of 91 players (76%) from 1 NFL team were studied before the 2008 preseason training camp. Cardiometabolic syndrome markers, body mass index (BMI), waist-height ratio, and triglycerides/high-density lipoprotein cholesterol ratio were compared between 69 players and an age-and gender-matched reference population from NHANES (1999 to 2002) and by player position of linemen versus nonlinemen. Blood pressure ≥130/85 mm Hg, glucose ≥100 mg/dl, and BMI ≥30 kg/m^2 were significantly more prevalent in the 69 players than the NHANES cohort (28% vs 17%, $p = 0.032$; 19% vs 7%, $p = 0.002$; and 51% vs 21%, $p < 0.001$, respectively), although cardiometabolic syndrome prevalence was similar in both groups. However, cardiometabolic syndrome prevalence, BMI ≥30 kg/m^2, and waist-height ratio >0.5 were significantly more common in the linemen versus the nonlinemen subgroup (22% vs 0%, $p = 0.004$; 100% vs 32%, $p < 0.001$, and 95% vs 36%, $p < 0.001$ respectively). In conclusion, cardiometabolic syndrome and its individual

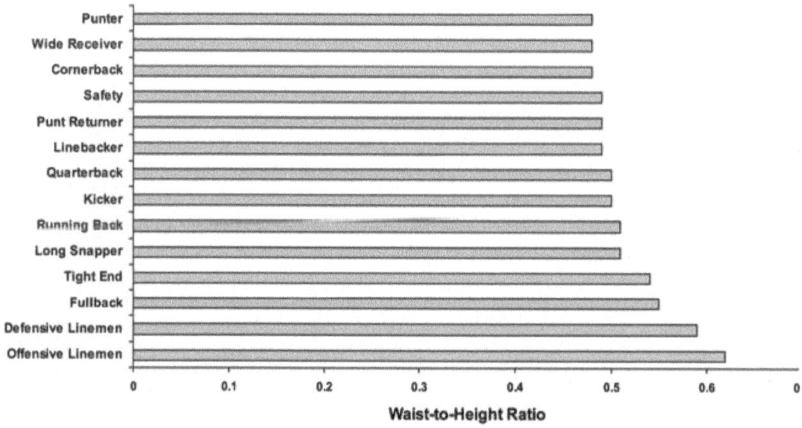

FIGURE 1.—Waist-height ratio by position in NFL players. (Reprinted from Selden MA, Helzberg JH, Waeckerle JF, et al. Cardiometabolic abnormalities in current national football league players. *Am J Cardiol.* 2009;103:969-971, with permission from Elsevier Inc.)

components were noted in current NFL players, particularly linemen (Fig 1).

▶ Previous studies and reports have shown that retired football linemen had an increased prevalence of disease risk factors and a substantially increased risk of dying of heart disease when compared with the general population.[1,2] In this study of current National Football League (NFL) team athletes, heavier NFL players had an elevated prevalence of cardiovascular risk factors and cardiometabolic syndrome. Fig 1 compares the waist-to-height ratio between players by position. The authors urged that careful medical evaluation of active players is warranted. Current players found to be at risk of future cardiovascular complications can undergo interventions to reduce their risk. These interventions may include both behavioral and medical therapy, particularly after their playing careers have concluded.

D. C. Nieman, DrPH

References

1. National Institute for Occupational Safety and Health. NFL mortality study, http://www.cdc.gov/niosh/pdfs/nflfactsheet.pdf.
2. Miller MA, Croft LB, Belanger AR, et al. Prevalence of metabolic syndrome in retired National Football League players. *Am J Cardiol.* 2008;101:1281-1284.

Pregame Urine Specific Gravity and Fluid Intake by National Basketball Association Players During Competition

Osterberg KL, Horswill CA, Baker LB (Gatorade Sports Science Inst, Barrington, IL)
J Athl Train 44:53-57, 2009

Context.—Urine specific gravity (USG) has been used to estimate hydration status in athletes on the field, with increasing levels of hypohydration indicated by higher USG measurements (eg, greater than 1.020). Whether initial hydration status based on a urine measure is related to subsequent drinking response during exercise or athletic competition is unclear.

Objective.—To determine the relationship between pregame USG and the volume of fluid consumed by players in a professional basketball game.

Design.—Cross-sectional study.

Setting.—Basketball players were monitored during Summer League competition.

Patients or Other Participants.—Players (n = 29) from 5 teams of the National Basketball Association agreed to participate.

Main Outcome Measure(s).—Pregame USG was measured for each player on 2 occasions. Athletes were given ad libitum access to fluid during each game and were unaware of the purpose of the study. Volume of fluid intake was measured for each player. To assess sweat loss, athletes were weighed in shorts before and after each game.

Results.—Sweat loss ranged from 1.0 to 4.6 L, with a mean sweat loss of 2.2 ± 0.8 L. Fluid intake ranged from 0.1 to 2.9 L, with a mean fluid intake of 1.0 ± 0.6 L. Pregame USG was greater than 1.020 in 52% of the urine samples collected and was not correlated with fluid volume consumed during either of the games ($r = 0.15$, $P = .48$, and $r = 0.15$, $P = .52$, respectively).

Conclusions.—Approximately half of the players began the games in a hypohydrated state, as indicated by USG. Fluid intake during the game did not compensate for poor hydration status before competition. Furthermore, sweat losses in these players during games were substantial (greater than 2 L in approximately 20 minutes of playing time). Therefore, both pregame and during-game hydration strategies, such as beverage availability and player education, should be emphasized.

▶ These are useful descriptive data, and confirm earlier reports that about half of individual and team-sport athletes are hypohydrated at the start of competition, with pregame urine specific gravity (USG) levels greater than 1.020.[1,2] Additionally, the average amount of fluid consumed during the National Basketball Association (NBA) basketball games (1.0 L) was less than half of the volume required to match sweat losses. Several factors may influence fluid replacement, including provision of individual bottles, proximity to bottles, duration and number of opportunities to drink, and awareness of personal sweating rates.[3] Together these data indicate that fluid replacement remains a challenge for some athletes and that positive hydration strategies should be employed by team trainers.

D. C. Nieman, DrPH

References

1. Bergeron MF, Waller JL, Marinik EL. Voluntary fluid intake and core temperature responses in adolescent tennis players: sports beverages versus water. *Br J Sports Med.* 2006;40:406-410.
2. Stover EA, Zachwieja JJ, Stofan JR, Murray R, Horswill CA. Consistently high urine specific gravity in adolescent American football players and the impact of an acute drinking strategy. *Int J Sports Med.* 2006;27:330-335.
3. Broad EM, Burke LM, Cox GR, Heeley P, Riley M. Body weight changes and voluntary fluid intakes during training and competition sessions in team sports. *Int J Sport Nutr.* 1996;6:307-320.

Plasma Vitamins, Amino Acids, and Renal Function in Postexercise Hyperhomocysteinemia

Venta R, Cruz E, Valcárcel G, et al (Hosp San Agustín, Avilés, Principado de Asturias, Spain; et al)

Med Sci Sports Exerc 41:1645-1651, 2009

Several studies have assessed the effect of the physical activity on plasma homocysteine (Hcy) concentrations, although the findings have been

TABLE 2.— Plasma or Serum Concentrations of Aminothiols, Vitamins, Creatinine, and Ratios (×100) before and after Exercise

	Kayakers		Cyclists	
	Before	After	Before	After
rHcy (μmol·L^{-1})[a,b]	0.182 ± 0.013	0.197 ± 0.013	0.149 ± 0.006	0.167 ± 0.006
tHcy (μmol·L^{-1})[a]	6.97 ± 0.44	8.16 ± 0.48	6.68 ± 0.27	7.87 ± 0.33
rCys (μmol·L^{-1})[a]	4.79 ± 0.26	4.93 ± 0.21	4.76 ± 0.13	5.26 ± 0.20
tCys (μmol·L^{-1})[a,b]	176.4 ± 3.4	188.5 ± 5.1	187.6 ± 3.9	211.2 ± 5.5
rHcy/rCys[a,b]	3.86 ± 0.24	4.02 ± 0.22	3.17 ± 0.15	3.23 ± 0.16
tHcy/tCys[a,c]	3.94 ± 0.21	4.31 ± 0.22	3.57 ± 0.15	3.75 ± 0.15
PLP (nmol·L^{-1})[a]	81.5 (201.9)	89.9 (223.6)	74.5 (529.3)	92.1 (655.1)
Vitamin B_{12} (pmol·L^{-1})[a,b]	342 ± 21	375 ± 21	696 ± 77	745 ± 95
Folate (nmol·L^{-1})	15.4 (34.2)	15.9 (26.1)	19.9 (36.7)	19.9 (36.2)
Creatinine (μmol·L^{-1})[a]	87.7 ± 2.3	109.9 ± 4.2	89.2 ± 2.0	109.3 ± 1.8

Values are means ± SEM or median (P_{90}). Log-transformed data were used for PLP and folate.
PLP, pyridoxal-5′-phosphate; rCys, reduced Cys; rHcy, reduced Hcy; tCys, total Cys; tHcy, total Hcy.
[a]Significant main effects from ANOVA: acute exercise.
[b]Significant main effects from ANOVA: group.
[c]Significant main effects from ANOVA: exercise × group interaction.

contradictory, and the exact mechanism by which plasma Hcy concentrations varied after an acute intense exercise remains unknown.

Purpose.—We studied the effect of different acute aerobic intense exercises on plasma, reduced, and total Hcy (rHcy, tHcy) and cysteine (rCys, tCys) and on its metabolically related vitamins and amino acids. Parallel effects on renal function were assessed by plasma creatinine.

Methods.—Fifteen cyclists and 14 kayakers were examined before and 30 ± 5 min after a specific test to exhaustion during a low-intensity training period.

Results.—After a bout of specific exercise, the concentrations of aminothiols were increased regardless of the group considered. Plasma concentrations were higher than baseline values in tHcy (17.7 ± 1.5%; $P < 0.001$), rHcy (10.6 ± 1.6%; $P < 0.001$), tCys (9.9 ± 1.6%; $P < 0.001$), and rCys (7.6 ± 2.2%; $P < 0.01$). Both groups showed significant elevations of pyridoxal-5′-phosphate (PLP; $P < 0.01$), vitamin B_{12} ($P < 0.001$), and creatinine concentrations ($P < 0.001$) after acute exercises, but no changes were seen in folate. Changes in plasma aminothiols after exercise did not reach significant correlation with changes in free amino acids or baseline vitamins, but significant and positive correlations were observed with changes in plasma PLP, vitamin B_{12}, and creatinine concentrations, when the pooled data were considered.

Conclusions.—Our results show that higher plasma concentrations of tHcy after an acute intense exercise are associated to higher concentrations of rHcy, and this effect is independent of the type of exercise, vitamin status, or amino acid metabolic stress but could be related to potential changes in the renal function (Table 2).

▶ Given the wide range of metabolic benefits associated with acute and chronic exercise, it is interesting to find at least one apparently negative metabolic consequence of vigorous physical activity, namely a temporary increase in plasma homocysteine (Table 2). High concentrations of plasma homocysteine are associated with atherosclerosis through several mechanisms: a prothrombotic effect, a cytotoxic effect, and endothelial dysfunction.[1,2] One previous report has also commented on increases in homocysteine during acute exercise,[3] although the more long-term effect seems to be a drop in homocysteine levels.[4,5] The underlying mechanism thus remains the subject of debate. Possibilities include an increased production of reactive species, an increased turnover of substrates such as acetylcholine, a temporary catabolism of muscle protein, or possibly simply a temporary reduction in renal clearance. Parallel increases in creatine levels suggest that temporary suppression of renal clearance is likely the most important factor. Also, given the beneficial response to habitual exercise, it seems unlikely that small acute exercise-induced increases in homocysteine have adverse health consequences.

R. J. Shephard, MD (Lond) PhD, DPE

References

1. Lawrence de Koning AB, Werstuck GH, Zhou J, Austin RC. Hyperhomocysteinemia and its role in the development of atherosclerosis. *Clin Biochem.* 2003;36: 431-441.
2. Welch GN, Loscalzo J. Homocysteine and atherothrombosis. *N Engl J Med.* 1998; 338:1042-1050.
3. König D, Bissé E, Deibert P, Müller HM, Wieland H, Berg A. Influence of training volume and acute physical exercise on the homocysteine levels in endurance-trained men: interactions with plasma folate and vitamin B12. *Ann Nutr Metab.* 2003;47:114-118.
4. Refsum H, Nurk E, Smith AD, et al. The Hordaland Homocysteine Study: a community-based study of homocysteine, its determinants, and associations with disease. *J Nutr.* 2006;136:1731S-1740S.
5. Unt E, Zilmer K, Mägi A, Kullisaar T, Kairane C, Zilmer M. Homocysteine status in former top-level male athletes: possible effect of physical activity and physical fitness. *Scand J Med Sci Sports.* 2008;18:360-366.

Objectively Measured Moderate- and Vigorous-Intensity Physical Activity but Not Sedentary Time Predicts Insulin Resistance in High-Risk Individuals

Ekelund U, Brage S, Griffin SJ, et al (Med Res Council Epidemiology Unit, Cambridge, UK)

Diabetes Care 32:1081-1086, 2009

Objective.—Low levels of physical activity appear to be associated with insulin resistance. However, the detailed associations of these complex relationships remain elusive. We examined the prospective associations between self-reported TV viewing time, objectively measured time spent

TABLE 2.—Associations Between Objectively Measured Time Estimates of Physical Activity and Self-reported TV and Video Viewing at Baseline with the HOMA Score and Fasting Insulin in Adults with a Family History of Type 2 Diabetes

	Baseline HOMA Score	*P* Value	Baseline Fasting Insulin	*P* Value	Follow-up HOMA Score	*P* Value	Follow-up Fasting Insulin	*P* Value
Sedentary (min/day)	0.0004 (−0.0006 to 0.001)	0.42	0.0004 (−0.0006 to 0.001)	0.39	0.001 (−0.002 to 0.00004)	0.21	0.001 (−0.0013 to 0.00005)	0.07
Light (min/day)	0.0001 (−0.001 to 0.001)	0.83	0.0002 (−0.001 to 0.001)	0.73	−0.001 (−0.001 to 0.0002)	0.16	−0.001 (−0.0013 to 0.0002)	0.18
MVPA (min/day)	−0.004 (−0.008 to −0.00001)	0.048	−0.005 (−0.008 to −0.001)	0.017	−0.003 (−0.007 to 0.000002)	0.052	−0.004 (−0.007 to −0.001)	0.022
TV/video (h/week)	0.01 (0.004 to 0.019)	0.002	0.01 (0.004 to 0.017)	0.002	−0.001 (−0.007 to 0.006)	0.88	0.0002 (−0.006 to 0.006)	0.99

Data are β coefficients (95% CI). $n = 192$. Data are adjusted for sex, age, smoking status (current, former, or never), and waist circumference. Prospective data are additionally adjusted for baseline phenotypes and follow-up time.

sedentary, at light-intensity activity, and at moderate- and vigorous-intensity physical activity (MVPA) with insulin resistance.

Research Design and Methods.—In 192 individuals (81 men and 111 women) with a family history of type 2 diabetes, we measured physical activity and anthropometric and metabolic variables at baseline and after 1 year of follow-up in the ProActive UK trial. Physical activity was measured objectively by accelerometry. Insulin resistance was expressed as fasting insulin and the homeostasis model assessment score (HOMA-IR).

Results.—Baseline MVPA was a significant predictor of fasting insulin at follow-up ($\beta = -0.004$ [95% CI -0.007 to -0.0001], $P = 0.022$), and the association approached significance for HOMA-IR ($\beta = -0.003$ [-0.007 to 0.000002], $P = 0.052$), independent of time spent sedentary, at light-intensity activity, sex, age, smoking status, waist circumference, and self-reported TV viewing. Time spent sedentary and at light-intensity activity were not significantly associated with insulin resistance. The change in MVPA between baseline and follow-up was inversely related to fasting insulin ($\beta = -0.003$ [-0.007 to -0.0003], $P = 0.032$) and the HOMA-IR score ($\beta = -0.004$ [-0.008 to -0.001], $P = 0.015$) at follow-up, after adjustment for baseline phenotype in addition to the same confounders as above.

Conclusions.—These results highlight the importance of promoting moderate-intensity activity such as brisk walking for improving insulin sensitivity and possibly other metabolic risk factors to prevent type 2 diabetes (Table 2).

▶ Several articles have suggested correlations between the time a person allocates to sedentary pursuits and abnormal glucose metabolism, the metabolic syndrome, or obesity.[1-3] Some authors have thus attributed health importance to the slight, incidental, and not otherwise noticed activity that is abolished when sitting watching television. However, it has not been entirely clear in such studies whether the reporting of sedentary behavior and the resulting elimination of incidental movement was a metabolic risk factor in itself, or whether it was merely serving as an indirect indicator of the type of person who took little moderate physical activity or engaged in other unhealthy behaviors (including the snack foods consumed while watching the television).[4] This article looks prospectively at insulin resistance in middle-aged overweight adults with a family history of diabetes, obtaining reports on TV viewing and making independent objective accelerometer measures of light and moderate physical activity. Only the last of these variables was independently associated with insulin resistance (Table 2). Limitations of the study were simple assessments of obesity (waist circumference) and insulin resistance (fasting insulin and homeostatic model assessment score rather than glucose tolerance). The self-reported TV viewing time also had some puzzling features suggestive of inaccurate recording, and the sampling of accelerometry data (4 successive days) was less than optimal. Nevertheless, this article suggests a need for further examination of the usefulness of making independent examination of the time spent in sedentary pursuits.

R. J. Shephard, MD (Lond), PhD, DPE

References

1. Dunstan DW, Salmon J, Healy GN, et al. Association of television viewing with fasting and 2-h postchallenge plasma glucose levels in adults without diagnosed diabetes. *Diabetes Care*. 2007;30:516-522.
2. Dunstan DW, Salmon J, Owen N, et al. Associations of TV viewing and physical activity with the metabolic syndrome in Australian adults. *Diabetologia*. 2005;48: 2254-2261.
3. Hu FB, Li TY, Colditz GA, Willett WC, Manson JE. Television watching and other sedentary behaviours in relation to risk of obesity and type 2 diabetes mellitus in women. *JAMA*. 2003;289:1785-1791.
4. Gore SA, Foster JA, DiLillo VG, Kirk K, Smith West D. Television viewing and snacking. *Eat Behav*. 2003;4:399-405.

Effects of Exercise Training Intensity on Pancreatic β-Cell Function

Slentz CA, Tanner CJ, Bateman LA, et al (Duke Univ Med Ctr, Durham, NC; East Carolina Univ, Greenville, NC)

Diabetes Care 32:1807-1811, 2009

Objective.—Insulin resistance and β-cell dysfunction both are important contributors to the pathogenesis of type 2 diabetes. Exercise training improves insulin sensitivity, but its effects on β-cell function are less well studied.

Research Design and Methods.—Sedentary, overweight adults were randomized to control or one of three 8-month exercise programs: *1)* low amount/moderate intensity, *2)* low amount/vigorous intensity, or *3)* high amount/vigorous intensity. Of 387 randomized, 260 completed the study and 237 had complete data. Insulin sensitivity (S_i), acute insulin response to glucose (AIRg), and the disposition index ($DI = S_i \times AIRg$) were modeled from an intravenous glucose tolerance test.

Results.—Compared with control subjects, all three training programs led to increases in DI. However, the moderate-intensity group experienced a significantly larger increase in DI than either of the vigorous-intensity groups and through a different mechanism. The high-amount/vigorous-intensity group improved S_i and had a compensatory reduction in AIRg, whereas the moderate-intensity group had a similar improvement in S_i but almost no reduction in AIRg. Importantly, the inactive control group experienced a significant increase in fasting glucose.

Conclusions.—To the extent that the DI accurately reflects β-cell function, we observed that both moderate- and vigorous-intensity exercise training improved β-cell function, albeit through distinct mechanisms. It is not clear which of these mechanisms is preferable for maintenance of metabolic health. While moderate-intensity exercise led to a larger improvement in DI, which may reflect a transition toward a more normal

DI, longer-term investigations would be necessary to determine which was more effective at reducing diabetes risk.

▶ The epidemic of type-2 diabetes mellitus appears to reflect both a decrease in sensitivity to insulin and a malfunction of the pancreatic β-cells.[1-3] As insulin sensitivity falls in the obese person there is a compensatory hyperactivity of the β-cells until these eventually fail.[4,5] The disposal index, used in this study, is a measure of the individual's capacity to respond to a loss of insulin sensitivity. The volume and intensity of the 3 exercise regimens chosen for the present 8-month experiment reflect the treatment of obese subjects; the high intensity, high volume program was at 65% to 80% of peak oxygen intake, but corresponded to no more than 32 km of walking or jogging per week, a normal exercise routine for many active elderly people, and perhaps for this reason program adherence (67%) was relatively good. Somewhat surprisingly, although all 3 exercise groups tended to improve, the largest increase in the index of β-cell function was seen with the moderate intensity low volume group (Fig 1 in the original article). The authors caution that further, longer duration studies are needed to confirm that the moderate intensity low volume program has the greatest effect in reducing the risk of developing diabetes. The findings are puzzling, as traditional markers of success such as reductions in obesity were greater in the subjects taking more physical activity. One possible factor contributing to differences in response is that a greater proportion of fat is metabolized with lower intensity exercise, with less of a resultant tendency to lipotoxicity in the pancreas.[6]

R. J. Shephard, MD (Lond), PhD, DPE

References

1. Kahn S, Hull R, Utzschneider K. Mechanisms linking obesity to insulin resistance and to type 2 diabetes. *Nature.* 2006;444:840-846.
2. Ferrannini E, Gastaldelli A, Miayzaki Y, et al. Predominant role of reduced beta-cell sensitivity to glucose over insulin resistance in impaired glucose tolerance. *Diabetologia.* 2003;46:1211-1219.
3. Bergman R. Banting lecture 2006: orchestration of glucose homeostasis: from a small acorn to the California Oak. *Diabetes.* 2007;56:1489-1500.
4. Hong J, Gu W, Zhang Y, et al. The interplay of insulin resistance and beta-cell dysfunction involves the development of type 2 diabetes in Chinese obeses. *Endocrine.* 2007;31:93-99.
5. Kahn S. Clinical review 135: the importance of beta cell failure in the development and progression of type 2 diabetes. *J Clin Endocrinol Metab.* 2001;86:4047-4058.
6. Slentz C, Houmard J, Johnson J, et al. Inactivity, exercise training and detraining, and plasma lipoproteins: STRRIDE: a randomized, controlled study of exercise intensity and amount. *J Appl Physiol.* 2007;103:432-442.

Effects of Quercetin and EGCG on Mitochondrial Biogenesis and Immunity

Nieman DC, Henson DA, Maxwell KR, et al (Appalachian State Univ, Boone, NC)

Med Sci Sports Exerc 41:1467-1475, 2009

Purpose.—To test the influence of 1000 mg of quercetin (Q) with or without 120 mg of epigallocatechin 3-gallate (EGCG), 400 mg of isoquercetin, and 400 mg of eicosapentaenoic acid and docosahexaenoic acid (Q–EGCG) on exercise performance, muscle mitochondrial biogenesis, and changes in measures of immunity and inflammation before and after a 3-d period of heavy exertion.

Methods.—Trained cyclists ($N = 39$) were randomized to placebo (P), Q, or Q–EGCG and ingested supplements in a double-blinded fashion for 2 wk before, during, and 1 wk after a 3-d period in which subjects cycled for $3\ h\cdot d^{-1}$ at ~57% W_{max}. Blood, saliva, and muscle biopsy samples were collected before and after 2 wk of supplementation and immediately after the exercise bout on the third day. Blood and saliva samples were also collected 14 h after exercise.

Results.—Two-week supplementation resulted in a significant increase in plasma quercetin for Q and Q–EGCG and granulocyte oxidative burst activity (GOBA) in Q–EGCG. Immediately after the third exercise bout, significant decreases for C-reactive protein (CRP), and plasma interleukin 6 (IL-6) and interleukin 10 (IL-10) were measured in Q–EGCG compared with P. Granulocyte colony-stimulating factor and CRP were reduced in Q–EGCG 14 h after exercise. No group differences were measured in muscle messenger RNA expression for peroxisome proliferator-activated receptor γ coactivator α, citrate synthase, or cytochrome *c*.

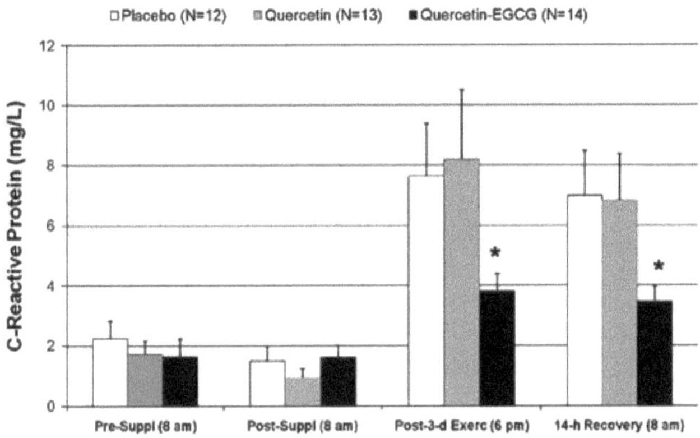

FIGURE 2.—Serum CRP before and after 2 wk of supplementation and immediately and 14 h after exercise. Group × time interaction P value = 0.023. *$P < 0.05$, change from before supplementation compared with placebo. (Reprinted from Nieman DC, Henson DA, Maxwell KR, et al. Effects of quercetin and EGCG on mitochondrial biogenesis and immunity. *Med Sci Sports Exerc.* 2009;41:1467-1475.)

Conclusions.—Two-week supplementation with Q–EGCG was effective in augmenting GOBA and in countering inflammation after 3 d of heavy exertion in trained cyclists (Fig 2).

▶ Quercetin exerts powerful anti-inflammatory and antioxidative effects in vitro, but a growing number of human studies indicate that 100 to 1000 mg of quercetin per day (in aglycone form) does not counter exercise-induced inflammation or chronic resting inflammation.[1] The bioavailability of quercetin is low (~25%), and what does pass through the small intestine and liver is extensively conjugated and thus metabolically transformed. However, when we gave athletes quercetin with green tea extract, fish oil, and isoquercetin (as found naturally in plants), postexercise inflammation was reduced (relative to placebo or quercetin alone) (Fig 2). These findings are in agreement with a growing number of in vitro and in vivo studies indicating that the pharma approach to nutritional supplements does not work, and that a flavonoid-food component cocktail supplement exerts the expected bioactive effects.[2,3] Future research will determine whether the addition of other polyphenols such as resveratrol and curcumin amplify quercetin's anti-inflammatory effects in athletes during and after heavy exertion.

D. C. Nieman, DrPH

References

1. Bae SC, Jung WJ, Lee EJ, Yu R, Sung MK. Effects of antioxidant supplements intervention on the level of plasma inflammatory molecules and disease severity of rheumatoid arthritis patients. *J Am Coll Nutr.* 2009;28:56-62.
2. Zamin LL, Filippi-Chiela EC, Dillenburg-Pilla P, Horn F, Salbego C, Lenz G. Resveratrol and quercetin cooperate to induce senescence-like growth arrest in C6 rat glioma cells. *Cancer Sci.* 2009;100:1655-1662.
3. Kale A, Gawande S, Kotwal S, et al. Studies on the effects of oral administration of nutrient mixture, quercetin and red onions on the bioavailability of epigallocatechin gallate from green tea extract. *Phytother Res. 2009.*

Coingestion of protein with carbohydrate during recovery from endurance exercise stimulates skeletal muscle protein synthesis in humans

Howarth KR, Moreau NA, Phillips SM, et al (McMaster Univ, Ontario, Canada)
J Appl Physiol 106:1394-1402, 2009

Coingestion of protein with carbohydrate (CHO) during recovery from exercise can affect muscle glycogen synthesis, particularly if CHO intake is suboptimal. Another potential benefit of protein feeding is an increased synthesis rate of muscle proteins, as is well documented after resistance exercise. In contrast, the effect of nutrient manipulation on muscle protein kinetics after aerobic exercise remains largely unexplored. We tested the hypothesis that ingesting protein with CHO after a standardized 2-h bout of cycle exercise would increase mixed muscle fractional synthetic rate (FSR) and whole body net protein balance (WBNB) vs. trials matched

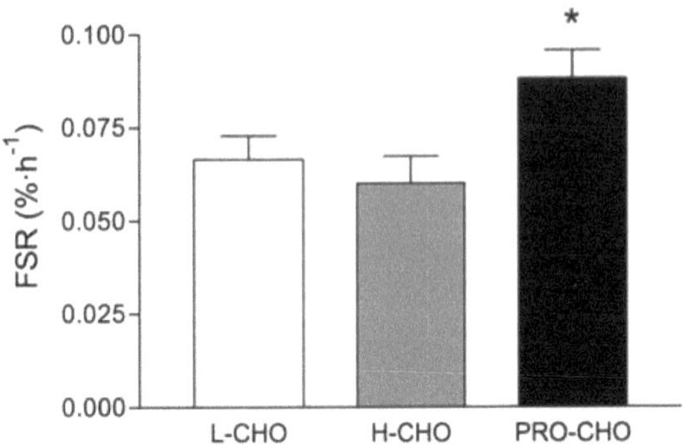

FIGURE 4.—Mixed muscle protein fractional synthetic rate (FSR) during 4 h of recovery from prolonged exercise while ingesting either 1.2 g CHO $\cdot$ kg^{-1} $\cdot$ h^{-1} (L-CHO), 1.6 g CHO $\cdot$ kg^{-1} $\cdot$ h^{-1} (H-CHO), or 1.2 g CHO + 0.4 g protein $\cdot$ kg^{-1} $\cdot$ h^{-1} (PRO-CHO). Values are means ± SE; $n = 6$. *$P < 0.05$ vs. other treatments. (Reprinted form Howarth KR, Moreau NA, Phillips SM, et al. Coingestion of protein with carbohydrate during recovery from endurance exercise stimulates skeletal muscle protein synthesis in humans. *J Appl Physiol.* 2009;106:1394-1402, with permission from American Physiological Society.)

for total CHO or total energy intake. We also examined whether postexercise glycogen synthesis could be enhanced by adding protein or additional CHO to a feeding protocol that provided 1.2 g CHO $\cdot$ kg^{-1} $\cdot$ h^{-1}, which is the rate generally recommended to maximize this process. Six active men ingested drinks during the first 3 h of recovery that provided either 1.2 g CHO $\cdot$ kg^{-1} $\cdot$ h^{-1} (L-CHO), 1.2 g CHO + 0.4 g protein $\cdot$ kg^{-1} $\cdot$ h^{-1} (PROCHO), or 1.6 g CHO $\cdot$ kg^{-1} $\cdot$ h^{-1} (H-CHO) in random order. Based on a primed constant infusion of L-[*ring*-$^{2}H_5$] phenylalanine, analysis of biopsies (vastus lateralis) obtained at 0 and 4 h of recovery showed that muscle FSR was higher ($P < 0.05$) in PRO-CHO (0.09 ± 0.01%/h) vs. both L-CHO (0.07 ± 0.01%/h) and H-CHO (0.06 ± 0.01%/h). WBNB assessed using [1-^{13}C]leucine was positive only during PRO-CHO, and this was mainly attributable to a reduced rate of protein breakdown. Glycogen synthesis rate was not different between trials. We conclude that ingesting protein with CHO during recovery from aerobic exercise increased muscle FSR and improved WBNB, compared with feeding strategies that provided CHO only and were matched for total CHO or total energy intake. However, adding protein or additional CHO to a feeding strategy that provided 1.2 g CHO $\cdot$ kg^{-1} $\cdot$ h^{-1} did not further enhance glycogen resynthesis during recovery (Fig 4).

▶ As summarized in Fig 4, coingestion of protein with carbohydrate (CHO) during recovery from 2-h endurance exercise increased mixed skeletal muscle fractional synthetic rate (FSR) and induced a more positive whole body net protein balance compared with drinks matched for total CHO or total energy intake. This is the first study to measure these effects using the needle biopsy technique, and the results are consistent with other studies using arterial-venous difference measurements.[1,2] As stated by the authors, "the higher FSR during recovery could promote muscle adaptation during recovery from acute exercise by stimulating the synthesis or repair of proteins that facilitate energy provision and force production." Whether or not using carbohydrate-protein beverages during exercise recovery promotes better muscle adaptation than simply eating regular meals at normal intervals has yet to be determined, but it is doubtful that a meaningful difference on performance will be found.

D. C. Nieman, DrPH

References

1. Levenhagen DK, Carr C, Carlson MG, Maron DJ, Borel MJ, Flakoll PJ. Postexercise protein intake enhances whole-body and leg protein accretion in humans. *Med Sci Sports Exerc.* 2002;34:828-837.
2. Levenhagen DK, Gresham JD, Carlson MG, Maron DJ, Borel MJ, Flakoll PJ. Post-exercise nutrient intake timing in humans is critical to recovery of leg glucose and protein homeostasis. *Am J Physiol Endocrinol Metab.* 2001;280:E982-E993.

Effects of resistance exercise and fortified milk on skeletal muscle mass, muscle size, and functional performance in middle-aged and older men: an 18-mo randomized controlled trial

Kukuljan S, Nowson CA, Sanders K, et al (Deakin Univ, Melbourne, Australia; The Univ of Melbourne, Geelong, Australia)

J Appl Physiol 107:1864-1873, 2009

Limited data have suggested that the consumption of fluid milk after resistance training (RT) may promote skeletal muscle hypertrophy. The aim of this study was to assess whether a milk-based nutritional supplement could enhance the effects of RT on muscle mass, size, strength, and function in middle-aged and older men. This was an 18-mo factorial design (randomized control trial) in which 180 healthy men aged 50–79 yr were allocated to the following groups: *1*) exercise + fortified milk, *2*) exercise, *3*) fortified milk, or *4*) control. Exercise consisted of progressive RT with weight-bearing impact exercise. Men assigned to the fortified milk consumed 400 ml/day of low-fat milk, providing an additional 836 kJ, 1000 mg calcium, 800 IU vitamin D_3, and 13.2 g protein per day. Total body lean mass (LM) and fat mass (FM) (dual-energy X-ray absorptiometry), midfemur muscle cross-sectional area (CSA) (quantitative computed tomography), muscle strength, and physical function were assessed. After 18 mo, there was no significant exercise by fortified milk interaction for total body LM, muscle CSA, or any functional measure. However, main effect analyses revealed that exercise significantly improved muscle strength (~20–52%, $P < 0.001$), LM (0.6 kg, $P < 0.05$), FM (−1.1 kg, $P < 0.001$), muscle CSA (1.8%, $P < 0.001$), and gait speed (11%, $P < 0.05$) relative to no exercise. There were no effects of the fortified milk on muscle size, strength, or function. In conclusion, the daily consumption of low-fat fortified milk does not enhance the effects of RT

on skeletal muscle size, strength, or function in healthy middle-aged and older men with adequate energy and nutrient intakes.

▶ Kukuljan and colleagues tested the hypothesis that progressive resistance exercise training combined with fortified milk would result in greater skeletal muscle strength, size, and function than either exercise or milk alone in middle-aged and older men (50-79 years). Fortified milk is a good source of dietary protein, vitamin D_3 (cholecalciferol), and calcium. The link between milk and resistance exercise is that muscle protein synthesis in response to a mechanical stimulus would be enhanced by the milk proteins casein and whey, whereas vitamin D_3 would support muscle function. Vitamin D deficiency has been associated with muscle weakness and poor physical function in older adults. The 400 mL per day milk supplement (approximately 13.5 oz) was fortified with 500 mg calcium and 400 IU of vitamin D_3 per 200 mL. The calcium fortification of the milk was more closely aligned with the companion study from Kukuljan et al,[1] which focused on changes in bone mineral density (BMD). In the United States, 8 oz of milk contains 290 mg calcium and is fortified with approximately 120 IU of vitamin D_3. The participants ($n = 180$) had not engaged in resistance training for at least 1 year and had normal to below average BMD but were not osteoporotic. They were in good health, and their diets were not deficient in protein or calcium. Serum 25-hydroxyvitamin D was, on average, in the normal range at baseline. The men were randomly assigned to 1 of 4 experimental groups: exercise, exercise and milk, milk alone, or control and were studied for 18 months. As expected, resistance exercise training resulted in significant increases in muscle strength, thigh muscle cross-sectional area (CSA), and total body lean tissue mass by 12 months and gait speed by 18 months. The fortified milk did not augment the effects of exercise on these outcomes. Fat and lean mass increased significantly in groups consuming milk compared with the other 2 groups. Notably, the timing of the ingestion of the milk was not controlled. Previous studies suggest that dietary protein stimulates skeletal muscle protein synthesis when consumed within a narrow time frame of the conclusion of exercise (eg, within 2 hours). Thus, a significant exercise and milk interaction may have been found if milk consumption was standardized to the exercise sessions. Furthermore, the modest exercise training intensity stimulated a small, albeit significant, increase in midthigh CSA (1.8%). Each session comprised 2 sets of exercises, one at 60% to 65% of the 1-repetition maximum (1-RM) and the second at an intensity of 80% to 85% 1-RM. The findings of the companion study of skeletal responses were similar to that of muscle, that is, a significant effect of exercise training on femoral neck and lumbar spine BMD but no additive benefits of fortified milk. Fortified milk may enhance the musculoskeletal adaptations to resistance training in men with compromised health or dietary deficiencies, such as those who are frail, osteoporotic, consume inadequate dietary protein, or are vitamin D deficient.

C. M. Jankowski, PhD

Reference

1. Kukuljan S, Nowson CA, Bass SL, et al. Effects of a multi-component exercise program and calcium-vitamin D3-fortified milk on bone mineral density in older men: a randomised controlled trial. *Osteoporosis Int.* 2009;20:1241-1251.

Effects of resistance exercise and fortified milk on skeletal muscle mass, muscle size, and functional performance in middle-aged and older men: an 18-mo randomized controlled trial

Kukuljan S, Nowson CA, Sanders K, et al (Deakin Univ, Melbourne, Australia; Univ of Melbourne, Geelong, Australia; et al)

J Appl Physiol 107:1864-1873, 2009

Limited data have suggested that the consumption of fluid milk after resistance training (RT) may promote skeletal muscle hypertrophy. The aim of this study was to assess whether a milk-based nutritional supplement could enhance the effects of RT on muscle mass, size, strength, and function in middle-aged and older men. This was an 18-mo factorial design (randomized control trial) in which 180 healthy men aged 50–79 yr were allocated to the following groups: *1*) exercise + fortified milk, *2*) exercise, *3*) fortified milk, or *4*) control. Exercise consisted of progressive RT with weight-bearing impact exercise. Men assigned to the fortified milk consumed 400 ml/day of low-fat milk, providing an additional 836 kJ, 1000 mg calcium, 800 IU vitamin D_3, and 13.2 g protein per day. Total body lean mass (LM) and fat mass (FM) (dual-energy X-ray absorptiometry), midfemur muscle cross-sectional area (CSA) (quantitative computed tomography), muscle strength, and physical function were assessed. After 18 mo, there was no significant exercise by fortified milk interaction for total body LM, muscle CSA, or any functional measure. However, main effect analyses revealed that exercise significantly improved muscle strength (~20–52%, $P < 0.001$), LM (0.6 kg, $P < 0.05$), FM (−1.1 kg, $P < 0.001$), muscle CSA (1.8%, $P < 0.001$), and gait speed (11%, $P < 0.05$) relative to no exercise. There were no effects of the fortified milk on muscle size, strength, or function. In conclusion, the daily consumption of low-fat fortified milk does not enhance the effects of RT on skeletal muscle size, strength, or function in healthy middle-aged and older men with adequate energy and nutrient intakes (Fig 2).

▶ This is a well-designed, long-term study with a large number of middle-aged and elderly male subjects. As supported in other investigations, resistance training (3 days/wk for 18 weeks) improved muscle strength and size in these older subjects (Fig 2). Contrary to expectations, however, drinking 1.5 glasses of milk per day increased protein intake by 16% but did not improve muscle strength or size outcome measures. Milk advocates urge that dairy foods, especially whole or fat-free milk, represent an ideal food source to enhance muscle protein synthesis and hypertrophy.[1,2] Proposed mechanisms

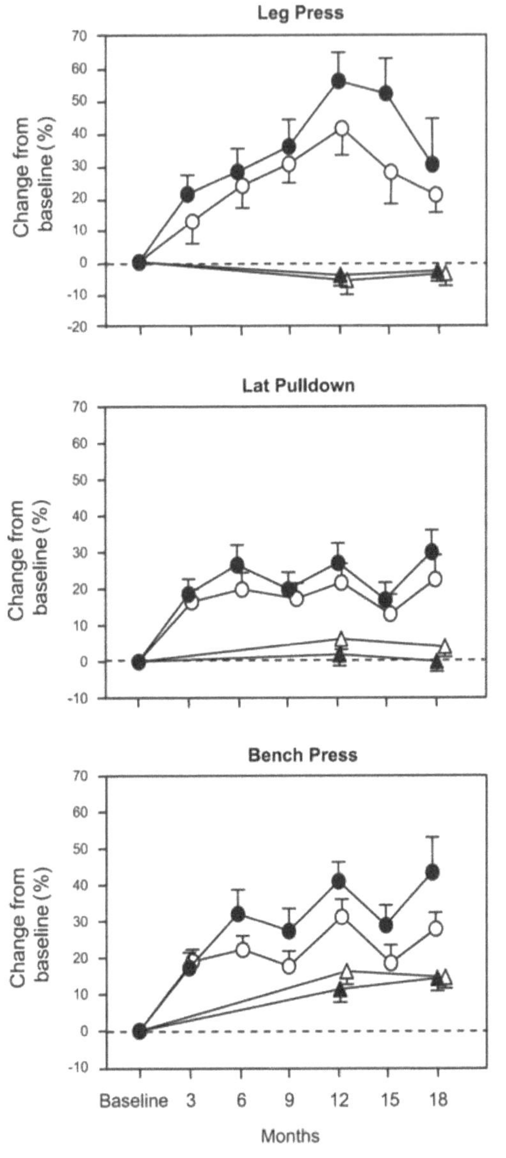

FIGURE 2.—Mean percentage changes (±SE) from baseline for upper body (bench press), back (lat pull down), and lower body (leg press) muscle strength according to group. Exercise resulted in significant increases in all muscle strength measures relative to both baseline and to the nonexercise group (main effects: all $P < 0.001$). Reprinted with permission from Kukuljan S, Nowson CA, Sanders K, et al. Effects of resistance exercise and fortified milk on skeletal muscle mass, muscle size, and functional performance in middle-aged and older men: an 18-mo randomized controlled trial. *J Appl Physiol*. 2009;107:1864-1873.)

include the mix of casein protein in milk, which is considered a slow protein that inhibits protein breakdown and whey protein, which is referred to as a fast protein that stimulates synthesis. Other factors present in whole milk (eg, vitamins, minerals, and carbohydrates) could add to these beneficial effects on muscle. However, as the data of this study demonstrate, the consumption of extra milk within the context of the total diet does not boost improvements in muscle strength and size beyond the stimulus provided from the resistance training program itself.

D. C. Nieman, DrPH

References

1. Elliot TA, Cree MG, Sanford AP, Wolfe RR, Tipton KD. Milk ingestion stimulates net muscle protein synthesis following resistance exercise. *Med Sci Sports Exer.* 2006;38:667-674.
2. Wilkinson SB, Tarnopolsky MA, Macdonald MJ, Macdonald JR, Armstrong D, Phillips SM. Consumption of fluid skim milk promotes greater muscle protein accretion after resistance exercise than does consumption of an isonitrogenous and isoenergetic soy-protein beverage. *Am J Clin Nutr.* 2007;85:1031-1040.

Dieting to win or to be thin? A study of dieting and disordered eating among adolescent elite athletes and non-athlete controls

Martinsen M, Bratland-Sanda S, Eriksson AK, et al (Norwegian School of Sport Sciences, Oslo; et al)

Br J Sports Med 44:70-76, 2010

Objective.—To examine the prevalence of dieting, reasons for dieting and prevalence of disordered eating among adolescent elite athletes and age-matched controls, and to examine the differences between athletes competing in leanness and non-leanness sports.

Methods.—First-year students of 16 different Norwegian Elite Sport High Schools (athlete group, n = 682) and two randomly selected ordinary high schools from a county representative of the general Norwegian population (control group, n = 423) were invited to participate in this cross-sectional study. A total of 606 athletes and 355 controls completed the questionnaire, giving a response rate of 89% and 84%, respectively. The questionnaire contained questions regarding training patterns, menstrual status and history, dieting, use of pathogenic weight control methods and the drive for thinness (DT) and body dissatisfaction (BD) subscales from the Eating Disorders Inventory.

Main Outcome Measure.—Disordered eating, defined as meeting one or more of the following criteria: DT score ≥15 (girls) and ≥10 (boys), BD score ≥14 (girls) and ≥10 (boys), body mass index <17.9 kg/m^2 (girls) and <17.5 kg/m^2 (boys), current and/or ≥3 previous efforts to lose weight, use of pathogenic weight control methods and self-reported menstrual dysfunction.

Results.—A higher prevalence of control subjects were dieting and classified with disordered eating compared with the athletes. An improvement of appearance was a more common reason for dieting among controls compared with athletes. No differences in dieting or disordered eating were found between leanness and nonleanness sports athletes.

Conclusions.—Self-reported disordered eating is more prevalent among controls than adolescent elite athletes, and losing weight to enhance performance is an important reason for dieting among adolescent elite athletes.

▶ In this study of nearly 1000 Norwegian adolescents, elite athletes had a lower frequency of disordered eating behavior than nonathletes. Previous studies have presented a mixed picture, but the best data support that disordered eating is less of a problem among adolescent athletes than it is in the community at large. The athletes' positive outlook of life and high self-efficacy may serve as protective factors for disordered eating.[1] Additionally, fewer athletes compared with controls are obese or dissatisfied with their bodies. Nonetheless, 11% of the adolescent athletes were dieting, with some using extreme methods such as diuretics, vomiting, and laxatives. The prevalence of disordered eating was 5 times higher for girl versus boy athletes, and performance and appearance were the primary objectives. In general, adolescents, whether athletic or not, need continued education and guidance regarding healthful lifestyle methods for controlling body weight.

D. C. Nieman, DrPH

Reference

1. Fulkerson JA, Keel PK, Leon GR, Dorr T. Eating-disordered behaviors and personality characteristics of high school athletes and nonathletes. *Int J Eat Disord.* 1999;26:73-79.

Dietary nitrate supplementation reduces the O_2 cost of low-intensity exercise and enhances tolerance to high-intensity exercise in humans

Bailey SJ, Winyard P, Vanhatalo A, et al (Univ of Exeter, UK)

J Appl Physiol 107:1144-1155, 2009

Pharmacological sodium nitrate supplementation has been reported to reduce the O_2 cost of submaximal exercise in humans. In this study, we hypothesized that dietary supplementation with inorganic nitrate in the form of beetroot juice (BR) would reduce the O_2 cost of submaximal exercise and enhance the tolerance to high-intensity exercise. In a double-blind, placebo (PL)-controlled, crossover study, eight men (aged 19–38 yr) consumed 500 ml/day of either BR (containing 11.2 ± 0.6 mM of nitrate) or blackcurrant cordial (as a PL, with negligible nitrate content) for 6 consecutive days and completed a series of "step" moderate-intensity and severe-intensity exercise tests on the last 3 days.

On *days* 4–6, plasma nitrite concentration was significantly greater following dietary nitrate supplementation compared with PL (BR: 273 ± 44 vs. PL: 140 ± 50 nM; $P < 0.05$), and systolic blood pressure was significantly reduced (BR: 124 ± 2 vs. PL: 132 ± 5 mmHg; $P < 0.01$). During moderate exercise, nitrate supplementation reduced muscle fractional O_2 extraction (as estimated using nearinfrared spectroscopy). The gain of the increase in pulmonary O_2 uptake following the onset of moderate exercise was reduced by 19% in the BR condition (BR: 8.6 ± 0.7 vs. PL: 10.8 ± 1.6 $ml \cdot min^{-1} \cdot W^{-1}$; $P < 0.05$). During severe

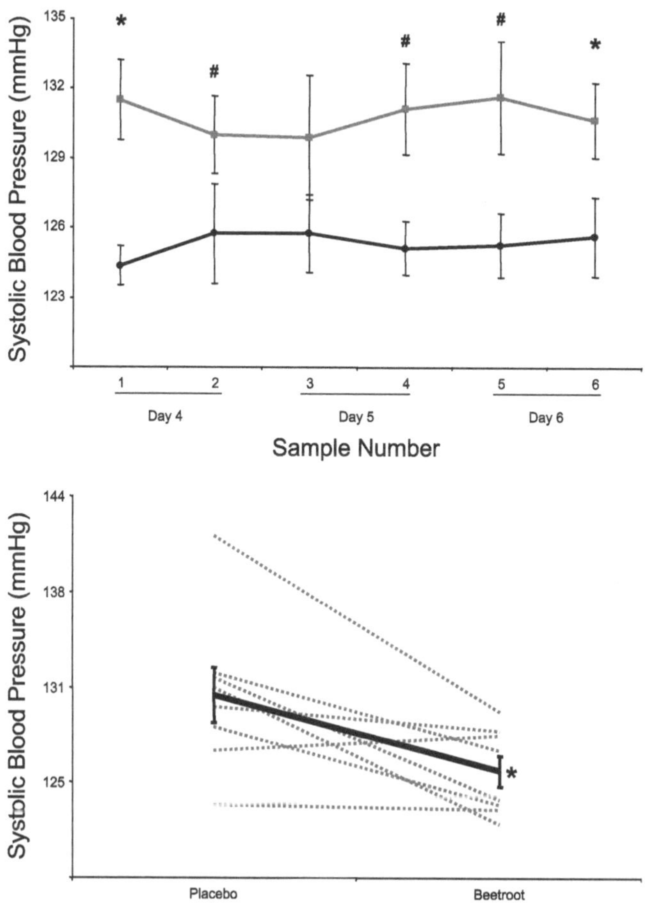

FIGURE 2.—Systolic blood pressure (SBP) following 4–6 days of dietary nitrate or placebo supplementation. *Top*: group mean (±SE) values of SBP on *days 4, 5,* and *6* of supplementation with either nitrate (solid circles) or placebo (shaded squares). Note the significantly lower SBP following dietary nitrate supplementation. Significant difference from placebo at corresponding time point at the #5% and *1% levels of significance are given. *Bottom*: individual (dotted shaded lines) and mean ± SE (solid line) values for SBP measured over *days 4, 5,* and 6. *$P < 0.01$. (Reprinted with permission from Bailey SJ, Winyard P, Vanhatalo A, et al. Dietary nitrate supplementation reduces the O_2 cost of low-intensity exercise and enhances tolerance to high-intensity exercise in humans. *J Appl Physiol.* 2009;107:1144-1155.)

exercise, the O_2 uptake slow component was reduced (BR: 0.57 ± 0.20 vs. PL: 0.74 ± 0.24 l/min; $P < 0.05$), and the time-to-exhaustion was extended (BR: 675 ± 203 vs. PL: 583 ± 145 s; $P < 0.05$). The reduced O_2 cost of exercise following increased dietary nitrate intake has important implications for our understanding of the factors that regulate mitochondrial respiration and muscle contractile energetics in humans (Fig 2).

▶ Vegetables account for 60% to 80% of daily nitrate intake. In the body, nitrate is converted to the bioactive nitrite, and then under favorable physiological conditions it is converted to nitric oxide (NO). NO is known to be an important endothelial relaxing factor. Beetroot juice is high in nitrate, and this study showed that drinking 0.5 L/day for 6 days doubled plasma nitrite levels, reduced the oxygen cost of cycling at a fixed submaximal work rate by 20% and systolic blood pressure by 6 mm Hg (Fig 2), and increased the time to fatigue during severe exercise. The authors suggested that their results mean that increased diet intake of nitrates through beetroot juice has the potential to enhance exercise tolerance during long duration endurance exercise. Additional research, however, is needed to understand underlying mechanisms.[1]

D. C. Nieman, DrPH

Reference

1. Larsen FJ, Ekblom B, Sahlin K, Lundberg JO, Weitzberg E. Effects of dietary nitrate on oxygen cost during exercise. *Acta Physiol (Oxf)*. 2007;191:59-66.

Dietary nitrate supplementation reduces the O_2 cost of low-intensity exercise and enhances tolerance to high-intensity exercise in humans

Bailey SJ, Winyard P, Vanhatalo A, et al (Univ of Exeter, UK)

J Appl Physiol 107:1144-1155, 2009

Pharmacological sodium nitrate supplementation has been reported to reduce the O_2 cost of submaximal exercise in humans. In this study, we hypothesized that dietary supplementation with inorganic nitrate in the form of beetroot juice (BR) would reduce the O_2 cost of submaximal exercise and enhance the tolerance to high-intensity exercise. In a double-blind, placebo (PL)-controlled, crossover study, eight men (aged 19–38 yr) consumed 500 ml/day of either BR (containing 11.2 ± 0.6 mM of nitrate) or blackcurrant cordial (as a PL, with negligible nitrate content) for 6 consecutive days and completed a series of "step" moderate-intensity and severe-intensity exercise tests on the last 3 days. On *days 4–6*, plasma nitrite concentration was significantly greater following dietary nitrate supplementation compared with PL (BR: 273 ± 44 vs. PL: 140 ± 50 nM; $P < 0.05$), and systolic blood pressure was significantly reduced (BR: 124 ± 2 vs. PL: 132 ± 5 mmHg; $P < 0.01$). During moderate exercise, nitrate supplementation reduced muscle fractional O_2 extraction (as estimated using near-infrared spectroscopy). The gain of the increase

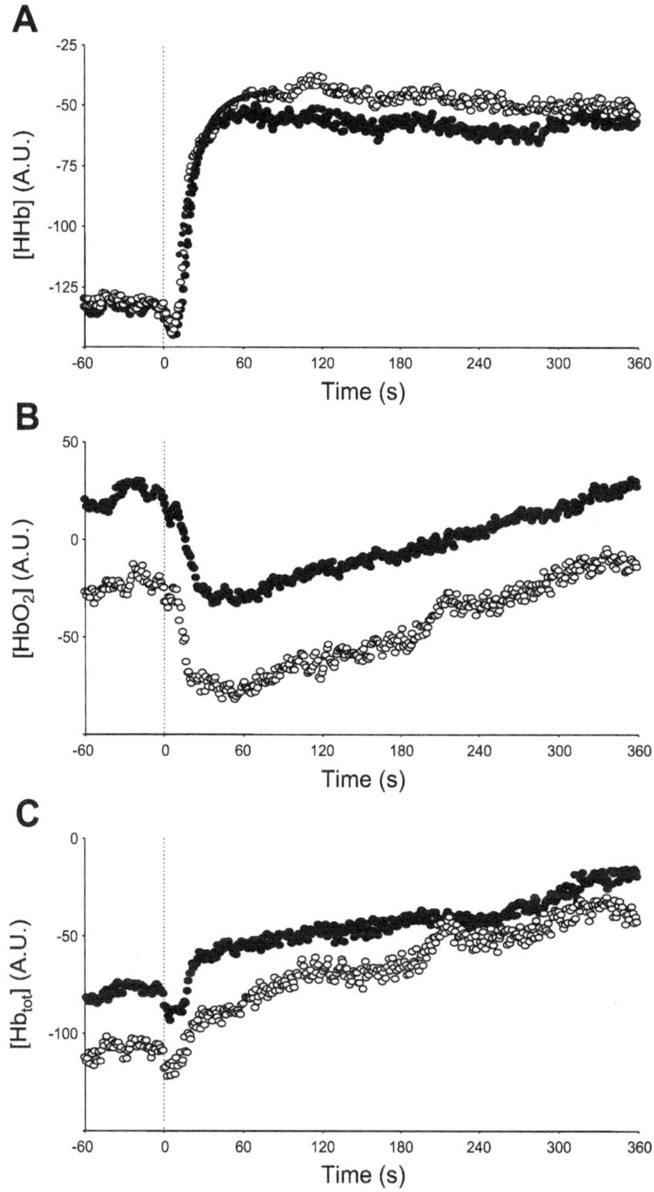

FIGURE 3.—Group mean changes in the parameters of muscle oxygenation following nitrate and placebo supplementation before and during a step increment to a moderate-intensity cycle work rate. Responses following nitrate supplementation are shown as solid circles, while the placebo responses are shown as open circles. The dotted vertical line represents the abrupt imposition of a moderate work rate from a baseline of "unloaded" cycling. *A*: deoxyhemoglobin concentration ([HHb]). *B*: oxyhemoglobin concentration ([HbO_2]). *C*: total hemoglobin concentration ([Hb_{tot}]). For each individual, the responses to four like-transitions were averaged together before analysis. Note the reduction in the amplitude of the [HHb] response and the greater [HbO_2] and [Hb_{tot}] before and during moderate exercise following dietary nitrate supplementation. Error bars are not shown for clarity, but see Table 1 in the original article for further details. AU, arbitrary units. (Reprinted from Bailey SJ, Winyard P, Vanhatalo A, et al. Dietary nitrate supplementation reduces the O_2 cost of low-intensity exercise and enhances tolerance to high-intensity exercise in humans. *J Appl Physiol.* 2009;107:1144-1155, with permission from the American Physiological Society.)

in pulmonary O_2 uptake following the onset of moderate exercise was reduced by 19% in the BR condition (BR: 8.6 ± 0.7 vs. PL: 10.8 ± 1.6 $ml \cdot min^{-1} \cdot W^{-1}$; $P < 0.05$). During severe exercise, the O_2 uptake slow component was reduced (BR: 0.57 ± 0.20 vs. PL: 0.74 ± 0.24 l/min; $P < 0.05$), and the time-to-exhaustion was extended (BR: 675 ± 203 vs. PL: 583 ± 145 s; $P < 0.05$). The reduced O_2 cost of exercise following increased dietary nitrate intake has important implications for our understanding of the factors that regulate mitochondrial respiration and muscle contractile energetics in humans (Fig 3).

▶ This article was sparked by a recent report from a group of well-respected investigators indicating that the provision of pharmacological sodium nitrate reduced the energy cost of cycle ergometer exercise performed at 45% to 80% of maximal oxygen intake.[1] This is a rather surprising finding, as the mechanical efficiency of cycle ergometer exercise is normally thought to be relatively constant. Given the absence of any change in lactate values, it appears that somehow the nitrate increased the efficiency of metabolism. Assuming that maximal oxygen intake remained unchanged, this would in turn enhance performance in vigorous exercise. The nitrate itself is relatively inactive in the human body, but it is probably converted to nitric oxide (NO). This might increase muscle vasodilatation, although this would only influence the efficiency of effort if anaerobic activity was reduced thereby. Other possibilities are that NO reduces slippage at the mitochondrial electron pumps,[2] or that NO_2^- serves as an alternative electron acceptor.[3]

Nitrate is ingested normally through vegetables (60%-80% of the total intake), and it was for this reason that the present small controlled trial compared 4 to 6 days of beetroot juice (in a dose sufficient to double plasma nitrite) versus blackcurrant juice. The only side effects were red stools and urine. Those taking the beetroot juice showed evidence of better muscle oxygenation (Fig 3), a reduced systolic blood pressure, and some reduction of oxygen cost for a standard exercise, as previously observed. The endurance of severe exercise was not tested, but presumably would have been increased. Given that beetroots are a normal component of diet, it would be difficult to regulate any resulting benefit in athletic competition. Maybe it is borscht that propels Russian competitors to victory?

R. J. Shephard, MD (Lond), PhD, DPE

References

1. Larsen FJ, Weitzberg E, Lundberg JO, Ekblom B. Effects of dietary nitrate on oxygen cost during exercise. *Acta Physiol (Oxf)*. 2007;191:59-66.
2. Clerc P, Rigoulet M, Leverve X, Fontaine E. Nitric oxide increases oxidative phosphorylation efficiency. *J Bioenerg Biomembr.* 2007;39:158-166.
3. Basu S, Azarova NA, Font MD, et al. Nitrite reductase activity of cytochrome c. *J Biol Chem.* 2008;283:32590-32597.

β-Alanine Improves Sprint Performance in Endurance Cycling

Van Thienen R, Van Proeyen K, Eynde BV, et al (Katholieke Universiteit Leuven, Belgium)

Med Sci Sports Exerc 41:898-903, 2009

Purpose.—Recent research has shown that chronic dietary β-alanine (βALA) supplementation increases muscle carnosine content, which is associated with better performance in short (1–2 min) maximal exercise. Success in endurance competitions often depends on a final sprint. However, whether βALA can be ergogenic in sprint performance at the end of an endurance competition is at present unknown. Therefore, we investigated the effect of 8-wk βALA administration in moderately to well-trained cyclists on sprint performance at the end of a simulated endurance cycling race.

Methods.—A double-blind study was performed, which consisted of two experimental test sessions interspersed by an 8-wk βALA (2–4 g d^{-1}; $n = 9$) or matched placebo (PL; $n = 8$) supplementation period. In the pretesting and the posttesting, subjects performed a 10-min time trial and a 30-s isokinetic sprint (100 rpm) after a 110-min simulated cycling race. Capillary blood samples were collected for determination of blood lactate concentration and pH.

Results.—Mean power output during the time trial was approximately 300 W and was similar between PL and βALA during either the pretesting or the posttesting. However, compared with PL, during the final sprint after the time trial, βALA on average increased peak power output by 11.4% (95% confidence interval = +7.8 to +14.9%, $P = 0.0001$), whereas mean power output increased by 5.0% (95% confidence interval = +2.0 to +8.1%, $P = 0.005$). Blood lactate and pH values were similar between groups at any time.

Conclusion.—Oral βALA supplementation can significantly enhance sprint performance at the end of an exhaustive endurance exercise bout (Table 2).

▶ Although subject numbers were small, the present crossover trial seems otherwise well designed and appears to show a substantial influence of

TABLE 2.—Effect of βALA Supplementation on 30-s Sprint Performance

	PL		βALA	
	Pretest	Posttest	Pretest	Posttest
Peak power output (W)	1095 ± 60	1070 ± 46	993 ± 58	1105 ± 57*
Mean power output (W)	717 ± 33	711 ± 24	693 ± 47	727 ± 45*
Final power output (W)	482 ± 19	512 ± 16	482 ± 29	535 ± 29*
% fatigue	55 ± 2	52 ± 2	51 ± 1	51 ± 2
Blood lactate ($mmol \cdot L^{-1}$)	7.61 ± 0.66	6.63 ± 0.60	6.93 ± 0.57	7.04 ± 0.57
Blood pH	7.25 ± 0.01	7.26 ± 0.01	7.27 ± 0.02	7.28 ± 0.03

Values are presented as mean ± SEM of either eight (PL) or nine (βALA) observations.
*Significant difference compared with the corresponding pretest value.

β-alanine (8 weeks at 2-4 g/day) on the final sprint performance of well-trained endurance competitive cyclists. There are 3 weaknesses in this proof: intramuscular buffering capacities were not determined, lactate concentrations were not increased, and much of the apparent benefit of the β-alanine rests on a low initial peak power output in the experimental trial (Table 2). Like many recently proposed ergogenic aids, β-alanine is essentially boosting the effects of a normal high-protein diet by increasing intramuscular levels of carnosine. The main benefit seems to arise from the endogenous buffering of hydrogen ions during anaerobic activity,[1] and in this regard β-alanine seems at least as effective as bicarbonate administration. It is a good question why β-alanine enhances function relative to a normal protein rich diet, but there seems consistent evidence that such supplements can substantially (> 50%) increase the carnitine content of both types I and II muscle fibers.[2,3,4] There are minor side effects such as flushing, but if the benefits are of the order suggested in this report, sports nutritionists will certainly need to consider use of this supplement. The mechanism is different from that of creatine, and there is thus a need to examine also the effects of creatine and β-alanine mixtures.

R. J. Shephard, MD (Lond), PhD, DPE

References

1. Parkhouse WS, McKenzie DC. Possible contribution of skeletal muscle buffers to enhanced anaerobic performance: a brief review. *Med Sci Sports Exerc.* 1984;16: 328-338.
2. Derave W, Ozdemir MS, Harris R, et al. Beta-alanine supplementation augments muscle carnosine content and attenuates fatigue during repeated isokinetic contraction bouts in trained sprinters. *J Appl Physiol.* 2007;103:1736-1743.
3. Harris RC, Tallon MJ, Dunnett M, et al. The absorption of orally supplied beta-alanine and its effect on muscle carnosine synthesis in human vastus lateralis. *Amino Acids.* 2006;30:279-289.
4. Hill CA, Harris RC, Kim HJ, et al. Influence of beta-alanine supplementation on skeletal muscle carnosine concentrations and high intensity cycling capacity. *Amino Acids.* 2007;32:225-233.

Vitamin C and E supplementation prevents mitochondrial damage of ileum myocytes caused by intense and exhaustive exercise training

Rosa EF, Ribeiro RF, Pereira FMT, et al (Universidade Federal de São Paulo-Campus São Paulo, Brazil)

J Appl Physiol 107:1532-1538, 2009

Intense and exhaustive exercise (IEE) is associated with oxidative stress in skeletal muscle, and we recently reported that intestine is sensitive to IEE. In the present study, we investigated the possible relationship between the effects of IEE on morphology and oxidative markers in the ileum and isolated mitochondria. C57BL/6 mice were ascribed either to a control group comprising two subgroups, one sedentary and another exercised for 10 days (E10), or to a corresponding supplemented control group again comprising two subgroups, one sedentary and another exercised

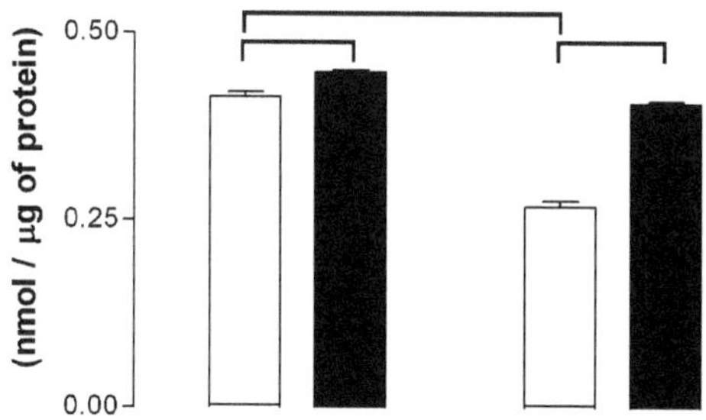

FIGURE 3.—Ileum total antioxidant capacity from CT ($n = 5$), CT-V ($n = 5$), E10 ($n = 5$), and E10-V ($n = 5$). Brackets indicate significant differences between indicated groups ($P < 0.05$). (Reprinted from Rosa EF, Ribeiro RF, Pereira FMT, et al. Vitamin C and E supplementation prevents mitochondrial damage of ileum myocytes caused by intense and exhaustive exercise training. *J Appl Physiol.* 2009;107:1532-1538, with permission from the American Physiological Society).

for 10 days (E10-V). The IEE program consisted of a single daily treadmill running session at 85% of V_{max}, until animal exhaustion. Vitamins C (10 mg/kg) and E (10 mg/kg) were concurrently intraperitoneally administered 2 h before the exercise sessions. IEE was shown to cause *1*) impairment of ileum internal membrane mitochondria verified by ultramicrography analysis; 2) increase in ileum carbonyl content (117%) and reduction in antioxidant capacity (36%); *3*) increase in mitochondria carbonyl content (38%), increase in the percentage of ruptured mitochondria (25.3%), increase in superoxide dismutase activity (186%), and reduction in citrate synthase activity (40.4%) compared with control animals. Observations in the vitamin-supplemented exercised animals (E10-V) were *1*) healthy appearance of myocyte mitochondria; 2) decrease in ileum carbonyl content (66%) and increase in antioxidant capacity (53%); *3*) decrease in mitochondria carbonyl content (43%), decrease in the percentage of ruptured mitochondria (30%), slight increase in superoxide dismutase activity (7%), and significant increase in citrate synthase activity (121%) compared with E10 animals. Therefore, the present results strongly corroborate the hypothesis that IEE leads to marked disturbances in intestinal mitochondria, mainly in redox status, and affects whole intestinal redox status (Fig 3).

▶ One of the problems associated with prolonged endurance exercise such as a marathon run is that the visceral blood flow is reduced by perhaps four-fifths; this limitation of visceral flow is particularly acute if the exercise bout is performed under conditions of heat stress. The resulting hypoxia in the gut wall may be sufficient to impair its barrier function, so that the endotoxins from intestinal gram-negative bacteria can enter the blood stream, causing a potentially fatal endotoxemia.[1] A second possible factor damaging tissues during exhausting exercise is oxidative stress arising from an increased production of free radicals. It is easy to envisage this occurring in the metabolically active skeletal and cardiac muscles, but it is less clear why such stress should develop in the gut during exhausting exercise. This study suggests that local hypoxia may have such an effect. The presence of oxidative stress in mice was evaluated in terms of a number of empirical indices, and its modulation was assessed in terms of the response to therapeutic intraperitoneal doses of vitamins C (10 mg/kg) and E (10 mg/kg). Controlled observations showed that mice receiving the antioxidants 2 hours before exercising showed reductions in a number of indices of oxidative stress (Fig 3). There have been previous reports of impaired redox status in the gut following exhausting exercise[2]; this may contribute to the gastrointestinal complaints of the distance runner, although the primary cause is likely an impaired regional blood flow and resulting local ischemia.[3,4] Despite the protection from the vitamins, I suspect that most sports physicians will seek to moderate the intensity of effort to avoid damaging the gut wall, rather than trying to counter it by the administration of antioxidants.

R. J. Shephard, MD (Lond), PhD, DPE

References

1. Shephard RJ. *Physical activity, training and the immune response.* Carmel, IN: Cooper Publications; 1997.
2. Rosa EF, Freymüller E, Ihara SS, Aboulafia J, Nouailhetas VL. Damaging effects of intense repetitive treadmill running on murine intestinal musculature. *J Appl Physiol.* 2008;104:1410-1417.
3. Peters HP, Bos M, Seebregts L, et al. Gastrointestinal symptoms in long-distance runners, cyclists, and triathletes: prevalence, medication, and etiology. *Am J Gastroenterol.* 1999;94:1570-1581.
4. Clark ET, Gewertz BL. Intermittent ischemia potentiates intestinal reperfusion injury. *J Vasc Surg.* 1991;13:601-606.

Glucose ingestion during endurance training does not alter adaptation

Akerstrom TCA, Fischer CP, Plomgaard P, et al (Univ of Copenhagen, Denmark)

J Appl Physiol 106:1771-1779, 2009

Glucose ingestion during exercise attenuates activation of metabolic enzymes and expression of important transport proteins. In light of this, we hypothesized that glucose ingestion during training would result in *1*) an attenuation of the increase in fatty acid uptake and oxidation during exercise, *2*) lower citrate synthase (CS) and β-hydroxyacyl-CoA dehydrogenase (β-HAD) activity and glycogen content in skeletal muscle, and *3*) attenuated endurance performance enhancement in the trained state. To investigate this we studied nine male subjects who performed 10 wk of one-legged knee extensor training. They trained one leg while ingesting a 6% glucose solution (Glc) and ingested a sweetened placebo while training the other leg (Plc). The subjects trained their respective legs 2 h at a time on alternate days 5 days a week. Endurance training increased peak power (P_{max}) and time to fatigue at 70% of P_{max} ~14% and ~30%, respectively. CS and β-HAD activity increased and glycogen content was greater after training, but there were no differences between Glc and Plc. After training the rate of oxidation of palmitate (R_{ox}) and

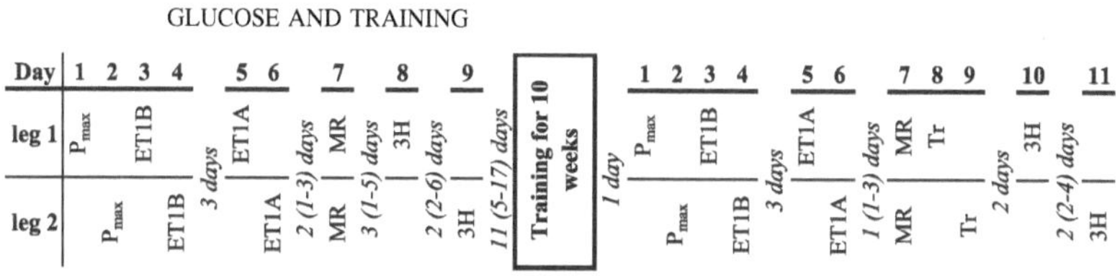

P_{max} P_{max}-test
ET1A End-test70%, subject ingests glucose drink
ET1B End-test70%, subject ingests placebo drink
MR MR-scanning
3H 3h-test
Tr Training

FIGURE 1.—Study outline. Outline of entire study over time with number of days between tests represented by means and ranges. P_{max}, peak power. (Reprinted with permission from Akerstrom TCA, Fischer CP, Plomgaard P, et al. Glucose ingestion during endurance training does not alter adaptation. *J Appl Physiol.* 2009;106:1771-1779.)

the % of rate of disappearance that was oxidized (%R_{dox}) changed. %R_{dox} was on average 16.4% greater during exercise after training whereas, after exercise %R_{dox} was 30.4% lower. R_{ox} followed the same pattern. However, none of these parameters were different between Glc and Plc. We conclude that glucose ingestion during training does not alter training adaptation related to substrate metabolism, mitochondrial enzyme activity, glycogen content, or performance (Fig 1).

▶ There is a belief among some physiologists that endurance athletes should train low on carbohydrate but compete while high on carbohydrates to augment training adaptations within the muscle. Other physiologists feel that training high on carbohydrate allows the athlete to push at a higher intensity for longer time periods, thus optimizing changes within the muscle for competition. The data from this study should put the train low, compete high theory to rest. After 10 weeks of training there was no apparent difference in substrate use, performance (Fig 1), glycogen content, or metabolic enzyme activity between carbohydrate and placebo condition. Thus, sugar ingestion during exercise training despite the acute effects on substrate use, enzyme activation, and gene expression does not alter the adaptation to 10 weeks of endurance training.

D. C. Nieman, DrPH

Antioxidants prevent health-promoting effects of physical exercise in humans

Ristow M, Zarse K, Oberbach A, et al (Univ of Jena, Germany; Univ of Leipzig, Germany; et al)

Proc Natl Acad Sci U S A 106:8665-8670, 2009

Exercise promotes longevity and ameliorates type 2 diabetes mellitus and insulin resistance. However, exercise also increases mitochondrial formation of presumably harmful reactive oxygen species (ROS). Antioxidants are widely used as supplements but whether they affect the health-promoting effects of exercise is unknown. We evaluated the effects of a combination of vitamin C (1000 mg/day) and vitamin E (400 IU/day) on insulin sensitivity as measured by glucose infusion rates (GIR) during a hyperinsulinemic, euglycemic clamp in previously untrained ($n = 19$) and pretrained ($n = 20$) healthy young men. Before and after a 4 week intervention of physical exercise, GIR was determined, and muscle biopsies for gene expression analyses as well as plasma samples were obtained to compare changes over baseline and potential influences of vitamins on exercise effects. Exercise increased parameters of insulin sensitivity (GIR and plasma adiponectin) only in the absence of antioxidants in

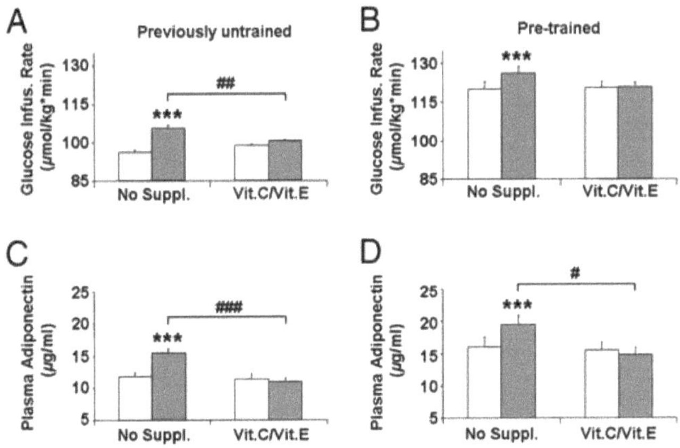

FIGURE 1.—Antioxidants prevent exercise-dependent induction of insulin sensitivity. *(A)* Glucose infusion rates (GIR) during euglycemic hyperinsulinemic clamps in previously untrained individuals before (white bars) and after (shaded bars) physical exercise over 4 weeks. (*Left pair of bars*) Individuals not taking any medication or placebo; (*Right pair of bars*) individuals taking both vitamin C (1000 mg/day) as well as vitamin E (400 IU/day). Bars depict means, error bars show standard error means (applies to all subsequent panels and figures). Significances (applies to all subsequent panels and Fig. 3): * indicates $0.01 < P < 0.05$ comparing data before and after 4 weeks of exercise, # indicates $0.01 < P < 0.05$ comparing "no suppl." with "Vit.C/Vit.E" groups after intervention, ** indicates $0.001 \leq P \leq 0.01$ comparing data before and after 4 weeks of exercise, ## indicates $0.001 \leq P \leq 0.01$ comparing "no suppl." with "Vit.C/Vit.E" groups after intervention, *** indicates $P < 0.001$ comparing data before and after 4 weeks of exercise, ### indicates $P < 0.001$ comparing "no suppl." with "Vit.C/Vit.E" groups after intervention. *(B)* The same set of data derived from a physically pretrained group of individuals. *(C)* Plasma adiponectin levels in the previously untrained and previously trained *(D)* state. (Reprinted from Ristow M, Zarse K, Oberbach A, et al. Antioxidants prevent health-promoting effects of physical exercise in humans. *Proc Natl Acad Sci U S A.* 2009;106:8665-8670)

both previously untrained ($P < 0.001$) and pretrained ($P < 0.001$) individuals. This was paralleled by increased expression of ROS-sensitive transcriptional regulators of insulin sensitivity and ROS defense capacity, peroxisome-proliferator-activated receptor gamma (PPARγ), and PPARγ coactivators PGC1α and PGC1β only in the absence of antioxidants ($P < 0.001$ for all). Molecular mediators of endogenous ROS defense (superoxide dismutases 1 and 2; glutathione peroxidase) were also induced by exercise, and this effect too was blocked by antioxidant supplementation. Consistent with the concept of mitohormesis, exercise-induced oxidative stress ameliorates insulin resistance and causes an adaptive response promoting endogenous antioxidant defense capacity. Supplementation with antioxidants may preclude these health-promoting effects of exercise in humans (Fig 1).

▶ Patients are often advised to take massive doses of antioxidants, not only to counter the increased production of reactive oxygen species during exercise, but also to prevent or minimize the effects of the common cold and to counter many of the effects of aging such as a deterioration of cerebral function and progressive macular degeneration of the retina. It is thus disturbing to consider the possibility that such therapy may not only counteract the production of endogenous antioxidases, but also reverse some of the more general benefits of regular exercise such as an improved glucose tolerance (Fig 1). The findings seem in keeping with several previous animal studies suggesting that some of the beneficial effects of regular exercise are dependent on the generation of reactive oxygen species.[1-5] Although findings to date are not entirely consistent, it is suggested that an increased endogenous production of reactive oxygen species induces genes that both increase insulin sensitivity and promote the endogenous production of antioxidases.[6] This study is based on a relatively small number of subjects and runs counter to a previous meta-analysis that found a beneficial effect of a high fruit and vegetable intake on the risk of diabetes.[7] In view of the importance of the issue, there is plainly need for a large randomized controlled trial of long-term antioxidant use.

R. J. Shephard, MD (Lond), PhD, DPE

References

1. McClung JP, Roneker CA, Mu W, et al. Development of insulin resistance and obesity in mice overexpressing cellular glutathione peroxidase. *Proc Natl Acad Sci USA.* 2004;101:8852-8857.
2. Goldstein BJ, Kalyankar M, Wu X. Redox paradox: Insulin action is facilitated by insulin-stimulated reactive oxygen species with multiple potential signaling targets. *Diabetes.* 2005;54:311-321.
3. Schulz TJ, Zarse K, Voigt A, Urban N, Birringer M, Ristow M. Glucose restriction extends Caenorhabditis elegans life span by inducing mitochondrial respiration and increasing oxidative stress. *Cell Metab.* 2007;6:280-293.
4. Birringer M, Kuhlow D, Pfluger PT, et al. Improved glucose metabolism in mice lacking alpha-tocopherol transfer protein. *Eur J Nutr.* 2007;46:397-405.
5. Gomez-Cabrera MC, Domenech E, Romagnoli M, et al. Oral administration of vitamin C decreases muscle mitochondrial biogenesis and hampers training-induced adaptations in endurance performance. *Am J Clin Nutr.* 2008;87:142-149.

6. St. Pierre J, Drori S, Uldry M, et al. Suppression of reactive oxygen species and neurodegeneration by the PGC-1 transcriptional coactivators. *Cell*. 2006;127: 397-408.
7. Hamer M, Chida Y. Intake of fruit, vegetables, and antioxidants and risk of type 2 diabetes: Systematic review and meta-analysis. *J Hypertens*. 2007;25: 2361-2369.

Dietary quercetin supplementation is not ergogenic in untrained men

Cureton KJ, Tomporowski PD, Singhal A, et al (Univ of Georgia, Athens, et al)
J Appl Physiol 107:1095-1104, 2009

Quercetin supplementation increases muscle oxidative capacity and endurance in mice, but its ergogenic effect in humans has not been established. Our study investigates the effects of short-duration chronic quercetin supplementation on muscle oxidative capacity; metabolic, perceptual, and neuromuscular determinants of performance in prolonged exercise; and cycling performance in untrained men. Using a double-blind, pretest-posttest control group design, 30 recreationally active, but not endurance-trained, young men were randomly assigned to quercetin and placebo groups. A noninvasive measure of muscle oxidative capacity (phosphocreatine recovery rate using magnetic resonance spectroscopy), peak oxygen uptake ($\dot{V}O_{2peak}$, metabolic and perceptual responses to submaximal exercise, work performed on a 10-min maximal-effort cycling test following the submaximal cycling, and voluntary and electrically evoked strength loss following cycling were measured before and after 7–16 days of supplementation with 1 g/day of quercetin in a sports hydration beverage or a placebo beverage. Pretreatment-to-posttreatment changes in phosphocreatine recovery time constant, $\dot{V}O_{2peak}$, substrate utilization, and perception of effort during submaximal exercise, total work done during the 10-min maximal effort cycling trial, and voluntary and electrically evoked strength loss were not significantly different ($P > 0.05$) in the quercetin and placebo groups. Short duration, chronic dietary quercetin supplementation in untrained men does not improve muscle oxidative capacity; metabolic, neuromuscular and perceptual determinants of performance in prolonged exercise; or cycling performance. The null findings indicate that metabolic and physical performance consequences of quercetin supplementation observed in mice should not be generalized to humans.

▶ Aerobic exercise increases muscle mitochondria anywhere between 20% and 100%, depending on the amount of training. An exciting finding from recent studies with animals is that ingestion of quercetin and other plant molecules can partially mimic the effects of exercise training in building muscle mitochondria and improving endurance performance. A study using sedentary mice showed that 7 days quercetin feeding (both 12.5 and 25 mg/kg) increased soleus muscle proliferator-activated receptor-γ coactivator-1α (PGC-1α) and sirtuin 1 (SIRT1) mRNA levels 2- to 3-fold, cytochrome C concentration between 18% to 32%, and treadmill run time to fatigue by 37%.[1] Results from a study of untrained males showed that supplementation with 1000 mg/day quercetin for 2 weeks resulted in a 3% improvement in performance and a 10% increase in muscle mitochondria when compared with placebo.[2] The quercetin effect on performance and muscle mitochondrial density in humans appears to be much smaller than reported in mice, and may only emerge when using untrained subjects and the strongest research designs. The quercetin supplementation regimen varied too widely in this study; each group only had 15 subjects, and the study did not use a cross-over design. The subject number was too low to detect a small performance difference, especially within the context of the research design. Muscle oxidative capacity was evaluated noninvasively from the rate of phosphocreatine (PCr) recovery following brief isometric quadriceps exercise using magnetic resonance spectroscopy (MRS). For unknown reasons, PCr recovery increased in both groups (without group differences). The authors state that failure to detect a difference between groups could be due to insensitivity of the measurement, lack of an effect, or inadequate statistical power. Future research on quercetin and performance should emphasize strong research designs, longer supplementation periods, and a mixed flavonoid approach.[3] There is increasing awareness that quercetin's bioactive effects are more apparent when quercetin is mixed with other flavonoids and food components.[3]

D. C. Nieman, DrPH

References

1. Davis JM, Murphy EA, Carmichael MD, Davis B. Quercetin increases brain and muscle mitochondrial biogenesis and exercise tolerance. *Am J Physiol Regul Integr Comp Physiol.* 2009;296:R1071-R1077.
2. Nieman DC, Williams AS, Shanely RA, et al. Quercetin's influence on exercise performance and muscle mitochondrial biogenesis. *Med Sci Sports Exerc. 2009 [Epub ahead of print].*
3. Nieman DC, Henson DA, Maxwell KR, et al. Effects of quercetin and EGCG on mitochondrial biogenesis and immunity. *Med Sci Sports Exerc.* 2009;41: 1467-1475.

Breaks in Sedentary Time: Beneficial associations with metabolic risk

Healy GN, Dunstan DW, Salmon J, et al (The Univ of Queensland, Brisbane, Australia; The International Diabetes Inst, Melbourne, Australia; Deakin Univ, Melbourne, Australia; et al)
Diabetes Care 31:661-666, 2008

Objective.—Total sedentary (absence of whole-body movement) time is associated with obesity, abnormal glucose metabolism, and the metabolic syndrome. In addition to the effects of total sedentary time, the manner in which it is accumulated may also be important. We examined the association of breaks in objectively measured sedentary time with biological markers of metabolic risk.

Research Design and Methods.—Participants ($n = 168$, mean age 53.4 years) for this cross-sectional study were recruited from the 2004–2005 Australian Diabetes, Obesity and Lifestyle study. Sedentary time was measured by an accelerometer (counts/minute^{-1} < 100) worn during waking hours for seven consecutive days. Each interruption in sedentary time (counts/min ≥ 100) was considered a break. Fasting plasma glucose, 2-h plasma glucose, serum triglycerides, HDL cholesterol, weight, height, waist circumference, and resting blood pressure were measured. Mat Lab was used to derive the breaks variable; SPSS was used for the statistical analysis.

Results.—Independent of total sedentary time and moderate-to-vigorous intensity activity time, increased breaks in sedentary time were beneficially associated with waist circumference (standardized $\beta = -0.16$, 95% CI −0.31 to −0.02, $P = 0.026$), BMI ($\beta = -0.19$, −0.35 to −0.02, $P = 0.026$), triglycerides $\beta = -0.18$, −0.34 to −0.02, $P = 0.029$), and 2-h plasma glucose ($\beta = -0.18$, −0.34 to −0.02, $P = 0.025$).

Conclusions.—This study provides evidence of the importance of avoiding prolonged uninterrupted periods of sedentary (primarily sitting) time. These findings suggest new public health recommendations regarding breaking up sedentary time that are complementary to those for physical activity (Table 2).

▶ Exercise scientists are now giving greater attention to sedentary behavior, such as television viewing, as a second adverse lifestyle characteristic that seems to operate independently of the individual's level of habitual physical activity.[1] The development of home and office devices that reduce the need for active behavior seems an important factor that has contributed to the current epidemic of obesity.[2] The accelerometer study of Mueller and associates suggests that a further issue may be not only total amount of sedentary time

TABLE 2.—Standardized Regression Coefficients of Total Breaks with Metabolic Risk Variables

Metabolic Risk Variable	β (95% CI)	P	Adjusted R^2
Waist circumference (cm)	−0.16 (−0.31 to −0.02)	0.027	0.26
BMI (kg/m^2)	0.19 (−0.35 to −0.02)	0.026	0.05
Triglycerides (log) (mmol/l)*	−0.18 (−0.34 to −0.02)	0.029	0.13
HDL cholesterol (mmol/l)*	0.03 (−0.12 to 0.18)	0.685	0.25
Systolic blood pressure (mmHg)†	−0.03 (−0.18 to 0.12)	0.697	0.21
Diastolic blood pressure (mmHg)†	0.03 (−0.12 to 0.19)	0.670	0.19
Fasting plasma glucose (mmol/l)	−0.09 (−0.25 to 0.07)	0.287	0.09
2-h plasma glucose (mmol/l)	−0.18 (−0.34 to −0.02)	0.025	0.14

Adjusted for age, sex, employment, alcohol intake, income, education, smoking, family history of diabetes, diet quality, moderate- to vigorous-intensity time, mean intensity of breaks, and total sedentary time.

Adjusted R^2 gives an estimate of explained variance, taking into account the sample size.

*Additional adjustment for lipid-lowering medication.

†additional adjustment for hypertensive medication.

during a day, but also how this is distributed. Individuals were considered as sedentary when accelerometer counts were less than 100 units/min. Most of the breaks in sedentary behavior were associated with light rather than vigorous physical activity (counts of 500/min), and they usually lasted less than 5 minutes. Nevertheless, the number of such breaks taken during the day was significantly correlated with several metabolic risk factors (Table 2). The underlying mechanisms remain to be elucidated; it may be the fidgety person differs in many respects from the person who works uninterrupted for several hours. Nevertheless, the data do suggest that there may be value in taking short breaks of light physical activity both when working at a desk and during commercial breaks on television.

R. J. Shephard, MD (Lond), PhD, DPE

References

1. Hamilton MT, Hamilton DG, Zderic TW. The role of low energy expenditure and sitting on obesity, metabolic syndrome, type 2 diabetes, and cardiovascular disease. *Diabetes*. 2007;56:2655-2667.
2. Zimmet P, Alberti KG, Shaw J. Global and societal implications of the diabetes epidemic. *Nature*. 2001;414:782-787.

Dual-process action of exercise on appetite control: increase in orexigenic drive but improvement in meal-induced satiety

King NA, Caudwell PP, Hopkins M, et al (Queensland Univ of Technology, Brisbane, Australia; Univ of Leeds, UK; Trinity and All Saints Colleges, Leeds, UK; et al)

Am J Clin Nutr 90:921-927, 2009

Background.—Exercise could contribute to weight loss by altering the sensitivity of the appetite regulatory system.

Objective.—The aim of this study was to assess the effects of 12 wk of mandatory exercise on appetite control.

Design.—Fifty-eight overweight and obese men and women [mean (±SD) body mass index (in kg/m^2) = 31.8 ± 4.5, age = 39.6 ± 9.8 y, and maximal oxygen intake = 29.1 ± 5.7 $mL \cdot kg^{-1} \cdot min^{-1}$] completed 12 wk of supervised exercise in the laboratory. The exercise sessions were designed to expend 2500 kcal/wk. Subjective appetite sensations and the satiating efficiency of a fixed breakfast were compared at baseline (week 0) and at week 12. An Electronic Appetite Rating System was used to measure subjective appetite sensations immediately before and after the fixed breakfast in the immediate postprandial period and across the whole day. The satiety quotient of the breakfast was determined by calculating the change in appetite scores relative to the breakfast's energy content.

Results.—Despite large variability, there was a significant reduction in mean body weight (3.2 ± 3.6 kg), fat mass (3.2 ± 2.2 kg), and waist circumference (5.0 ± 3.2 cm) after 12 wk. The analysis showed that

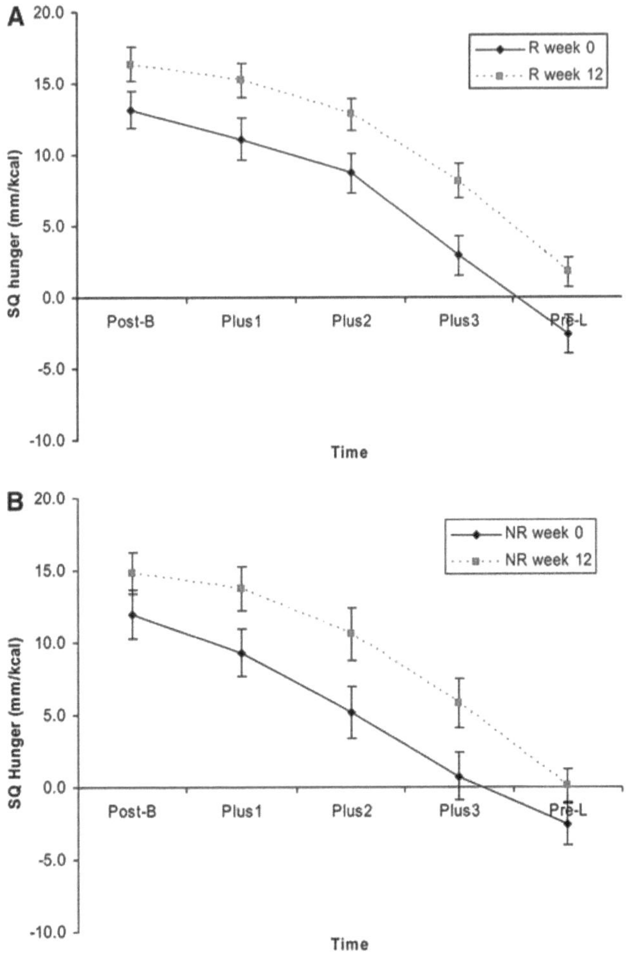

FIGURE 3.—Mean (±SEM) immediate and subsequent satiety quotients (SQs) in response to the fixed breakfast preloads at weeks 0 and 12 in responders (R; $n = 32$; A) and nonresponders (NR; $n = 26$; B). The SQ indicated a stronger suppression of hunger after the fixed breakfast at week 12 than at week 0. The SQ increased similarly in both R and NR. A mixed ANOVA showed a significant main effect of week ($F_{3,144} = 3.62$, $P < 0.0001$) and time ($F_{4,192} = 122.8$, $P < 0.0001$). There was no significant interaction between week and sex ($F_{3,144} = 1.004$, $P = 0.393$) and no significant main effect of sex ($F_{1,48} = 3.25$, $P = 0.08$). Post-B, immediately after breakfast; Plus1, 1 h after breakfast; Plus2, 2 h after breakfast; Plus3, 3 h after breakfast; Pre-L, 4 h after breakfast. (Reprinted from King NA, Caudwell PP, Hopkins M, et al. Dual-process action of exercise on appetite control: increase in orexigenic drive but improvement in meal-induced satiety. *Am J Clin Nutr.* 2009;90:921-927, with permission from the American Society for Nutrition.

a reduction in body weight and body composition was accompanied by an increase in fasting hunger and in average hunger across the day ($P < 0.0001$). Paradoxically, the immediate and delayed satiety quotient of the breakfast also increased significantly ($P < 0.05$).

Conclusions.—These data show that the effect of exercise on appetite regulation involves at least 2 processes: an increase in the overall (orexigenic) drive to eat and a concomitant increase in the satiating efficiency of a fixed meal (Fig 3).

▶ One objection that many obese people make to exercising is that it merely makes them more hungry.[1,2] I have maintained that much depends on the timing of the activity bout, and that if vigorous exercise is performed immediately before a meal, the resultant catecholamine release can raise blood sugar temporarily, thus curbing appetite—an important advantage relative to a simple curbing of food intake. However, there is plainly going to be a subsequent phase with replenishment of glycogen stores, and this will lower blood sugar and increase hunger. This study had subjects undertake a required volume of physical activity in the laboratory (2 MJ/day, 5 days/wk for 12 weeks) at an intensity equivalent to 70% of maximal heart rate, but unfortunately the timing of this activity in relation to meals does not seem to have been standardized. A visual analog device made electronic ratings of hunger, fullness, desire to eat, and prospective food consumption at varying points throughout the day.[3] A satiety quotient related sensations to the amount of food consumed. The program achieved a modest average 3.2 kg decrease of fat mass, but when subjects were divided into responders and nonresponders at the end of the 12 week period, responders were the individuals with an increase in satiety following ingestion of a standard meal (Fig 3). This may be contrasted with dietary induced weight loss, where satiety is often decreased following weight reduction.[4] The authors of this report suggest that the change in satiety is important to a program of exercise-induced weight loss.

R. J. Shephard, MD (Lond), PhD, DPE

References

1. Blundell JE, King NA. Effects of exercise on appetite control: loose coupling between energy expenditure and energy intake. *Int J Obes Relat Metab Disord.* 1998;22:S22-S29.
2. Martins C, Morgan L, Truby H. A review of the effects of exercise on appetite regulation: an obesity perspective. *Int J Obes.* 2008;32:1337-1347.
3. Rogers PJ, Blundell JE. Separating the actions of sweetness and calories: effects of saccharin and carbohydrates on hunger and food intake in human subjects. *Physiol Behav.* 1989;45:1093-1099.
4. Leidy HJ, Carnell NS, Mattes RD, Campbell WW. Higher protein intake preserves lean mass and satiety with weight loss in pre-obese and obese women. *Obesity (Silver Spring).* 2007;15:421-429.

Nutrition and Exercise Prevent Excess Weight Gain in Overweight Pregnant Women

Mottola MF, Giroux I, Gratton R, et al (The Univ of Western Ontario, London, Canada; Brescia Univ College, London, Ontario, Canada; et al)
Med Sci Sports Exerc 42:265-272, 2010

Purpose.—To determine the effect of a Nutrition and Exercise Lifestyle Intervention Program (NELIP) for overweight (OW) and obese (OB) pregnant women on pregnancy weight gain, birth weight, and maternal weight retention at 2 months postpartum.

Methods.—This is a single-arm intervention matched by prepregnant body mass index, age, and parity to a historical cohort (4:1). Women with a prepregnancy body mass index of $\geq$25.0 kg·m^{-2} ($N = 65$) participated in a NELIP starting at 16–20 wk of pregnancy, continuing until delivery. NELIP consisted of an individualized nutrition plan with total energy intake of approximately 2000 kcal·d^{-1} (8360 kJ·d^{-1}) and 40%–55% of total energy intake from carbohydrate. Exercise consisted of a walking program (30% HR reserve), three to four times per week, using a pedometer to count steps. Matched historical cohort (MC; $N = 260$) was from a large local perinatal database.

Results.—Weight gained by women on the NELIP was 6.8 ± 4.1 kg (0.38 ± 0.2 kg·wk^{-1}), with a total pregnancy weight gain of 12.0 ± 5.7 kg. Excessive weight gain occurred before NELIP began at 16 wk of gestation. Eighty percent of the women did not exceed recommended pregnancy weight gain on NELIP. Weight retention at 2 months postpartum was 2.2 ± 5.6 kg with no difference between the OW and the OB women on NELIP. Mean birth weight was not different between NELIP (3.59 ± 0.5 kg) and MC (3.56 ± 0.6 kg, $P > 0.05$).

Conclusions.—NELIP reduces the risk of excessive pregnancy weight gain with minimal weight retention at 2 months postpartum in OW and OB women. This intervention may assist OW and OB women in successful weight control after childbirth.

▶ Maternal obesity increases multiple health risks for women and their infants. For mothers, excess weight gain during pregnancy and postpartum weight retention increases the risk of long-term obesity, cardiovascular disease, and type 2 diabetes. Maternal weight gain has been positively associated with birth weight, and maternal obesity is an independent risk factor for macrosomic infants (> 4.0 kg) who, in turn, are at greater risk for obesity and comorbidities later in life. Therefore, it is important to prevent excessive gestational weight gain and promote postpartum weight loss in overweight and obese mothers. In this study, overweight (body mass index [BMI] $\geq$25.0-29.9 kg/m^2) and obese (BMI $\geq$30.0 kg/m^2) women were enrolled in the Nutrition and Exercise Lifestyle Intervention Program (NELIP) beginning in weeks 16 to 20 of gestation. The NELIP included meal plans to meet total calorie and nutrient goals and a low intensity progressive walking program. The goal of the intervention program was to prevent excessive pregnancy weight gain ($\leq$10.6 kg) and minimize weight retention at 2 months postpartum. One of the many challenges to intervention studies in pregnant women is establishing an appropriate control group. These authors used medical records of women who delivered singleton births in the same geographic area as the intervention. The controls were matched to the NELIP group by prepregnancy BMI, maternal age, and parity. All participants had the same access to health care. The goals of NELIP were achieved with 80% of women experiencing weight gain less than 10.6 kg and postpartum weight retention of 2.2 ± 5.6 kg. Approximately, half of the 65 women in NELIP were within 2 kg of prepregnancy body mass at 2 months postpartum. The NELIP women doubled the number of steps taken per day, from 5678 ± 1738 steps/d (sedentary) to more than 10 000 steps per day (active) by the time of delivery. Birth weight outcomes were not significantly different between NELIP and controls although, in a subanalysis, fewer macrosomic infants (4.0-4.5 kg) were born to overweight NELIP mothers than to overweight controls (3.2 % vs 18% of all infants). Fewer small babies (< 2.5 kg) were born to NELIP mothers than controls (0% vs 3.5%). Low birth weight also increases the risk for obesity later in life. Together, the NELIP demonstrates that optimal nutrition and mild regular exercise during pregnancy for overweight and obese women prevents excessive pregnancy weight gain and is more likely to result in healthy infants.

C. M. Jankowski, PhD

Ultrasound Techniques Applied to Body Fat Measurement in Male and Female Athletes

Pineau J-C, Filliard JR, Bocquet M (Centre Natl de Recherche Scientifique, Paris, France; Institut Natl des Sports et de l'Education Physique (INSEP), Paris, France; Ecole Nationale Supérieure d'Arts et Metiers, Paris, France)
J Athl Train 44:142-147, 2009

Context.—For athletes in disciplines with weight categories, it is important to assess body composition and weight fluctuations.

Objective.—To evaluate the accuracy of measuring body fat percentage with a portable ultrasound device possessing high accuracy and reliability versus fan-beam, dual-energy X-ray absorptiometry (DEXA).

Design.—Cross-validation study.

Setting.—Research laboratory.

Patients or Other Participants.—A total of 93 athletes (24 women, 69 men), aged 23.5 ± 3.7 years, with body mass index = 24.0 ± 4.2 and body fat percentage via DEXA = 9.41 ± 8.1 participated. All participants were elite athletes selected from the Institut National des Sports et de l'Education Physique. These participants practiced a variety of weight-category sports.

Main Outcome Measure(s).—We measured body fat and body fat percentage using an ultrasound technique associated with anthropometric values and the DEXA reference technique. Cross-validation between the ultrasound technique and DEXA was then performed.

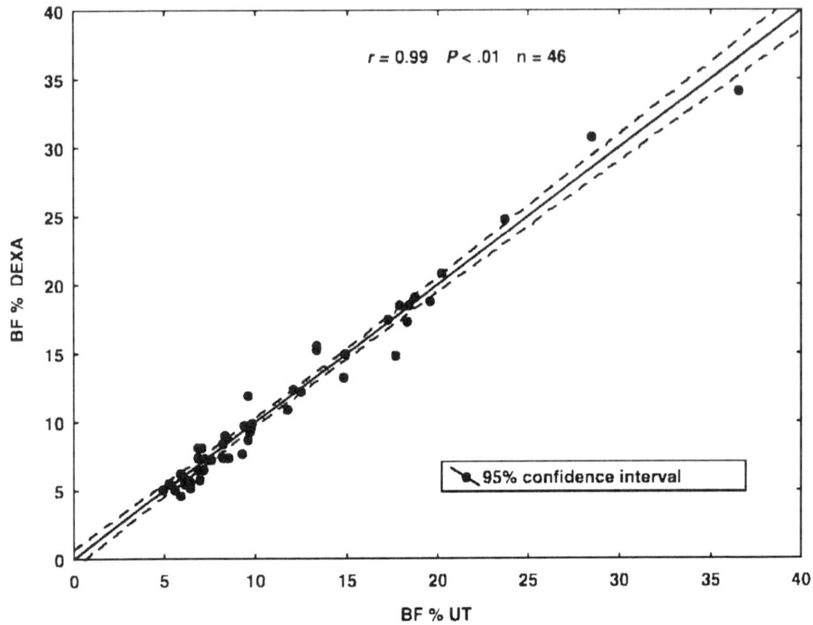

FIGURE 2.—Regression between body fat (BF) percentage estimates using dual-energy X-ray absorptiometry (DEXA) and portable ultrasound (UT) on 46 athletes. (Reprinted from Pineau J-C, Filliard JR, Bocquet M. Ultrasound techniques applied to body fat measurement in male and female athletes. *J Athl Train.* 2009;44:142-147.)

Results.—Ultrasound estimates of body fat percentage were correlated closely with those of DEXA in both females ($r = 0.97$, standard error of the estimate = 1.79) and males ($r = 0.98$, standard error of the estimate = 0.96). The ultrasound technique in both sexes had a low total error (0.93). The 95% limit of agreement was −0.06 ± 1.2 for all athletes and did not show an overprediction or underprediction bias. We developed a new model to produce body fat estimates with ultrasound and anthropometric dimensions.

Conclusions.—The limits of agreement with the ultrasound technique compared with DEXA measurements were very good. Consequently, the use of a portable ultrasound device produced accurate body fat and body fat percentage estimates in relation to the fan-beam DEXA technique (Fig 2).

▶ The use of ultrasound technique (UT) to measure body fat in athletes is gaining interest due to the greater portability and lower cost of UT compared with dual-energy X-ray absorptiometry (DEXA). Clinicians and trainers may be getting more questions from athletes, coaches, and parents about the reliability of UT-derived measures of body fat. Pineau and colleagues conducted a small, but well-done cross validation study of young (aged 18-33 years) athletes in sports that have weight classes. The sports represented were judo, wrestling, tae kwon do, boxing, and rowing. One of the limitations of the study is that only 24 of the 93 athletes were women. UT measures the thickness of fat between the skin and muscle. The ultrasonic waves emitted by the transducer probe are partially reflected by the interface of fat and muscle. In this study, subcutaneous fat thickness was measured in the abdominal and thigh regions. Sex-specific regression equations of DEXA-derived percent body fat against UT fat thickness were generated. These equations also included body mass, height, and limb circumference factors. There was a very strong agreement between body fat percent measured by DEXA and UT, and the errors of estimating percent body fat using UT were very small in women and men (Fig 2). Although further validation is needed, UT measures of body fat may be a useful resource to help an athlete identify her/his most competitive weight class. It will be interesting to see if future research addresses the sensitivity of UT to measure changes in body fat in athletes.

C. M. Jankowski, PhD

Classification of Body Fatness by Body Mass Index–for-Age Categories Among Children

Freedman DS, Wang J, Thornton JC, et al (Ctrs for Disease Control and Prevention, Atlanta, GA; St Luke's–Roosevelt Hosp, NY; et al)
Arch Pediatr Adolesc Med 163:805-811, 2009

Objective.—To examine the ability of various body mass index (BMI)–for-age categories, including the Centers for Disease Control and Prevention's 85th to 94th percentiles, to correctly classify the body fatness of children and adolescents.

Design.—Cross-sectional.

Setting.—The New York Obesity Research Center at St Luke's-Roosevelt Hospital from 1995 to 2000.

Participants.—Healthy 5- to 18-year-old children and adolescents (N = 1196) were recruited in the New York City area through newspaper notices, announcements at schools and activity centers, and word of mouth.

Main Outcome Measures.—Percent body fat as determined by dual-energy x-ray absorptiometry. Body fatness cutoffs were chosen so that the number of children in each category (normal, moderate, and elevated fatness) would equal the number of children in the corresponding BMI-for-age category (<85th percentile, 85th-94th percentile, and ≥95th percentile, respectively).

Results.—About 77% of the children who had a BMI for age at or above the 95th percentile had an elevated body fatness, but levels of body fatness among children who had a BMI for age between the 85th and 94th percentiles (n = 200) were more variable; about one-half of these children had a moderate level of body fatness, but 30% had a normal body fatness and 20% had an elevated body fatness. The prevalence of normal levels of body fatness among these 200 children was highest

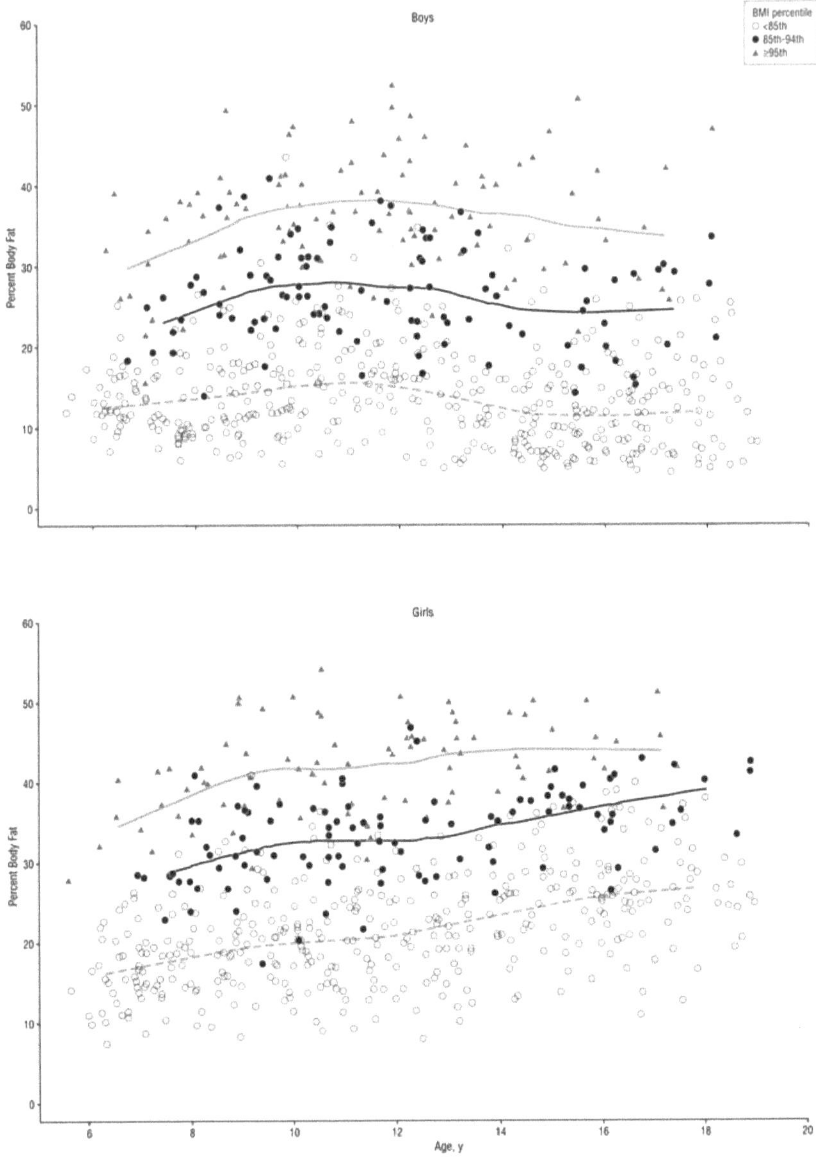

FIGURE.—Percent body fat by age among boys and girls who have body mass index (BMI)–for-age levels lower than the 85th percentile, between the 85th and 94th percentiles, and at or above the 95th percentile. Each point represents an individual boy or girl, and the 3 lines represent smoothed (Lowess) levels of body fatness by age in each BMI group. (Reprinted from Freedman DS, Wang J, Thornton JC, et al. Classification of body fatness by body mass index-for-age categories among children. *Arch Pediatr Adolesc Med.* 2009;163:805-811, with permission from the American Medical Association.)

among black children (50%) and among those within the 85th to 89th percentiles of BMI for age (40%).

Conclusion.—Body mass index is an appropriate screening test to identify children who should have further evaluation and follow-up, but it is not diagnostic of level of adiposity (Fig).

▶ Body mass index (BMI)-for-age cutoffs are rated overweight (85th-94th percentile) and obese (≥95th percentile) by pediatric medical experts.[1] However, the ability of these cutoffs to correctly identify children and adolescents who have high body fatness is questionable. Fig 1 shows that despite the large differences in mean body fatness across the BMI categories, the body fatness of individual children and adolescents overlapped substantially. Overall, BMI was a fairly good indicator of body fatness among most children and adolescents, especially when BMI for age was at or above the 95th percentile. There was more misclassification among children and adolescents who had a BMI for age between the 85th and 94th percentiles, with only about one-half having a moderate body fatness. BMI was almost useless as an estimator of percentage of body fat in normal weight children and adolescents, with only 42% correctly classified. The bottom line is that BMI for age cannot be considered diagnostic for body fatness in children and adolescents. Thus, dual energy X-ray absorptiometry (DEXA) measurement of body fat in youth is recommended to double check BMI classification, especially when medical follow-up is indicated.

D. C. Nieman, DrPH

Reference

1. Barlow SE, Expert Committee. Expert committee recommendations regarding the prevention, assessment, and treatment of child and adolescent overweight and obesity: summary report. *Pediatrics*. 2007;120:S164-S192.

Effect of Android to Gynoid Fat Ratio on Insulin Resistance in Obese Youth

Aucouturier J, Meyer M, Thivel D, et al (Blaise Pascal Univ, Aubière; Univ Hosp, Clermont-Ferrand; et al)

Arch Pediatr Adolesc Med 163:826-831, 2009

Background.—Upper body fat distribution is associated with the early development of insulin resistance in obese children and adolescents.

Objective.—To determine if an android to gynoid fat ratio is associated with the severity of insulin resistance in obese children and adolescents, whereas peripheral subcutaneous fat may have a protective effect against insulin resistance.

Setting.—The pediatric department of University Hospital, Clermont-Ferrand, France.

Design.—A retrospective analysis using data from medical consultations between January 2005 and January 2007.

Participants.—Data from 66 obese children and adolescents coming to the hospital for medical consultation were used in this study.

Main Outcome Measures.—Subjects were stratified into tertiles of android to gynoid fat ratio determined by dual-energy x-ray absorptiometry. Insulin resistance was assessed by the homeostasis model of insulin resistance (HOMA-IR) index.

Results.—There were no differences in weight, body mass index, and body fat percentage between tertiles. Values of HOMA-IR were significantly increased in the 2 higher tertiles (mean [SD], tertile 2, 2.73 [1.41]; tertile 3, 2.89 [1.28]) compared with the lower tertile (tertile 1, 1.67 [1.24]) of android to gynoid fat ratio ($P < .001$). The HOMA-IR value was significantly associated with android to gynoid fat ratio ($r = 0.35$; $P < .01$).

Conclusions.—Android fat distribution is associated with an increased insulin resistance in obese children and adolescents. An android to gynoid fat ratio based on dual-energy x-ray absorptiometry measurements is a useful and simple technique to assess distribution of body fat associated with an increased risk of insulin resistance.

▶ An increased incidence of prediabetes and type 2 diabetes mellitus has been reported in obese children and adolescents.[1] Visceral fat content is related to glucose intolerance independently of total fat mass and subcutaneous abdominal adipose tissue.[2] Interestingly, peripheral subcutaneous fat may represent a metabolic sink for the storage of excess energy.[3] When peripheral fat depots fail to expand to store excess energy intake, fat accumulates in liver, pancreas, and skeletal muscles, leading to metabolic alterations that cause type 2 diabetes. For example, among individuals with similar waist circumferences, those with thick thigh skinfolds have a more favorable lipoprotein-lipid profile.[4] In this study, obese children and adolescents were given dual energy x-ray absorptiometry (DEXA) scans, with the percentage of abdominal fat determined manually by drawing a rectangular box between vertebral bodies L1 and L4. Gynoid fat deposition was assessed by lower limb fat percentage. Android to gynoid fat ratio was determined by using fat percentages in lower limbs and in the abdominal region. As summarized in Fig 1 in the original article, a positive relationship was found between insulin resistance and the android to gynoid fat ratio. Thus, a simple index of android to gynoid fat distribution from DEXA scans can identify obese youth at the highest risk for metabolic disorders. The next and more difficult challenge is helping these youth lose their excess visceral fat through lifestyle changes.

D. C. Nieman, DrPH

References

1. Weiss R, Dufour S, Taksali SE, et al. Prediabetes in obese youth: a syndrome of impaired glucose tolerance, severe insulin resistance, and altered myocellular and abdominal fat partitioning. *Lancet.* 2003;362:951-957.
2. Despre's JP. Cardiovascular disease under the influence of excess visceral fat. *Crit Pathw Cardiol.* 2007;6:51-59.

3. Okura T, Nakata Y, Yamabuki K, Tanaka K. Regional body composition changes exhibit opposing effects on coronary heart disease risk factors. *Arterioscler Thromb Vasc Biol.* 2004;24:923-929.
4. Terry RB, Stefanick ML, Haskell WL, Wood PD. Contributions of regional adipose tissue depots to plasma lipoprotein concentrations in overweight men and women: possible protective effects of thigh fat. *Metabolism.* 1991;40: 733-740.

Effect of school-based physical activity interventions on body mass index in children: a meta-analysis

Harris KC, Kuramoto LK, Schulzer M, et al (BC Children's Hosp, Vancouver; Vancouver General Hosp, BC)

CMAJ 180:719-726, 2009

Background.—The prevalence of childhood obesity is increasing at an alarming rate. Many local governments have enacted policies to increase physical activity in schools as a way to combat childhood obesity. We conducted a systematic review and meta-analysis to determine the effect of school-based physical activity interventions on body mass index (BMI) in children.

Methods.—We searched MEDLINE, EMBASE, CINAHL and the Cochrane Central Register of Controlled Trials up to September 2008. We also hand-searched relevant journals and article reference lists. We included randomized controlled trials and controlled clinical trials that had objective data for BMI from before and after the intervention, that involved school-based physical activity interventions and that lasted for a minimum of 6 months.

Results.—Of 398 potentially relevant articles that we identified, 18 studies involving 18 141 children met the inclusion criteria. The participants were primarily elementary school children. The study duration ranged from 6 months to 3 years. In 15 of these 18 studies, there was some type of cointervention. Meta-analysis showed that BMI did not improve with physical activity interventions (weighted mean difference -0.05 kg/m^2, 95% confidence interval -0.19 to 0.10). We found no consistent changes in other measures of body composition.

Interpretation.—School-based physical activity interventions did not improve BMI, although they had other beneficial health effects. Current population-based policies that mandate increased physical activity in schools are unlikely to have a significant effect on the increasing prevalence of childhood obesity.

▶ The results of this meta-analysis are rather disappointing, but perhaps at least instructive. We continue to be in grave need of effective interventions that can be generally applied and are documented to be effective in combating childhood obesity, but we don't seem to have defined them yet. There are a number of considerations regarding this study, which may be of importance, This investigation looked at the results of studies designed to treat rather than prevent obesity. The age group addressed included only young children, and this review only included school-based programs. Thus, one cannot conclude that increasing physical activity is of no use in our efforts to stem the tide of increasing obesity. However, it seems we need to better pinpoint how, in what setting, and by whom such interventions can best be applied.

T. Rowland, MD

Comparison of Weight-Loss Diets with Different Compositions of Fat, Protein, and Carbohydrates

Sacks FM, Bray GA, Carey VJ, et al (Harvard School of Public Health, Boston, MA; Pennington Biomedical Res Ctr of the Louisiana State Univ System, Baton Rouge, LA; Brigham and Women's Hosp and Harvard Med School, Boston, MA; et al)

N Engl J Med 360:859-873, 2009

Background.—The possible advantage for weight loss of a diet that emphasizes protein, fat, or carbohydrates has not been established, and there are few studies that extend beyond 1 year.

Methods.—We randomly assigned 811 overweight adults to one of four diets; the targeted percentages of energy derived from fat, protein, and carbohydrates in the four diets were 20, 15, and 65%; 20, 25, and 55%; 40, 15, and 45%; and 40, 25, and 35%. The diets consisted of similar foods and met guidelines for cardiovascular health. The participants were offered group and individual instructional sessions for 2 years. The primary outcome was the change in body weight after 2 years in two-by-two factorial comparisons of low fat versus high fat and average protein versus high protein and in the comparison of highest and lowest carbohydrate content.

Results.—At 6 months, participants assigned to each diet had lost an average of 6 kg, which represented 7% of their initial weight; they began to regain weight after 12 months. By 2 years, weight loss remained similar in those who were assigned to a diet with 15% protein and those assigned to a diet with 25% protein (3.0 and 3.6 kg, respectively); in those assigned to a diet with 20% fat and those assigned to a diet with 40% fat (3.3 kg for both groups); and in those assigned to a diet with 65% carbohydrates and those assigned to a diet with 35% carbohydrates (2.9 and 3.4 kg, respectively) ($P > 0.20$ for all comparisons). Among the 80% of participants who completed the trial, the average weight loss was 4 kg; 14 to 15% of the participants had a reduction of at least 10% of their initial body weight. Satiety, hunger, satisfaction with the diet, and attendance at group sessions were similar for all diets; attendance was strongly associated with weight loss (0.2 kg per session attended). The diets improved lipid-related risk factors and fasting insulin levels.

Conclusions.—Reduced-calorie diets result in clinically meaningful weight loss regardless of which macronutrients they emphasize. (ClinicalTrials.gov number, NCT00072995.)

► As emphasized nearly a half-century ago, a calorie is a calorie is a calorie, and whether the source is protein, fat, or carbohydrate, total energy intake and balance is by far the primary issue for weight loss.[1] In the discussion, the authors urged that these divergent results suggest that any type of diet, when taught for the purpose of weight loss with enthusiasm and persistence, can be effective. When nonnutritional influences are minimized, as they were in our study, the specific macronutrient content is of minor importance. This 2-year study not only showed that the varied diets were equally successful in promoting weight loss, but also that satiety did not differ between groups, and improvements in disease risk factors were in the directions that would be expected on the basis of macronutrient content. So in the end, diets can be individualized according to cultural and personal preferences, with an emphasis on tight control of energy balance.

D. C. Nieman, DrPH

Reference

1. Kinsell LW, Gunning B, Michaels GD, Richardson J, Cox SE, Lemon C. Calories do count. *Metabolism.* 1964;13:195-204.

Aerobic and Strength Training Reduces Adiposity in Overweight Latina Adolescents

Davis JN, Tung A, Chak SS, et al (Univ of Southern California, Los Angeles; et al)

Med Sci Sports Exerc 41:1494-1503, 2009

Purpose.—To date, no study has examined the synergistic effects of a nutrition and combination of aerobic and strength training (CAST) on both adiposity and metabolic parameters in overweight Latina adolescent females. The goal was to assess if a 16-wk nutrition plus CAST pilot study had stronger effects on reducing adiposity and on improving glucose/insulin indices compared with control (C), nutrition only (N), and a nutrition plus strength training (N + ST) groups.

Methods.—In a 16-wk randomized trial, 41 overweight Latina girls (15.2 ± 1.1 yr) were randomly assigned to C ($n = 7$), N ($n = 10$), N + ST ($n = 9$), or N + CAST (n = 15). All intervention groups received modified carbohydrate nutrition classes (once a week), whereas the N + ST also received strength training (twice a week) and the N + CAST received a combination of strength and aerobic training (twice a week). The following were measured before and after intervention: strength by one repetition maximum, physical activity by the 7-d accelerometry and the 3-d physical activity recall, dietary intake by 3-d records, body composition by dual-energy x-ray absorptiometry (DEXA), glucose/insulin indices by oral glucose tolerance test, and intravenous glucose tolerance test with minimal modeling. Across intervention group, effects were tested using ANCOVA with *post hoc* pairwise comparisons.

Results.—There were significant overall intervention effects for all adiposity measures (weight, body mass index [BMI], BMI *z*-scores, and DEXA total body fat), with a decrease of 3% in the N + CAST group compared with a 3% increase in the N + ST group ($P \leq 0.05$). There was also an intervention effect for fasting glucose with the N group increasing by 3% and the N + CAST group decreasing by 4% ($P \leq 0.05$).

Conclusion.—The CAST was more effective than nutrition alone or nutrition plus strength training for reducing multiple adiposity outcomes and fasting glucose in overweight Latina girls. However, further research investigating and identifying intervention approaches that improve both adiposity and insulin indices, particularly in high-risk populations, are warranted.

▶ As we continue the battle against childhood obesity it is important that we gain an understanding of the most effective strategies at our disposal. Indeed, lack of insights regarding what works has hampered the adoption of any generalized management approach to treating overly fat youth. In terms of exercise, there has been growing attention to resistance exercise programs as being efficacious for obese youth instead of overly stressful, weight-bearing aerobic exercise that is poorly tolerated. This is one of few studies that has actually tried to compare the 2 approaches. This report is weakened by the low number of subjects in each of the treatment groups (as well as the lack of an aerobic exercise only arm to the study design), but the findings interestingly suggest that a combination of both forms of exercise might be the best approach for both reducing body fat and improving glucose tolerance. We are in need of more studies like this one if we are going to identify the best therapeutic approaches for obese youth.

T. Rowland, MD

Aerobic Exercise Increases Peripheral and Hepatic Insulin Sensitivity in Sedentary Adolescents

van der Heijden G-J, Toffolo G, Manesso E, et al (Baylor College of Medicine, Houston, TX; Univ of Padova, Italy; et al)
J Clin Endocrinol Metab 94:4292-4299, 2009

Context.—Data are limited on the effects of controlled aerobic exercise programs (without weight loss) on insulin sensitivity and glucose metabolism in children and adolescents.

Objective.—To determine whether a controlled aerobic exercise program (without weight loss) improves peripheral and hepatic insulin sensitivity and affects glucose production (GPR), gluconeogenesis and glycogenolysis in sedentary lean and obese Hispanic adolescents.

Patients and Design.—Twenty-nine post-pubertal adolescents (14 lean: 15.1 ± 0.3y; 20.6 ± 0.8 kg/m^2; 18.9 ± 1.5% body fat and 15 obese: 15.6 ± 0.4y; 33.2 ± 0.9 kg/m^2; 38.4 ± 1.4% body fat) (mean ± SE), completed a 12 wk aerobic exercise program (4 × 30 min/week at ≥70% of VO_2 peak). Peripheral and hepatic insulin sensitivity and glucose kinetics were quantified using GCMS pre- and post-exercise.

Results.—No weight loss occurred. Lean and obese participants complied well with the program (~90% of the exercise sessions attended, resulting in ~15% increase in fitness in both groups). Peripheral and hepatic insulin sensitivity were higher in lean than obese adolescents but increased in both groups; peripheral insulin sensitivity by 35 ± 14% (lean) ($p < 0.05$) and 59 ± 19% (obese) ($p < 0.01$) and hepatic insulin sensitivity by 19 ± 7% (lean) ($p < 0.05$) and 23 ± 4% (obese) ($p < 0.01$). GPR, gluconeogenesis and glycogenolysis did not differ between the groups. GPR decreased slightly, 3 ± 1% (lean) ($p < 0.05$) and 4 ± 1% (obese) ($p < 0.01$). Gluconeogenesis remained unchanged, while glycogenolysis decreased slightly in the obese group ($p < 0.01$).

Conclusion.—This well accepted aerobic exercise program, without weight loss, is a promising strategy to improve peripheral and hepatic insulin sensitivity in lean and obese sedentary adolescents. The small decrease in GPR is probably of limited clinical relevance.

▶ This article is just one of numerous articles that have appeared recently giving us a picture of the role of physical exercise in improving insulin sensitivity in young persons, particularly the obese. Of course, this research focus is a reflection of the increasing concern regarding the negative health implications of the dramatic rise in incidence of obesity and type 2 diabetes in this age group. This study is particularly important because it suggests that regular exercise, by itself, may be efficacious in improving insulin sensitivity independent of changes in body fat. Previous investigations have indicated that, because body fat and insulin resistance are typically directly related, exercise might prove useful to improve insulin sensitivity by reducing body fat content. In this case, we see evidence for an independent action of exercise. This bears significance to the role of exercise in promoting metabolic and vascular health in the general pediatric population, lean and obese alike.

T. Rowland, MD

Blood and Urinary Concentration of Salbutamol in Asthmatic Subjects

Elers J, Pedersen L, Henninge J, et al (Bispebjerg Hosp, Copenhagen, Denmark; Aker Univ Hosp, Oslo, Norway)

Med Sci Sports Exerc 42:244-249, 2010

Purpose.—Data on blood and urinary concentrations of salbutamol after inhalation and oral administration in healthy subjects are scarce. Accordingly, we examined the pharmacokinetics of inhaled and oral salbutamol in asthmatic subjects.

Methods.—We enrolled 10 men aged 18–45 yr in an open-label study in which 0.8 mg of inhaled or 8 mg of systemic salbutamol was administered in a crossover design. All subjects had doctor-diagnosed asthma, used β_2 agonist when needed, and abstained from any medicine, β_2 agonist inclusive, for 14 d before visit. Urine was collected from all subjects (0–4, 4–8, and 8–12 h), and blood samples were taken at 0, 0.5, 1, 2, 3, 4, and 6 h after salbutamol administration.

Results.—Maximum urine concentration was reached during the first 4 h after administration of both inhaled and oral salbutamol. We found differences in median urinary concentrations (C_{max}) of 260.9 and 2422.2 $ng \cdot mL^{-1}$, respectively ($P < 0.005$). Urinary concentrations show high individual variability irrespective of the route of administration. Blood analyses showed a systemic exposure of salbutamol after both inhaled and oral salbutamol with peak concentration after inhalation before the oral intake ($P < 0.05$). A difference in median C_{max} after inhalation and oral treatment was found: 1.75 and 18.77 $ng \cdot mL^{-1}$, respectively ($P < 0.05$).

Conclusions.—Median urinary concentrations after oral administration of 8 mg of salbutamol were significantly higher than those after inhalation of 0.8 mg of salbutamol.

▶ The World Anti-Doping Agency (WADA) allows the inhalation of β_2-agonists (terbutaline, salbutamol, formoterol, and salmeterol) to those athletes who have been given a "therapeutic use exemption" by their physicians. However, it is important to distinguish such legitimate use from the oral ingestion of the same substances in the hope of gaining a competitive advantage. To distinguish such use, the WADA has set a limiting urinary concentration of 1000 ng/mL (free salbutamol plus glucuronide); preferably, this should be corrected for urinary specific gravity in case there has been an attempt to mask doping by ingesting a large volume of water. One criticism of present data is that limits were set based mainly on experiments in healthy nonasthmatic subjects.[1-4] Elers and associates thus examined pharmacodynamics in a small sample of asthmatic individuals (10) who were regular users of β_2-agonists. Results showed considerable inter-individual variation, but in no case did nasal inhalation of 0.8 mg salbutamol (4 times the recommended therapeutic dose) yield peak levels greater than 500 ng/mL (590 ng/mL if not corrected for urinary specific gravity), whereas with oral ingestion of 8 mg, all subjects had levels >1000 ng/mL 4 to 8 hours after ingestion, and 9 of 10 subjects also exceeded the threshold 0 to 4 hours after ingestion (Fig 4 in the original article). Although others have suggested ceilings of 250[2] or 500 ng/mL,[5] the present data support the exiting threshold of 1000 ng/mL.

R. J. Shephard, MD (Lond), PhD, DPE

References

1. Anderson PJ. Pharmacokinetics of (R, S)-albuterol after aerosol inhalation in healthy adult volunteers. *J Pharm Sci.* 1998;87:841-844.
2. Pichon A, Venisse N, Krupka E, et al. Urinary and blood concentrations of A-2-agonists in trained subject: comparison between routes of use. *Int J Sports Med.* 2006;27:187-192.
3. Sporer BC, Sheel AW, McKenzie DC. Dose response of inhaled salbutamol on exercise performance and urine concentrations. *Med Sci Sports Exerc.* 2008;40: 149-157.
4. Sporer BC, Sheel AW, Taunton J, et al. Inhaled salbutamol and doping control: effects of dose on urine concentrations. *Clin J Sport Med.* 2008;18:282-285.
5. Ventura R, Segura J, Berges R, et al. Distinction of inhaled and oral salbutamol by urine analysis using conventional screening procedures for doping control. *Ther Drug Monit.* 2000;22:277-282.

Androgenic anabolic steroids also impair right ventricular function

Kasikcioglu E, Oflaz H, Umman B, et al (Istanbul Univ, Turkey)

Int J Cardiol 134:123-125, 2009

Chronic anabolic steroid use suppresses left ventricular functions. However, there is no information regarding the chronic effects of anabolic steroids on right ventricular function which also plays a key role in global cardiac function. The main objective of the present study was to investigate the effects of androgenic anabolic steroids usage among athletes on remodeling the right part of the heart. Androgenic–anabolic steroids-using bodybuilders had smaller diastolic velocities of both ventricles than drug-free bodybuilders and sedentary counterparts. This study shows that androgenic anabolic steroids-using bodybuilders exhibited depressed diastolic functions of both ventricles (Table 1).

► There are many good reasons to avoid the abuse of anabolic steroids, from the viewpoint of both ethics and health. Previous authors have noted a suppression of left ventricular function in those abusing anabolic steroids,[1] and the present small cross-sectional study suggests that there are also substantial adverse changes in right ventricular performance (Table 1). However, there are problems with this sort of study; one cannot administer mega-doses of steroids experimentally, so it is necessary to rely on such cross-sectional data. Moreover, the steroid abusers have taken a wide variety of drugs of uncertain purity, and dosage and the scheduling of dosage is far from clear. It seems that the disturbances of right ventricular function is greater than that for the left ventricle, but further studies are needed to assess how there are myocardial

TABLE 1.—Subjects Characteristics, Standard and Tissue Doppler Data of Left and Right Ventricle.

	AAS-using bodybuilders (n=12)	AAS-not using bodybuilders (n=14)	Controls (n=15)	p value
Age (years)	27 ± 1	26 ± 1	26 ± 1	0.59
Height (cm)	170 ± 2	172 ± 2	175 ± 2	0.44
Weight (kg) *†	80 ± 3	67 ± 3	69 ± 3	0.04
Body surface area (m^2)	1.91 ± 0.05	1.80 ± 0.04	1.83 ± 0.04	0.31
Heart rate (beats/min) ‡	60 ± 2	55 ± 2	64 ± 2	0.03
Systolic blood pressure (mmHg)	120 ± 3	112 ± 3	111 ± 2	0.07
Diastolic blood pressure (mmHg)	79 ± 2	73 ± 2	74 ± 2	0.14
Left ventricle (LV)				
LV mass (g)*†	240 ± 10	184 ± 10	156 ± 9	<0.001
LV mass index (g/m^2) *†‡	124 ± 4	102 ± 4	85 ± 4	<0.001
E-wave (cm/s) †‡	62 ± 4	77 ± 4	92 ± 4	<0.001
A-wave (cm/s) *†	81 ± 4	44 ± 4	56 ± 4	<0.001
E/A*†	0.94 ± 0.13	1.77 ± 0.12	1.67 ± 0.12	<0.001
Deceleration time (ms)	179 ± 9	182 ± 9	166 ± 9	0.43
Isovolumetric relaxation time (ms)†	105 ± 4	98 ± 3	87 ± 3	0.006
E_m (cm/s) *†‡	9.63 ± 0.41	13.27 ± 0.38	11.66 ± 0.36	<0.001
A_m (cm/s) *	8.88 ± 0.44	7.23 ± 0.41	8.32 ± 0.39	0.03
E_m/A_m*†‡	1.09 ± 0.09	1.91 ± 0.08	1.45 ± 0.08	<0.001
S_m (cm/s)	11.01 ± 0.57	12.07 ± 0.52	12.22 ± 0.51	0.25
Right ventricle (RV)				
RV diameter †‡	3.65 ± 0.10	3.72 ± 0.09	3.03 ± 0.09	<0.001
E-wave (cm/s)	60 ± 5	79 ± 5	75 ± 5	0.06
A-wave (cm/s)	39 ± 2	43 ± 2	37 ± 2	0.32
E/A	1.58 ± 0,17	1.91 ± 0.15	2.10 ± 0.15	0.09
E_m (cm/s) *†‡	5.77 ± 0.27	8.41 ± 0.25	7.39 ± 0.24	<0.001
A_m (cm/s)	6.77 ± 0.33	6.58 ± 0.31	6.36 ± 0.29	0.65
E_m/A_m*†	0.85 ± 0.05	1.31 ± 0.05	1.18 ± 0.05	<0.001
S_m (cm/s)	9.61 ± 0.42	9.54 ± 0.39	9.41 ± 0.38	0.94

Values are mean ± SE. AAS, androgenic anabolic steroids; S_m, myocardial systolic wave; E_m, early myocardial diastolic wave; A_m, late myocardial diastolic wave. Symbols; *, significantly different between AAS-using bodybuilders and controls; †, significantly different between AAS-using bodybuilders and AAS-not using bodybuilders; ‡, significantly different between AAS-not using bodybuilders and controls.

changes,[2] and how far steroid-induced hypertension or changes in the vasculature are responsible.[3]

R. J. Shephard, MD (Lond), PhD, DPE

References

1. Urhausen A, Albers T, Kindermann W. Are the cardiac effects of anabolic steroid abuse in strength athletes reversible? *Heart.* 2004;90:496-501.
2. Nottin S, Nguyen LD, Terbah M, Obert P. Cardiovascular effects of androgenic anabolic steroids in male bodybuilders determined by tissue Doppler imaging. *Am J Cardiol.* 2006;15:912-915.
3. Kasikcioglu E, Oflaz H, Arslan A, et al. Aortic elastic properties in athletes using anabolic–androgenic steroids. *Int J Cardiol.* 2007;114:132-134.

Detection of testosterone administration based on the carbon isotope ratio profiling of endogenous steroids: international reference populations of professional soccer players

Strahm E, Emery C, Saugy M, et al (Univ Ctr of Legal Medicine, West Switzerland; et al)

Br J Sports Med 43:1041-1044, 2009

Background and Objectives.—The determination of the carbon isotope ratio in androgen metabolites has been previously shown to be a reliable, direct method to detect testosterone misuse in the context of antidoping testing. Here, the variability in the $^{13}C/^{12}C$ ratios in urinary steroids in a widely heterogeneous cohort of professional soccer players residing in different countries (Argentina, Italy, Japan, South Africa, Switzerland and Uganda) is examined.

Methods.—Carbon isotope ratios of selected androgens in urine specimens were determined using gas chromatography/ combustion/isotope ratio mass spectrometry (GCC-IRMS).

Results.—Urinary steroids in Italian and Swiss populations were found to be enriched in ^{13}C relative to other groups, reflecting higher consumption of C3 plants in these two countries. Importantly, detection criteria based on the difference in the carbon isotope ratio of androsterone and pregnanediol for each population were found to be well below the established threshold value for positive cases.

Conclusions.—The results obtained with the tested diet groups highlight the importance of adapting the criteria if one wishes to increase the sensitivity of exogenous testosterone detection. In addition, confirmatory tests might be rendered more efficient by combining isotope ratio mass spectrometry with refined interpretation criteria for positivity and subject-based profiling of steroids.

▶ Testosterone doping cannot be detected simply by measuring blood levels of this steroid. However, a method of detecting exogenous administration of testosterone has been developed based on the proportions of the ^{13}C isotope of carbon found on mass spectrometry. Endogenous steroids are synthesized from cholesterol, which in turn is based on compounds synthesized from atmospheric carbon dioxide by plants that use either ^{3}C or ^{4}C pathways. The 2 types of plants (^{3}C and ^{4}C) yield steroids containing differing proportions of the ^{13}C isotope.[1,2] Pharmaceutical preparations are synthesized from phytosterols of ^{13}C depleted (^{3}C) plants (typically soy and Mexican yam). The levels of ^{13}C observed in athletes depend on their diet: ^{3}C plants (wheat, barley, oats, sugar beet, rye, cotton, corn, millet, sugar cane, and sorghum) yield ^{13}C levels of −22% to −35% relative to the expected content, and ^{4}C plants show a deficit of −8% to −20% relative to standards. When trying to detect exogenous steroid use, it might thus be thought necessary to take account of interindividual differences in an athlete's diet. However, this difficulty can be solved by looking at intraindividual differences in ^{13}C content between anabolic steroids and reference endogenous compounds; a difference of more than 3% is currently

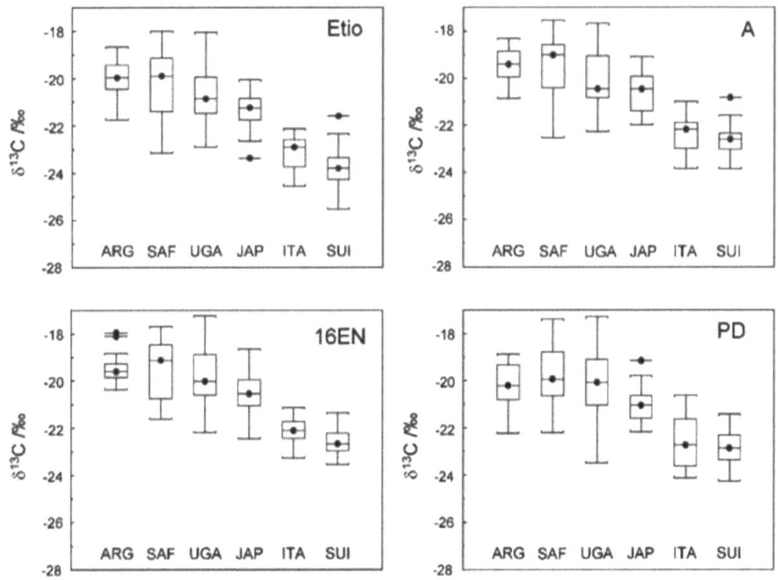

FIGURE 2.—Distribution of d13C values obtained for etiocholanolone (Etio), androsterone (A), 16(5α)-androstenol (16EN) and 5β-pregnanediol (PD) in the urine specimens of the top-level soccer players residing in the six surveyed countries. (Reprinted from Strahm E, Emery C, Saugy M, et al. Detection of testosterone administration based on the carbon isotope ratio profiling of endogenous steroids: international reference populations of professional soccer players. *Br J Sports Med.* 2009;43:1041-1044, with permission from the BMJ Publishing Group.)

accepted as evidence of doping.[3] The present report looked at C13 content in both androgens and reference compounds in athletes where the prevalence of doping was assumed to be low, and the C13 relationship between androgenic and reference compounds was sustained over quite a wide range of diets (Fig 2). However, in some comparisons (eg, 5β-pregnanediol vs androsterone), the 3% doping detection margin appeared to be somewhat too permissive, and a little too restrictive for etiocholanolone versus reference compounds.

R. J. Shephard, MD (Lond), PhD, DPE

References

1. Smith BN, Epstein S. Two categories of $^{13}C/^{12}C$ ratios for higher plants. *Plant Physiol.* 1971;47:380-384.
2. O'Leary MH. Carbon isotope fractionation in plants. *Phytochem.* 1981;20: 553-567.
3. WADA. WADA technical document -T2004EAAS: reporting and evaluation guidance for testosterone, epitestosterone, T/E ratio and other endogenous steroids, 2004. http://www.wada-ama.org. Accessed January 2010.

The use of growth hormone (GH)-dependent markers in the detection of GH abuse in sport: Physiological intra-individual variation of IGF-I, type 3 pro-collagen (P-III-P) and the GH-2000 detection score

Erotokritou-Mulligan I, Eryl Bassett E, Cowan DA, et al (Univ of Southampton, UK; Univ of Kent, UK; Drug Control Centre, London, UK; et al)

Clin Endocrinol 72:520-526, 2010

Background.—Growth Hormone is abused by athletes for its lipolytic and anabolic properties. Its use is prohibited by the World Anti-Doping Agency. The GH-2000 project developed a methodology to detect its abuse using the concentrations of two GH-dependent biomarkers, IGF-I and type 3 procollagen (P-III-P). The sensitivity of this method may be improved by considering intra-individual variability.

Aim.—The aim of this study was to examine the intra-individual variability of IGF-I, P-III-P and the GH-2000 score.

Subjects and Methods.—IGF-I, P-III-P and GH-2000 score were evaluated in four longitudinal studies involving 303 elite and 78 amateur athletes. Samples were collected over a period of up to 12 months from a total of 238 men and 143 women aged between 17 and 53 years (mean 24·2).

Results.—The four studies showed good agreement with no apparent difference in within-individual variation between amateur and elite athletes. The intra-individual variability for IGF-I ranged between 14–16% while the variability for P-III-P was 7–18%. No athlete tested positive for growth hormone during any of the studies. The overall

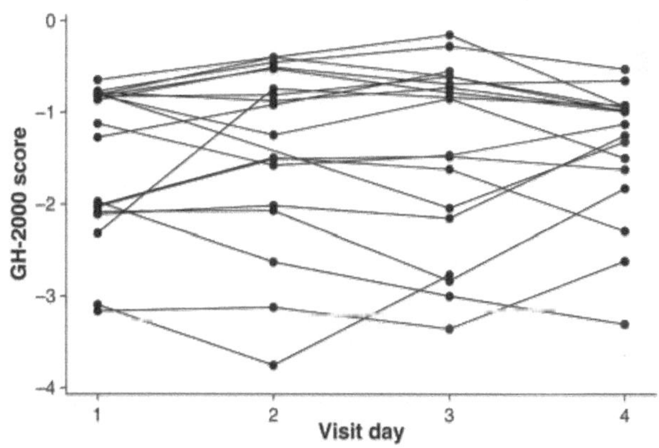

FIGURE 3.—Calculated GH-2000 scores for each female individual at each visit day participating in the GH-2004 longitudinal study. Visits were approximately 1 month apart. Each line connects the samples connected for each individual; each symbol represents the calculated GH-2000 score at each visit. (Reprinted from Erotokritou-Mulligan I, Eryl Bassett E, Cowan DA, et al. The use of growth hormone (GH)-dependent markers in the detection of GH abuse in sport: Physiological intra-individual variation of IGF-I, type 3 pro-collagen (P-III-P) and the GH-2000 detection score. *Clin Endocrinol.* 2010;72:520-526, with permission from Blackwell Publishing Ltd.)

mean intra-individual variability of the GH-2000 score was less than 0·6 units in all studies.

Conclusions.—The high stability of marker levels suggests that concentrations are largely genetically determined. Adopting a test based on the concept of an athlete's 'passport' or 'profiling' would take advantage of this and most likely increase the sensitivity of the test. These data also provide strong evidence that a positive test result for GH abuse would not occur as a result of chance variability (Fig 3).

▶ The detection of growth hormone (GH) abuse is difficult, in part because of its pulsatile release under normal conditions.[1] However, it is encouraging that the tests are now emerging that can detect some, if not all, athletes who engage in the abuse of GH. The necessary tests are based on the measurement of 2 GH-dependent markers: insulin-like growth factor-I (IGF-I) and type III procollagen (P-III-P).[2] Even after the application of age- and gender-specific discriminant formulae, there remain substantial (possibly genetic) interindividual differences in blood levels of the IGF-1 and P-III-P markers. However, the intra-individual differences at repeat testing are relatively small (Fig 3), allowing a profile or athletic passport to be developed for each competitor,[3,4] showing the anticipated levels of biomarkers in the absence of doping.

R. J. Shephard, MD (Lond), PhD, DPE

References

1. Holt RI, Sonksen PH. Growth hormone, IGF-I and insulin and their abuse in sport. *Br J Pharmacol.* 2008;154:542-556.
2. Powrie JK, Bassett EE, Rosen T, et al. Detection of growth hormone abuse in sport. *Growth Horm IGF Res.* 2007;17:220-226.
3. Sottas PE, Saudan C, Schweizer C, Baume N, Mangin P, Saugy M. From population-to subject-based limits of T/E ratio to detect testosterone abuse in elite sports. *Forensic Sci Internat.* 2008;174:166-172.
4. Strahm E, Sottas PE, Schweizer C, Saugy M, Dvorak J, Saudan C. Steroid profiles of professional soccer players: an international comparative study. *Br J Sports Med.* 2009;43:1126-1130.

Desmopressin and Hemodilution: Implications in Doping

Sanchis-Gomar F, Martinez-Bello VE, Nascimento AL, et al (Univ of Valencia, Spain; et al)

Int J Sports Med 31:5-9, 2010

Blood doping improves physical performance in sport. This is the reason why the antidoping authorities subject athletes to blood tests. Plasma volume expanders are prohibited agents used to reduce an artificial increase in hematological values using different illegal practices. The aim of our study was to test whether desmopressin (DDAVP)-induced hemodilution would alter the concentration of hematological parameters used to detect blood doping in sports. This was an intra-subject crossover study. Venous blood samples were obtained from eight physically active

TABLE 2.—Hemoglobin, Hematocrit, Reticulocyte and Values of the OFF-Hr Score in Water and Water + DDAVP Groups

Time	Water + DDAVP	Mean Levels Water	Mean Difference
Hemoglobin (g/dL)			
basal	15.2 (0.5)	15.6 (0.5)	−0.4 (0.3, 1.6)
after Treatment	13.8 (0.5)#	15.5 (0.6)	−1.8 (−11.8, 13.8)*
Hematocrit (%)			
basal	45.8 (1.5)	46.8 (1.8)	−1.0 (−3.0, 1.0)
after treatment	42.0 (1.3)#	46.4 (1.9)	−4.4 (−38.2, 40.2)*
Reticulocytes (%)			
basal	0.8 (0.2)	0.8 (0.2)	0.0 (0.7, 1.2)
after treatment	0.6 (0.2)	0.7 (0.2)	−0.1 (0.3, 1.7)
OFF-Hr Score			
basal	100.8 (0.7)	100.4 (5.2)	−3.2 (−6.8, 8.8)
after treatment	90.9 (5.9)#	104.1 (4.2)	−13.2 (−84.8, 86.8)*

Data presented as mean (SD) and mean differences (95 % CI) of different hematological parameters in five physically active humans (n = 5).

*Indicates significant difference ($p < 0.05$) between Water + DDAVP vs. Water groups using the non-parametric Mann-Whitney U test.

#Indicates significant difference ($p < 0.05$) between Basal and After Treament extractions using the non-parametric Wilcoxon Test.

males on two occasions. On the first occasion the subjects ingested 1.5 L of mineral water and 4.3 μg/kg of DDAVP. On the second occasion the subjects ingested 1.5 L of mineral water. The samples were analyzed for hematocrit, hemoglobin, reticulocytes, OFF Hr-Score, glucose, albumin, creatinine and total proteins. After treatment with DDAVP we found a significant decrease in the hematocrit, hemoglobin and in the OFF Hr-Score values. We also found a significant decrease in glucose, albumin, creatinine and total proteins concentration; however, in this case, all the values were significantly below the physiological levels. Treatment with DDAVP has a very effective hemodilution effect. We consider that this substance should be included in the WADA's prohibited list (Table 2).

▶ A number of Olympic competitors have admitted to using blood doping, notably the United States cycling team at the Los Angeles Olympics,[1] and the International Olympic Committee (IOC) officially prohibited the use of erythropoietin in 1990. The technique of detection used by the Union Cycliste Internationale is to measure the hemoglobin, hematocrit, and reticulocyte count, if the athlete exceeds a specified threshold for any of these 3 variables, he or she is banned from competition for 15 days. Unfortunately, it appears that a rapid and temporary hemodilution induced by the ingestion of desmopressin (4.3 g/kg) can allow an athlete to avoid detection of this type of doping (Table 2). One of the key indices that is distorted is the Off-Hr score, the combination of a high hemoglobin and a low reticulocyte count that is seen when erythropoietin treatment is stopped.[2] Other plasma volume expanders such as albumin, dextran, or hydroxyethyl starch are already banned[3,4] because of both masking effects and their own ability to enhance endurance performance.

It seems that the time has come to add desmopressin to the list of banned substances.

R. J. Shephard, MD (Lond), PhD, DPE

References

1. Cooper CE, Beneke RE. *Drugs and Ergogenic Aids to Improve Sport Performance.* London: Portland Press; 2008. 1–152.
2. Souillard A, Audran M, Bressolle F, Gareau R, Duvallet A, Chanal JL. Pharmacokinetics and pharmacodynamics of recombinant human erythropoietin in athletes. Blood sampling and doping control. *Br J Clin Pharmacol.* 1996;42:355-364.
3. Guddat S, Thevis M, Schanzer W. Identication and quantification of the plasma volume expander dextran in human urine by liquid chromatography-tandem mass spectrometry of enzymatically derived isomaltose. *Biomed Chromatogr.* 2005;19:743-750.
4. Gutierrez GR, Segura J. Rapid screening of plasma volume. *Clin Pharmacol.* 1996; 42:355-364.

Identification of Darbepoetin Alfa in Human Plasma by Liquid Chromatography Coupled to Mass Spectrometry for Doping Control

Guan F, Uboh CE, Soma LR, et al (Univ of Pennsylvania, Kennett Square; West Chester Univ, PA)

Int J Sports Med 30:80-86, 2009

Darbepoetin alfa (DPO) or Novel Erythropoiesis Erythropoiesis Stimulating Protein (NESP), an analog of recombinant human erythropoietin (rhEPO), is abused as a blood doping agent along with the latter in human sports. This paper describes a new method for unequivocal identification of DPO in human plasma. The analyte was extracted from plasma by immunoaffinity separation with anti-rhEPO antibodies, digested by trypsin followed by PNGase F, and analyzed by liquid chromatography coupled to tandem mass spectrometry. The deglycosylated tryptic peptide, T_9, was employed in DPO identification using liquid chromatographic retention time and major product ions of the T_9 peptide. The limit of detection of this method for DPO was 0.1 ng/mL in plasma, and that of identification was 0.2 ng/mL. This method is definitive and devoid of false positive results, providing "mass fingerprints" for identification of DPO in human plasma samples. Although this method is not applicable to identification of rhEPO in human plasma because it cannot differentiate rhEPO from endogenous EPO, it is the first successful attempt towards establishing a reliable and selective method for definitive identification of exogenously administered EPOs in doping control analyses (Fig 4).

▶ The detection of the administration of recombinant erythropoietin and its analog darbepoetin alpha remains one of the major challenges in doping control. Current screening techniques based on western blotting[1] are limited by false positive results. The alternative approach of liquid chromatography has previously lacked adequate sensitivity, but the technique of a preliminary

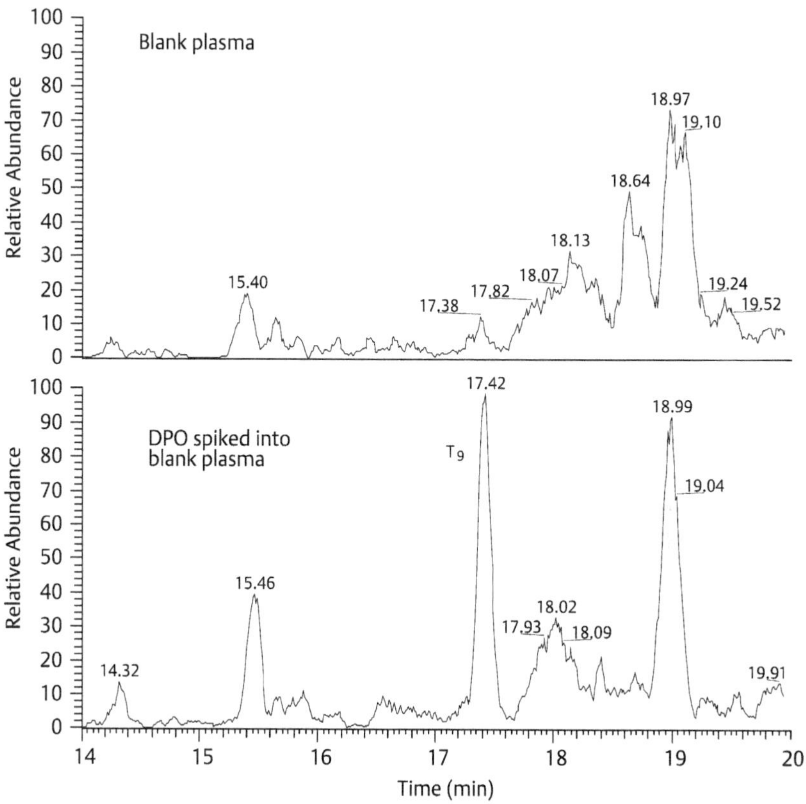

FIGURE 4.—LC-MS/MS chromatograms of blank human plasma and DPO (0.2 ng/mL) spiked into blank human plasma showing detection of DPO via the deglycosylated tryptic peptide T_9 at 17.42 min. The chromatograms were reconstructed using product ions of the T_9 peptide, *m/z* 857.6, 907, 963.5, 1020.1, and 1055.8. The small peak at t_R of 17.38 min in the chromatogram of blank human plasma does not relate to the T_9 peptide and interfere with the identification of DPO, as indicated by MS/MS spectrum of the peak shown in Fig. 5 of the original article. (Reprinted from Guan F, Uboh CE, Soma LR, et al. Identification of darbepoetin alfa in human plasma by liquid chromatography coupled to mass spectrometry for doping control. *Int J Sports Med.* 2009;30:80-86.)

separation by erythropoietin antibodies as described in this article gives promise of an unequivocal demonstration of the presence of darbepoetin alpha (Fig 4). However, further research seems needed to confirm the claims of adequate sensitivity and an absence of false positive results.

R. J. Shephard, MD (Lond), PhD, DPE

Reference

1. Lamon S, Robinson N, Mangin P, Saugy M. Detection window of Darbepoetin-a following one single subcutaneous injection. *Clin Chim Acta.* 2007;379: 145-149.

Urinary di-(2-ethylhexyl)phthalate metabolites in athletes as screening measure for illicit blood doping: a comparison study with patients receiving blood transfusion

Monfort N, Ventura R, Latorre A, et al (IMIM- Hosp Del Mar, Spain; Universitat Pompeu Fabra, Spain; Hosp del Mar, Barcelona, Spain)
Transfusion 50:145-149, 2010

Background.—Subjects submitted to intravenous (IV) blood transfusions for medical reasons or blood doping to increase athletic performance are potentially exposed to the plasticizer di-(2-ethylhexyl)phthalate (DEHP) found in IV bags. Exposure to DEHP has been evaluated by measuring DEHP metabolites in selected groups of subjects.

Study Design and Methods.—Urinary DEHP metabolites, mono-(2-ethylhexyl)phthalate, mono-(2-ethyl-5-hydroxyhexyl)phthalate (MEHHP), and mono-(2-ethyl-5-oxohexyl)phthalate (MEOHP) were measured in a control group with no explicit known exposure to DEHP (n = 30), hospitalized patients receiving blood transfusions (n = 25), nontransfused hospitalized patients receiving other medical care involving plastic materials (n = 39), and athletes (n = 127). Patients were tested in the periods 0 to 24 and 24 to 48 hours after exposition.

Results.—Urinary concentrations of all three DEHP metabolites were significantly higher in patients receiving blood transfusion than in nontransfused patients and the control group, except for MEHHP and MEOHP in the period 24 to 48 hours. Samples from four athletes showed increased concentrations of DEHP metabolites comparable to urinary concentrations of patients receiving blood transfusion.

Conclusion.—Elevated concentrations of urinary DEHP metabolites represent increased exposure to DEHP. High concentrations of DEHP metabolites present in urine collected from athletes may suggest illegal blood transfusion and can be used as a qualitative screening measure for blood doping (Table 2).

▶ The plasticizer DEHP leaks from transfusion bags into the blood stored in such packaging,[1-3] and is subsequently excreted in the urine as a conjugate with glucuronic acid.[4,5] This has 2 practical consequences. Firstly, it offers

TABLE 2.—Distribution of Concentrations of DEHP Metabolites Among the Athletes Group

			Concentrations (ng/mL)								
			Percentile					Outliers*			
Group	Number	Metabolite	10th	25th	50th	75th	90th	A†	B†	C†	D†
Athletes		MEHP	0.3	3.8	7.1	11.5	19.7	38.7	40.0	58.6	119.2
	127	MEHHP	4.7	8.8	18.4	27.5	49.8	102.0	161.1	155.9	119.2
		MEOHP	5.1	11.4	18.4	30.0	51.7	100.3	226.8	154.2	243.2

*Concentrations above the 75th percentile plus three times the interquartile (75th-25th) range.
†A code (A, B, C, D) was assigned to each subject with outlier concentrations.

a simple qualitative test for blood doping for up to 2 days following transfusion (Table 2). In contrast with most available techniques, it works for both autologous and allogenic blood, and does not require blood samples (not always available from athletes). Competitors detected by this form of triage can subsequently be subjected to more definitive blood testing. Secondly, the plasticizers are toxic, and thus repeated blood doping could have adverse consequences for the health of an athlete.

R. J. Shephard, MD (Lond), PhD, DPE

References

1. FDA Public Health Notification [monograph on the Internet]. Safety assessment of di(2-ethylhexyl)phthalate (DEHP) released from polyvinyl chloride (PVC) medical devices, http://www.fda.gov/cdrh/ost/dehp-pvc.pdf. Updated 2001. Accessed November 6, 2008.
2. European Commission Health & Consumer Protection DG Brussels. Scientific Committee on Emerging and Newly-Identified Health Risks (SCENIHR). The safety of medical devices containing DEHP plasticized PVC or other plasticizers on neonates and other groups possibly at risk. European Commission [Updated 2008. Accessed November 6, 2008].
3. Inoue K, Kawaguchi M, Yamanaka R, et al. Evaluation and analysis of exposure levels of di-(2-ethylhexyl)phthalate from blood bags. *Clin Chim Acta.* 2005;358: 159-166.
4. Silva MJ, Slakman AR, Reidy JA, et al. Analysis of human urine for fifteen phthalate metabolites using automated solid-phase extraction. *J Chromatogr B.* 2004; 805:161-167.
5. Koch H, Bolt H, Preuss R, Angerer J. New metabolites of di(2-ethylhexyl)phthalate(DEHP) in human urine and serum after single oral doses of deuterium-labelled DEHP. *Arch Toxicol.* 2005;79:367-376.

Caffeine Supplementation and Multiple Sprint Running Performance

Glaister M, Howatson G, Abraham CS, et al (St Mary's Univ College, Twickenham, UK; UWIC, Cardiff, UK)

Med Sci Sports Exerc 40:1835-1840, 2008

Purpose.—The aim of this study was to examine the effects of caffeine supplementation on multiple sprint running performance.

Methods.—Using a randomized double-blind research design, 21 physically active men ingested a gelatin capsule containing either caffeine ($5\ \mathrm{mg\,kg^{-1}}$ body mass) or placebo (maltodextrin) 1 h before completing an indoor multiple sprint running trial (12×30 m; repeated at 35-s intervals). Venous blood samples were drawn to evaluate plasma caffeine and primary metabolite concentrations. Sprint times were recorded via twin-beam photocells, and earlobe blood samples were drawn to evaluate pretest and posttest lactate concentrations. Heart rate was monitored continuously throughout the tests, with RPE recorded after every third sprint.

Results.—Relative to placebo, caffeine supplementation resulted in a 0.06-s (1.4%) reduction in fastest sprint time (95% likely range = 0.04–0.09 s), which corresponded with a 1.2% increase in fatigue (95% likely range = 0.3–2.2%). Caffeine supplementation also resulted in a 3.4-bpm increase in mean heart rate (95% likely range = 0.1–6.6 bpm) and elevations in pretest (+0.7 $mmol \cdot L^{-1}$; 95% likely range = 0.1–1.3 $mmol \cdot L^{-1}$) and posttest (+1.8 $mmol \cdot L^{-1}$; 95% likely range = 0.3–3.2 $mmol \cdot L^{-1}$) blood lactate concentrations. In contrast, there was no significant effect of caffeine supplementation on RPE.

Conclusion.—Although the effect of recovery duration on caffeine-induced responses to multiple sprint work requires further investigation, the results of the present study show that caffeine has ergogenic properties with the potential to benefit performance in both single and multiple sprint sports.

▶ This study showed that an acute caffeine dose (the amount found in 3 cups of coffee) improved performance during intermittent sprinting. However, the underlying mechanism was not established, and the ergogenic benefit was offset by an overall increase in fatigue. Additionally, although participants sprinted faster in the early stages of the test and showed a greater rate of fatigue, individual perceptions of exertion were the same as those of baseline and placebo. Nonetheless, the authors concluded that the results of this study suggest that caffeine has ergogenic properties with the potential to benefit performance in both single and multiple sprint sports. In general, most studies support a small but important enhancement in repeated bouts of sprinting.[1]

D. C. Nieman, DrPH

Reference

1. Carr A, Dawson B, Schneiker K, Goodman C, Lay B. Effect of caffeine supplementation on repeated sprint running performance. *J Sports Med Phys Fitness*. 2008 Dec;48:472-478.

Substrate Metabolism and Exercise Performance with Caffeine and Carbohydrate Intake

Hulston CJ, Jeukendrup AE (Univ of Birmingham, UK)

Med Sci Sports Exerc 40:2096-2104, 2008

Purpose.—1) To investigate the effect of caffeine on exogenous carbohydrate (CHO) oxidation and glucose kinetics during exercise; and 2) to determine whether combined ingestion of caffeine and CHO enhanced cycling performance compared with CHO alone.

Methods.—Ten endurance-trained cyclists performed three experimental trials consisting of 105 min steady-state (SS) cycling at 62% $\dot{V}O_{2max}$ followed by a time trial (TT) lasting approximately 45 min. During exercise, subjects ingested either of the following: a 6.4% glucose solution (GLU), a 6.4% glucose plus caffeine solution providing 5.3 $mg \cdot kg^{-1}$ of caffeine (GLU + CAF), or a placebo (PLA). Glucose solutions contained a trace amount of [U-^{13}C]glucose, and eight subjects received a primed continuous [6,6-$^{2}H_2$]glucose infusion.

Results.—Peak exogenous CHO oxidation rates were not significantly different between GLU and GLU + CAF trials (52.6 ± 2.7 and 49.1 ± 2.1 $\mu mol \cdot kg^{-1} \cdot min^{-1}$, respectively). Rates of appearance (R_a) and disappearance (R_d) of glucose were significantly higher with CHO ingestion than PLA ($P < 0.01$) but were not significantly different between GLU and GLU + CAF trials. Performance times were 43.45 ± 0.86, 45.45 ± 1.07, and 47.40 ± 1.30 min for GLU + CAF, GLU, and PLA, respectively. Therefore, GLU + CAF ingestion enhanced TT performance by 4.6% ($P < 0.05$) compared with GLU and 9% ($P < 0.05$) compared with PLA.

Conclusion.—The coingestion of caffeine (5.3 $mg \cdot kg^{-1}$) with CHO during exercise enhanced TT performance by 4.6% compared with CHO and 9.0% compared with water placebo. However, caffeine did not influence exogenous CHO oxidation or glucose kinetics during SS exercise.

▶ Caffeine ingestion improves endurance performance, and this was originally related to enhanced mobilization of free fatty acids from adipose tissue.[1] This theory has not held up under scrutiny, and it appears that caffeine exerts its positive effects through the central nervous system.[2] Caffeine may also increase the intestinal absorption and oxidation of carbohydrate when both are ingested during exercise.[3] In this study, the coingestion of glucose and caffeine enhanced performance when compared with glucose alone or placebo. However, caffeine did not influence exogenous carbohydrate oxidation or glucose kinetics during exercise. Instead, subjects experienced a reduced perception of effort with caffeine ingestion, which allowed the subjects to adopt a higher work rate. There is increasing support for the use of energy drinks containing carbohydrate and caffeine to enhance performance, and most sports drink companies will probably start adding caffeine to their sugar-based beverages.[4]

D. C. Nieman, DrPH

References

1. Costill DL, Dalsky GP, Fink WJ. Effects of caffeine ingestion on metabolism and exercise performance. *Med Sci Sports.* 1978;10:155-158.
2. Tarnopolsky MA. Effect of caffeine on the neuromuscular system–potential as an ergogenic aid. *Appl Physiol Nutr Metab.* 2008;33:1284-1289.
3. Van Nieuwenhoven MA, Brummer RM, Brouns F. Gastrointestinal function during exercise: comparison of water, sports drink, and sports drink with caffeine. *J Appl Physiol.* 2000;89:1079-1085.
4. Ivy JL, Kammer L, Ding Z, et al. Improved cycling time-trial performance after ingestion of a caffeine energy drink. *Int J Sport Nutr Exerc Metab.* 2009;19:61-78.

Effects of exercise on cravings to smoke: The role of exercise intensity and cortisol

Scerbo F, Faulkner G, Taylor A, et al (Univ of Toronto, Ontario, Canada; Univ of Exeter, UK)

J Sports Sci 28:11-19, 2009

Research consistently demonstrates that a bout of moderate exercise alleviates cravings to smoke among abstaining smokers. The aims of this study were to examine whether doses of exercise (moderate or vigorous) reduced cravings differently, and whether reductions in cravings were associated with changes in cortisol concentration. Using a within-participant, crossover design, 18 participants conducted three 15-min treatment sessions on separate days: passive, walking (45–50% heart rate reserve), and running (80–85% heart rate reserve) conditions. Participants rated cravings at baseline, mid-treatment, and 0, 10, 20, and 30 min after each treatment. Salivary cortisol samples were collected at baseline, immediately after, and 30 min after each condition. Significant group × time interactions were identified, demonstrating significant reductions in craving items after the walking and running conditions compared with the passive control. No significant differences in craving reductions were found between walking and running conditions. *Post hoc* comparisons found that running condition cravings to smoke scores were reduced for a longer duration post-treatment than post-walking condition scores. The decline in cortisol concentration was attenuated in the running group only. Vigorous exercise has a similar effect to moderate exercise in terms of the magnitude of craving reduction. However, performing bouts of moderate-intensity exercise may be a better recommendation for reducing cravings.

▶ Despite its importance to preventive medicine, there has been relatively little study of the benefits of exercise in controlling addiction to cigarettes,[1-5] although there have been some reports that cravings were reduced by participation in low and moderate intensity exercise, both rhythmic and isometric. Distraction and expectancy do not seem to be the primary mechanisms of benefit, and in this study Scerbo and associates look at the potential role of exercise-induced changes in cortisol concentration. Cortisol concentrations are known to be higher in smokers, and to fall substantially within the first 12 hours of smoking cessation.[6] A cross-over trial here compared the effects of high intensity exercise (15 minutes of running at 80%-85% of heart rate reserve, where there was likely a substantial release of cortisol) with moderate intensity exercise (walking for 15 minutes at 45%-50% of heart rate reserve) in a group of recently abstinent strongly nicotine-dependent smokers (normally smoking at least 10 cigarettes per day and abstinent for 3 hours). Cravings to smoke were assessed on two 7-point Likert scales, and as would be anticipated from a cortisol release hypothesis, cravings were reduced for longer, but not to a greater extent by running than by walking (Fig 1 in the original article); however, changes in serum cortisol did not entirely match the altered cravings, casting some doubt on cortisol as a mechanism; possibly, there is a ceiling effect for hormone-induced benefits. The present data suggest that either moderate or vigorous intensity exercise can help in smoking withdrawal, although there remains a need to conduct similar studies on subjects who are in the process of smoking withdrawal. There is also a need to evaluate how far changes in cravings translate into less recidivism among such a group. Finally, the subjects tested by Scerbo and associates were relatively active, and there is a need to repeat observations on more typical sedentary smokers.

R. J. Shephard, MD (Lond), PhD, DPE

References

1. Taylor AH, Ussher MH. Effects of exercise on smoking cessation and coping with withdrawal symptoms and nicotine cravings. In: Faulkner GEJ, Taylor AH, eds. *Exercise, Health and Mental Health: Emerging Relationships*. Abingdon, UK: Routledge; 2005:135-158.
2. Taylor AH, Ussher MH, Faulkner G. The acute effects of exercise on smoking behaviour, cravings, withdrawal symptoms and affect: a systematic review. *Addiction*. 2007;102:534-543.
3. Ussher MH, Nunziata P, Cropley M, West R. Effect of a short bout of exercise on tobacco withdrawal symptoms and desire to smoke. *Psychopharmacol*. 2001;158: 66-72.
4. Ussher M, West R, Doshi R, Sampuran AK. Acute effect of isometric exercise on desire to smoke and tobacco withdrawal symptoms. *Human Psychopharmacol*. 2006;21:39-46.
5. Everson ES, Daley AJ, Ussher M. The effects of moderate and vigorous exercise on desire to smoke, withdrawal symptoms and mood in abstaining young adult smokers. *Mental Health Phys Activ*. 2008;1:26-31.
6. Pomerleau CS, Garcia AW, Pomerleau OF, Cameron OG. The effects of menstrual phase and nicotine abstinence on nicotine intake and on biochemical and subjective measures in women smokers: a preliminary report. *Psychoneuroendocrinol*. 1992;17:627-638.

Ergogenic and Antioxidant Effects of Spirulina Supplementation in Humans

Kalafati M, Jamurtas AZ, Nikolaidis MG, et al (Ctr for Res and Technology–Thessaly, Trikala, Greece; et al)

Med Sci Sports Exerc 42:142-151, 2010

Purpose.—Spirulina is a popular nutritional supplement that is accompanied by claiMSS for antioxidant and performance-enhancing effects. Therefore, the aim of the present study was to examine the effect of spirulina supplementation on (i) exercise performance, (ii) substrate metabolism, and (iii) blood redox status both at rest and after exercise.

Methods.—Nine moderately trained males took part in a double-blind, placebo-controlled, counterbalanced crossover study. Each subject received either spirulina ($6\ g \cdot d^{-1}$) or placebo for 4 wk. Each subject ran on a treadmill at an intensity corresponding to 70%–75% of their $\dot{V}O_{2max}$ for 2 h and then at 95% $\dot{V}O_{2max}$ to exhaustion. Exercise performance and respiratory quotient during exercise were measured after both placebo and spirulina supplementation. Blood samples were drawn before, immediately after, and at 1, 24, and 48 h after exercise. Reduced glutathione (GSH), oxidized glutathione (GSSG), GSH/GSSG, thiobarbituric acid-reactive substances (TBARS), protein carbonyls, catalase activity, and total antioxidant capacity (TAC) were determined.

Results.—Time to fatigue after the 2-h run was significantly longer after spirulina supplementation (2.05 ± 0.68 vs 2.70 ± 0.79 min). Ingestion of spirulina significantly decreased carbohydrate oxidation rate by 10.3% and increased fat oxidation rate by 10.9% during the 2-h run compared with the placebo trial. GSH levels were higher after the spirulina supplementation compared with placebo at rest and 24 h after exercise. TBARS levels increased after exercise after placebo but not after spirulina supplementation. Protein carbonyls, catalase, and TAC levels increased similarly immediately after and 1 h after exercise in both groups.

Conclusions.—Spirulina supplementation induced a significant increase in exercise performance, fat oxidation, and GSH concentration and attenuated the exercise-induced increase in lipid peroxidation.

▶ Spirulina is a microscopic blue-green algae living both in sea and fresh water. Spirulina is cultivated around the world and is used as an animal and human dietary supplement. Most cultivated spirulina is produced in open-channel raceway ponds, with paddle wheels used to agitate the water. Spirulina is 55% to 77% protein by dry weight and contains essential fatty acids, numerous vitamins, and minerals. As is common with food supplements, such as spirulina, the hype far outweighs the evidence, and well-designed human trials are needed to confirm potential ergogenic and health benefits.[1] In this study, ingestion of 6 g/d spirulina for 4 weeks had a small but significant effect in improving performance after a 2-hour preload (Fig 2 in the original article). The authors admitted that the reasons behind the enhanced performance are poorly understood but suggested that spirulina consumption may increase fat oxidation and reduced glutathione (GSH) levels during exercise. Most human studies use 6 to 8 g/d spirulina, and this amount provides small amounts of protein, vitamins, and minerals, and, thus, is unlikely to increase GSH, despite the authors' speculation on this point. At 6 g/d, spirulina only provides 3.5 g protein, 34 UI vitamin A, and 0.3 mg vitamin E, which when balanced against total diet intake is negligible.

D. C. Nieman, DrPH

Reference

1. Park HJ, Lee YJ, Ryu HK, Kim MH, Chung HW, Kim WY. A randomized double-blind, placebo-controlled study to establish the effects of spirulina in elderly Koreans. *Ann Nutr Metab*. 2008;52:322-328.

Influence of acetaminophen on performance during time trial cycling

Mauger AR, Jones AM, Williams CA (Univ of Exeter, Devon, UK)

J Appl Physiol 108:98-104, 2010

To establish whether acetaminophen improves performance of self-paced exercise through the reduction of perceived pain, 13 trained male cyclists performed a self-paced 10-mile (16.1 km) cycle time trial (TT) following the ingestion of either acetaminophen (ACT) or a placebo (PLA), administered in randomized double-blind design. TT were completed in a significantly faster time ($t_{12} = 2.55$, $P < 0.05$) under the ACT condition (26 min 15 s ± 1 min 36 s vs. 26 min 45 s ± 2 min 2 s). Power output (PO) was higher during the middle section of the TT in the ACT condition, resulting in a higher mean PO ($P < 0.05$) (265 ± 12 vs. 255 ± 15 W). Blood lactate concentration (B[La]) and heart rate (HR) were higher in the ACT condition (B[La] = 6.1 ± 2.9 mmol/l; HR = 87 ± 7%max) than in the PLA condition (B[La] = 5.1 ± 2.6 mmol/l; HR = 84 ± 9%max) ($P < 0.05$). No significant difference in rating of perceived exertion (ACT = 15.5 ± 0.2; PLA = 15.7 ± 0.2) or perceived pain (ACT = 5.6 ± 0.2; PLA = 5.5 ± 0.2) ($P > 0.05$) was observed. Using acetaminophen, participants cycled at a higher mean PO, with an increased HR and B[La], but without changes in perceived pain or exertion. Consequently, completion time was significantly faster. These findings support the notion that exercise is regulated by pain perception, and increased pain tolerance can improve exercise capacity (Fig 1).

▶ Even if one is not an athlete, it is only necessary to look at some of the sculptures of Tait McKenzie to realize that tolerance of pain is a part of athletic success.[1,2] Such peripheral pain, rather than the loudly proposed "Central

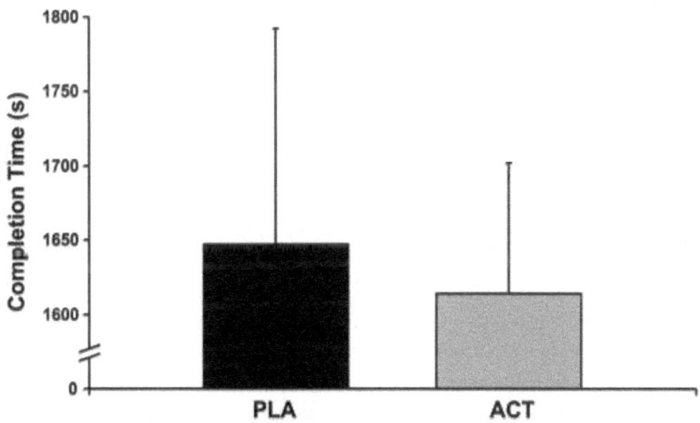

FIGURE 1.—Mean change in completion time from placebo (PLA) to acetaminophen (ACT) condition for all participants. Participants completed the ACT condition in a significantly quicker time than in the PLA condition ($P = 0.05$). Twelve of 13 participants completed the ACT quicker than the PLA condition. (Reprinted from Mauger AR, Jones AM, Williams CA, Influence of acetaminophen on performance during time trial cycling. *J Appl Physiol.* 2010;108:98-104.)

Governor" is the usual determinant of peak effort.[3] Distance cyclists have long recognized this fact, and at one period some of them were attempting to enhance their performance by the use of opiates. However, it seems logical that performance might also be enhanced by more readily available pain remedies, and indeed many athletes do use simple pain killers.[4] A previous study showed that performance was enhanced by administration of the peripheral analgesic fentanyl,[5] although at the expense of severe muscle fatigue late in an event. Acetominophen is one of the safest non-opiod analgesics; it acts by inhibiting cyclooxygenase. The present small-scale randomized controlled trial demonstrates that it can indeed improve performance in a cycling time trial by as much as 2% (Fig. 1). The bettering of performance by the relief of the warning symptom of pain is of some medical and ethical concern; the resulting greater level of effort may damage the visceral organs that the symptom of pain is intended to prevent. Like other ergogenic aids, analgesics also lead to unfair competition, and the question of "over the counter" pain medication may need to be considered more carefully by anti-doping agencies.

R. J. Shephard, MD (Lond), PhD, DPE

References

1. O'Connor PJ, Cook DB. Exercise and pain: the neurobiology, measurement, and laboratory study of pain in relation to exercise in humans. *Exerc Sport Sci Rev.* 1999;27:119-166.
2. O'Connor PJ. Psychological aspects of endurance performance. In: Shephard RJ, Åstrand PO, eds. *Endurance in Sport.* Blackwell Science; 1992:139-148.
3. Atkinson G, Brunskill A. Pacing strategies during a cycling time trial with simulated headwinds and tailwinds. *Ergonomics.* 2000;43:1449-1460.
4. Garcin M, Mille-Hamard L, Billat V, Imbenotte M, Humbert L, Lhermitte Z. Use of acetaminophen in young subelite athletes. *J Sports Med Phys Fitness.* 2005;45: 604-607.
5. Amann M, Proctor LT, Sebranek JJ, Pegelow DF, Dempsey JA. Opioid-mediated muscle afferents inhibit central motor drive and limit peripheral muscle fatigue development in humans. *J Physiol.* 2009;15:271-283.

Influence of acetaminophen on performance during time trial cycling

Mauger AR, Jones AM, Williams CA (Univ of Exeter, Devon, UK)

J Appl Physiol 108:98-104, 2010

To establish whether acetaminophen improves performance of self-paced exercise through the reduction of perceived pain, 13 trained male cyclists performed a self-paced 10-mile (16.1 km) cycle time trial (TT) following the ingestion of either acetaminophen (ACT) or a placebo (PLA), administered in randomized double-blind design. TT were completed in a significantly faster time ($t_{12} = 2.55$, $P < 0.05$) under the ACT condition (26 min 15 s ± 1 min 36 s vs. 26 min 45 s ± 2 min 2 s). Power output (PO) was higher during the middle section of the TT in the ACT condition, resulting in a higher mean PO ($P < 0.05$) (265 ± 12 vs. 255 ± 15 W). Blood lactate concentration (B[La]) and heart rate

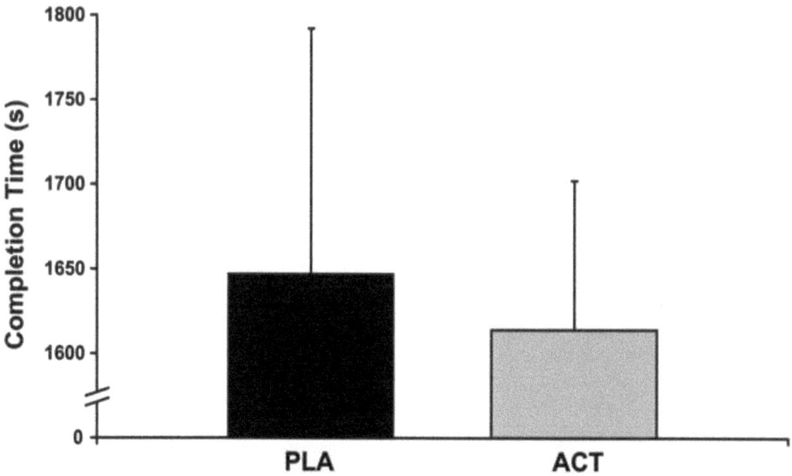

FIGURE 1.—Mean change in completion time from placebo (PLA) to acetaminophen (ACT) condition for all participants. Participants completed the ACT condition in a significantly quicker time than in the PLA condition ($P < 0.05$). Twelve of 13 participants completed the ACT quicker than the PLA condition. (Reprinted with permission from Mauger AR, Jones AM, Williams CA. Influence of acetaminophen on performance during time trial cycling. *J Appl Physiol.* 2010;108:98-104.)

(HR) were higher in the ACT condition (B[La] = 6.1 ± 2.9 mmol/l; HR = 87 ± 7%max) than in the PLA condition (B[La] = 5.1 ± 2.6 mmol/l; HR = 84 ± 9%max) ($P < 0.05$). No significant difference in rating of perceived exertion (ACT = 15.5 ± 0.2; PLA = 15.7 ± 0.2) or perceived pain (ACT = 5.6 ± 0.2; PLA = 5.5 ± 0.2) ($P > 0.05$) was observed. Using acetaminophen, participants cycled at a higher mean PO, with an increased HR and B[La], but without changes in perceived pain or exertion. Consequently, completion time was significantly faster. These findings support the notion that exercise is regulated by pain perception, and increased pain tolerance can improve exercise capacity (Fig 1).

▶ The ability of an athlete to tolerate exercise-induced pain is a critical factor in successful performance in endurance sports. Pain moderates the exercise intensity that athletes can withstand, thus any mechanism that reduces pain or increases tolerance to it may theoretically serve to enhance performance. Acetaminophen, also known as paracetamol, is a commonly used nonprescription analgesic and antipyretic. Its main mechanism of action is the inhibition of cyclooxygenase (COX), similar to that of nonsteroidal antiinflammatories (NSAIDs). Acetaminophen relieves pain by elevating the pain threshold, allowing a greater amount of pain to develop before it is felt. Despite acetaminophen's action on COX, its mechanism of action is different from that of NSAIDs, affecting central not peripheral pain pathways. For these reasons, the authors hypothesized that ingestion of 1.5 g acetaminophen would reduce perceived pain and the rating of perceived exertion during a 10-mile time trial, resulting in improved times relative to placebo. As depicted in Fig 1, this hypothesis was confirmed in this study, with subjects improving in completion time by 2% while on acetaminophen. Athletes were able to exercise at a greater intensity and power output for the same level of perceived pain and exertion. The authors speculated that the increased tolerance of pain with acetaminophen allowed exercise intensity to be set closer to the actual physiological limit or critical threshold, which would otherwise be limited by a central regulator. If these results are confirmed in other athletic settings and endeavors, regulations will soon follow.

D. C. Nieman, DrPH

The effects of inhaled L-methamphetamine on athletic performance while riding a stationary bike: a randomised placebo-controlled trial

Dufka F, Galloway G, Baggott M, et al (APRL-California Pacific Med Ctr Res Inst, San Francisco)

Br J Sports Med 43:832-835, 2009

Objective.—L-methamphetamine (the non-abused isomer of methamphetamine) is banned in athletic competition because it may improve athletic performance, but there are no studies assessing its effects on performance. In the United States L-methamphetamine is formulated in the non-prescription Vick's Vapor Inhaler (VVI) nasal decongestant. VVIs sold elsewhere (we used ones from the UK) contain similar inactive ingredients (menthol, camphor and Siberian pine oil) but no L-methamphetamine. This study tested the effects of inhaled L-methamphetamine delivered from a widely available non-prescription product on athletic performance.

Design.—In a 2-session double-blind placebo-controlled study 12 participants (ages 14–17) were dosed with 4 (session 1) and 12 (session 2) inhalations from VVIs with (USA) or without (UK) L-methamphetamine and then performed two 20 minute rides on a stationary bike with rides separated by a 30 minute rest.

Outcome Measure.—The main outcome measure was miles travelled during each 20 minute ride. Secondary outcome measures included post-ride urine toxicology; heart rate and blood pressure before, 1, 5 and 10 minutes postride; energy, performance, endurance, and ability to breathe; and VVI preference. Data were analysed using Excel statistical macros.

Results.—After ~16 μg L-methamphetamine distance travelled was 5.26 (SD 0.53) miles vs 5.30 (0.55) with placebo; $p = 0.81$. After ~48 μg L-methamphetamine distance travelled was 5.30 (0.51) vs 5.35 (0.43) with placebo; $p = 0.85$. The ~16 μg dose increased systolic blood pressure from 72.6 (4.3) to 79.6 (6.6) mm Hg ($p = 0.03$) at 5 minutes postride but there were no other differences in outcomes.

Conclusions.—Modest doses of inhaled L-methamphetamine probably do not improve athletic performance but do minimally raise diastolic blood pressure.

▶ Use of L-methamphetamine is prohibited by most sports agencies. All Vick's inhalers contain menthol, camphor, and Siberian pine oil, but only those sold in the United States contain L-methamphetamine. Use of the Vick's Vapor Inhaler by Alain Baxter, a downhill skier, resulted in a positive urine test and the loss of his Olympic Bronze medal in 2002. Only L-methamphetamine was detected, but the International Olympic Committee (IOC) does not distinguish between isomers.[1] In this study, modest doses of L-methamphetamine delivered from the Vick's nasal inhaler did not alter distance covered during 2 20-minute cycle ergometer sessions, even at 3 times the recommended dose. The authors question the inclusion of L-methamphetamine as a performance enhancing drug.

D. C. Nieman, DrPH

Reference

1. Mace A, Smith R, Sandhu G. How we do it: ENT prescribing to competitive athletes—a review of current regulations. *Clin Otolaryngol.* 2005;30:201-205.

6 Cardiorespiratory Disorders

Adherence to Guidelines for Cardiovascular Screening in Current High School Preparticipation Evaluation Forms

Rausch CM, Phillips GC (The Children's Hosp, Aurora, CO; Univ of Iowa Children's Hosp)

J Pediatr 155:584-586, 2009

We compared the content of the cardiac screening questions on US state high school athletic association preparticipation evaluation forms with current consensus recommendations. We reviewed the high school athletic association's approved, recommended, or required sports preparticipation form from each of the 50 US states and the District of Columbia, and compared the content of the personal and family history components with current recommendations for cardiac screening questions. We found that 85% of the preparticipation forms in current use contain all elements of the formerly recommended guidelines, but only 17% contain all elements of the new consensus guidelines. We conclude that although there appears to be some improvement in the content of the preparticipation forms in current use compared with previous studies, the vast majority of these forms are incomplete compared with current consensus guidelines.

▶ This kind of news is, of course, distressing. There is currently considerable debate concerning the appropriate content of preparticipation medical screening of athletes to prevent unexpected cardiac deaths in sport play. But this controversy surrounds the use of supplementary testing, including the electrocardiogram, echocardiogram, and exercise stress testing. All are in agreement that a good medical history probing past symptoms with exercise (chest pain, syncope) and a family history of sudden death is an important part of this assessment. Positive information is detected in perhaps 20% to 30% of youth with hypertrophic cariomyopathy or congenital coronary artery anomalies, the 2 most common causes of these tragedies in the United States. Given that the cardiac physical examination is typically unremarkable in both of these conditions, the medical history takes on particular importance, even if not providing a high yield of detection. Given that most are reluctant to suggest routine electrocardiogram and echocardiograms in this screening process (at least in the United States), it would seem critical that physicians follow guidelines for an appropriate medical history 100% of the time. If nothing else, this study highlights the need for continuing education on this matter.

T. Rowland, MD

Sudden Deaths in Young Competitive Athletes: Analysis of 1866 Deaths in the United States, 1980–2006

Maron BJ, Doerer JJ, Haas TS, et al (Minneapolis Heart Inst Found and Abbott Northwestern Hosp, Minn; et al)

Circulation 119:1085-1092, 2009

Background.—Sudden deaths in young competitive athletes are highly visible events with substantial impact on the physician and lay communities. However, the magnitude of this public health issue has become a source of controversy.

Methods and Results.—To estimate the absolute number of sudden deaths in US competitive athletes, we have assembled a large registry over a 27-year period using systematic identification and tracking strategies. A total of 1866 athletes who died suddenly (or survived cardiac arrest), 19 ± 6 years of age, were identified throughout the United States from 1980 to 2006 in 38 diverse sports. Reports were less common during 1980 to 1993 (576 [31%]) than during 1994 to 2006 (1290 [69%], $P<0.001$) and increased at a rate of 6% per year. Sudden deaths were predominantly due to cardiovascular disease (1049 [56%]), but causes also included blunt trauma that caused structural damage (416 [22%]), commotio cordis (65 [3%]), and heat stroke (46 [2%]). Among the 1049 cardiovascular deaths, the highest number of events in a single year was 76 (2005 and 2006), with an average of 66 deaths per year (range 50 to 76) over the last 6 years; 29% occurred in blacks, 54% in high school students, and 82% with physical exertion during competition/training, whereas only 11% occurred in females (although this increased with time; $P=0.023$). The most common cardiovascular causes were hypertrophic cardiomyopathy (36%) and congenital coronary artery anomalies (17%).

Conclusions.—In this national registry, the absolute number of cardiovascular sudden deaths in young US athletes was somewhat higher than previous estimates but relatively low nevertheless, with a rate of <100 per year. These data are relevant to the current debate surrounding preparticipation screening programs with ECGs and also suggest the need for systematic and mandatory reporting of athlete sudden deaths to a national registry (Table 1).

▶ The Canadian Society of Exercise Physiology has previously underlined one of the points made in this report – the need for a mandatory reporting of adverse events during exercise testing and training. Only in this way will the true risks be known, either for healthy individuals or for those with well-defined clinical conditions. The incidence of sudden death in apparently healthy competitors

TABLE 1.—Demographics of Sudden Death in Young Athletes

Sport	No. (%)	Age, y	Male, n (%)	Female, n (%)	Race, n			Survivors, n (%)	Cause of Death, n (%)		
					White	Black	Other*		Trauma Injury	Commotio Cordis	CV Diseases†
Football	565 (30)	17 ± 4	564 (99.8)	1 (0.2)	280	205	80	13 (2)	140 (25)	12 (2)	281 (50)
Basketball	405 (22)	17 ± 4	364 (90)	41 (10)	142	243	20	30 (7)	4 (1.0)	0	349 (86)
Soccer	115 (6)	16 ± 4	93 (81)	22 (19)	81	14	20	7 (6)	11 (10)	4 (4)	80 (70)
Baseball	111 (6)	16 ± 4	111 (100)	0	95	5	11	14 (13)	16 (14)	30 (27)	54 (49)
Motor vehicle racing‡	104 (6)	28 ± 8	103 (99)	1 (1)	102	0	2	0	97 (93)	0	5 (5)
Track and field	96 (5)	17 ± 4	74 (77)	22 (23)	62	22	12	3 (3)	25 (26)	0	61 (64)
Wrestling	69 (4)	22 ± 8	69 (100)	0	56	4	9	2 (3)	7 (10)	1 (1.4)	37 (54)
Boxing	56 (3)	25 ± 6	55 (98)	1 (2)	21	19	16	0	42 (75)	0	11 (1.8)
Swimming§	46 (2)	17 ± 4	30 (65)	16 (35)	43	1	2	1 (2)	0	0	35 (76)
Cross country	38 (2)	17 ± 4	29 (76)	9 (24)	30	6	2	2 (5)	0	0	29 (76)
Hockey	29 (1.5)	18 ± 5	29 (100)	0	28	1	0	3 (10)	4 (14)	7 (24)	11 (38)
Horse riding‖	27 (1.4)	27 ± 8	17 (63)	10 (37)	21	1	5	0	24 (89)	0	2 (7)
Softball	22 (1.2)	19 ± 6	6 (27)	16 (73)	19	0	3	2 (9)	3 (14)	1 (5)	12 (55)
Marathon	20 (1.1)	28 ± 7	15 (75)	5 (25)	16	0	4	3 (15)	0	0	13 (65)
Lacrosse	19 (1.0)	18 ± 2	19 (100)	0	18	1	0	2 (11)	1 (5)	8 (24)	9 (47)
Skiing¶	19 (1.0)	25 ± 8	14 (74)	5 (26)	19	0	0	0	15 (79)	0	1 (5)
Triathlon	17 (0.9)	32 ± 5	15 (88)	2 (12)	16	0	1	0	3 (18)	0	8 (47)
Rugby	16 (0.9)	21 ± 3	16 (100)	0	13	2	1	0	3 (19)	0	7 (44)
Martial arts	15 (0.8)	23 ± 7	14 (93)	1 (7)	12	3	0	0	5 (33)	2 (13)	2 (13)
Others#	14 (0.8)	26 ± 9	12 (86)	2 (14)	14	0	0	2 (14)	3 (21)	0	5 (36)
Rowing	11 (0.6)	22 ± 6	8 (73)	3 (27)	10	0	1	0	0	0	9 (82)
Cycling	10 (0.5)	29 ± 8	8 (80)	2 (20)	7	2	1	0	7 (70)	0	3 (30)
Tennis	10 (0.5)	19 ± 4	8 (80)	2 (20)	8	0	2	0	0	0	8 (80)
Volleyball	10 (0.5)	18 ± 5	1 (10)	9 (90)	5	3	2	1 (10)	0	0	10 (100)
Gymnastics	9 (0.5)	15 ± 3	5 (56)	4 (44)	6	0	3	0	4 (44)	0	3 (33)
Surfing	9 (0.5)	23 ± 8	9 (100)	0	7	0	2	0	2 (22)	0	1 (11)
Figure skating	2 (0.1)	24 ± 6	2 (100)	0	2	0	0	0	0	0	1 (50)

(*Continued*)

TABLE 1. *(continued)*

Sport	No. (%)	Age, y	Male, n (%)	Female, n (%)	Race, n White	Race, n Black	Race, n Other*	Survivors, n (%)	Cause of Death, n (%) Trauma Injury	Cause of Death, n (%) Commotio Cordis	Cause of Death, n (%) CV Diseases†
Golf	2 (0.1)	18 ± 0.7	2 (100)	0	2	0	0	0	0	0	2 (100)
Totals	1866	19 ± 6	1692	174	1135	532	199	85	416	65	1049

CV Indicates cardiovascular.
*Hispanic (n = 103); Asian (n = 20); Native American (n = 5); Pacific Islander (n = 5); Middle Eastern (n = 3); Indian (n = 1); Japanese (n = 1); mixed (n = 6); unknown (n = 55).
†Documented by autopsy and/or clinical findings.
‡Includes automobile (n = 63) and motorcycle (n = 41) racing.
§Swimming (n = 40); water polo (n = 6).
‖Jockey (n = 16); equestrian (n = 11).
¶Skiing (n = 12); snowboarding (n = 5); ski-jumping (n = 2).
#Skateboarding (n = 5); jai-alai (n = 4); field hockey (n = 2); bobsledding (n = 1); bowing (n = 1); riflery (n = 1).

has particular relevance to cost-benefit analyses of pre-participation screening[1] and the wider availability of cardiac defibrillators.[2] The present incidence data (Table 1) is based on a rather comprehensive search of 18 000 newspapers, public and legal records, internet searches, consumer safety reports, the National Center for Catastrophic Sports Injury Research, NHI archives, Minneapolis Heart Institute files, and personal communications; it is thus likely to be close to the actual incidence. The search found 1866 cases of exercise-related deaths in mainly young United States athletes (average age 18 years) between 1980 and 2006; 1049 of these were thought to be cardiac in type, and 690 were presumed to be so on the basis of autopsy or clinical history (Table 1). Perhaps because of growing public knowledge of the various registries, the number of reported cases has increased steadily over the study period. There has been much talk among cardiologists concerning the risks of exercise in those with Hypertrophic cardiomyopathy; this condition was diagnosed in only 251 cases, less than 10 incidents per year, despite an estimated annual participation rate approaching 11 million. Probably because of the popularity of these 2 sports in the United States, football and baseball participants accounted for a major fraction of the reported deaths; the majority of incidents also occurred in a high school rather than a more advanced sport setting. Although the occasional death of an athlete is very distressing to those involved, it seems to have a frequency similar to that of a fatal lightning strike. Plainly, the primary focus of public health agencies should be on more common causes of death in young adults, such as automobile accidents and suicides.

R. J. Shephard, MD (Lond), PhD, DPE

References

1. Shephard RJ. Preparticipation screening of young athletes: an effective investment?. In: Year Book of Sports Medicine, 2005. Philadelphia, PA: Elsevier; 2006:xix-xxv.
2. Myerburg RJ, Estes NAM, Fontaine JM, et al. Task force 10: automatic external defibrillators. *J Am Coll Cardiol.* 2005;45:1369-1371.

Comparison of U.S. and Italian Experiences With Sudden Cardiac Deaths in Young Competitive Athletes and Implications for Preparticipation Screening Strategies

Maron BJ, Haas TS, Doerer JJ, et al (Minneapolis Heart Inst Foundation, Minneapolis, MN; et al)
Am J Cardiol 104:276-280, 2009

Controversy has evolved over the most practical and effective strategy for preparticipation cardiovascular screening of competitive athletes to detect unsuspected cardiovascular disease and prevent sudden death on the athletic field. Athlete screening in the Veneto region of Italy is part of a national program (with 12-lead electrocardiography) that has reported the detection of previously undiagnosed hypertrophic cardiomyopathy and a decrease in the cardiovascular death rate in young athletes.

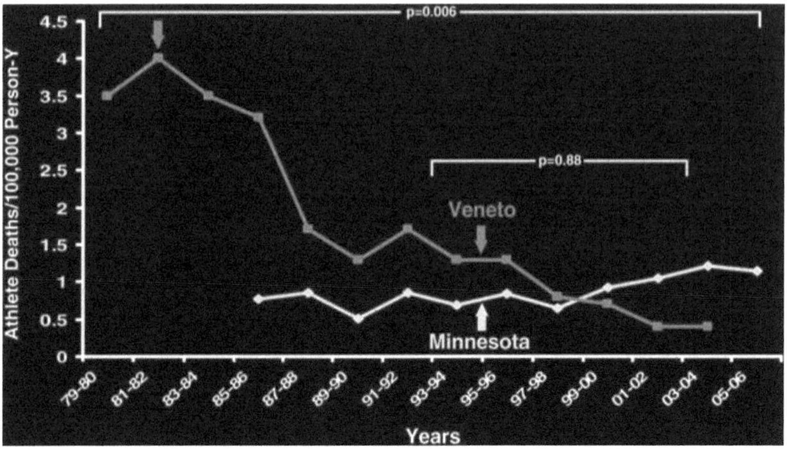

FIGURE 2.—Plot comparing annual athlete mortality per 100,000 person-years in Veneto region and Minnesota. Italian national preparticipation screening began in 1981 (*arrow*). (Reprinted from Maron BJ, Haas TS, Doerer JJ, et al. Comparison of U.S. and Italian experiences with sudden cardiac deaths in young competitive athletes and implications for preparticipation screening strategies. *Am J Cardiol*. 2009;104:276-280, with permission from Elsevier Inc.)

In this study, over time periods of similar length, cardiovascular-related mortality rates in Veneto athletes were compared with those of a demographically similar region of the United States (Minnesota) in which screening is limited to history and physical examination. There were 55 sudden cardiovascular deaths reported in Veneto over 26 years (2.1/year), compared with 22 deaths in 23 years (0.96/year) in Minnesota. Over the recent and comparable 11-year period, 1993 to 2004, 12 deaths were reported in Veneto and 11 in Minnesota. When analyzed as deaths per 100,000 person-years, Veneto exceeded Minnesota for all years combined (1.87 for 1979 to 2004 vs 1.06 for 1985 to 2007, respectively, $p = 0.006$), although the 2 regions did not differ significantly for 1993 to 2004 (0.87 vs 0.93, respectively, $p = 0.88$) or most recently for 2001 to 2004 (0.43 vs 0.90, respectively, $p = 0.38$). In conclusion, sudden cardiovascular deaths in young competitive athletes occurred at a low rate in both Veneto and Minnesota. Despite different preparticipation screening strategies, athlete sudden death rates in these demographically similar regions of the United States and Italy have not differed significantly in recent years. These data do not support a lower mortality rate associated with preparticipation screening programs involving routine electrocardiography and examinations by specially trained personnel (Fig 2).

▶ In 2005 I observed that there was no objective evidence of benefit from the mandatory preparticipatory screening of Italian athletes; the incidence of sudden death during exercise was, if anything, higher in Italy than in the United States, where ECG and echocardiographic screening of young athletes was rarely undertaken, and the norm was a history plus physical examination. The number of incidents of sudden exercise-related death in Italy has dropped in recent years, and it might be possible to argue that as Italian physicians have gained experience in ECG interpretation, their program has yielded some benefits (Fig 2), although the current analysis by Maron and associates shows that there was still no statistically significant diminution of risk of sudden exercise deaths relative to United States athletes for the period from 1993-2004. Caution is necessary in making this comparison between the 2 countries, because it is difficult to be certain that person-years of exposure to sport were comparable; moreover, the sports that were played undoubtedly differed (soccer with largely uninterrupted play vs American football, for example), and despite the investigators' best efforts, it is difficult to be certain that participation rates and hours of play were comparable in the 2 countries. One point that Maron does not underline is that if rates are now comparable, the Italian athletes are worse off, both financially and in terms of the health costs of false positive diagnoses. It is finally interesting to note from the probable causes of death that Maron's claim of cardiomyopathy as the most common cause of sudden exercise-related death appears to be fading, with only 17% of incidents now attributed to this cause.

R. J. Shephard, MD (Lond), PhD, DPE

Diagnostic accuracy of extended-length electrocardiogram in differentiating between athlete's heart and hypertrophic cardiomyopathy

Caselli L, Galanti G, Padeletti L, et al (Univ of Florence, Italy; et al)

J Electrocardiol 42:636-641, 2009

Background.—Standard 12-lead electrocardiogram (ECG) has several limitations in solving the differential diagnosis between physiologic left ventricular hypertrophy (PLVH) and hypertrophic cardiomyopathy (HCM), given the high rate of false-positive results in athletes. The aim of this study was to assess the usefulness of several arrhythmic risk indexes in differentiating PLVH from HCM.

Methods.—A multiparametric ECG analysis (extended-length ECG) was performed on 30 male athletes with PLVH and 30 male patients with HCM, with homogeneous age distribution.

Results.—The combination of 4 extended-length ECG variables, namely, corrected QT interval (Bazett), QT dispersion, mean resting heart rate, and low-amplitude signal duration at 25 Hz (low-amplitude signal duration at the end of filtered QRS) displayed remarkable diagnostic accuracy (area under receiver operating characteristic curve, 94%). The same accuracy was obtained replacing QT dispersion with T-wave complexity index.

TABLE 2.—Echocardiographic Indexes in 30 Athletes with PLVH and in 30 Patients with HCM

	PLVH Mean (SD) N = 30	HCM Mean (SD) N = 30	*P*
LVM (g)	285.0 (21.8)	326.8 (72.9)	.0039
LVMi (g/m^2)	148.7 (13.4)	174.8 (42.1)	.0020
IVS (mm)	11.3 (0.7)	18.3 (3.4)	<.0001
PWT (mm)	10.9 (0.6)	10.8 (1.9)	.7150
LVDd (mm)	54.2 (2.4)	45.9 (4.6)	<.0001
LA (mm)	38.8 (3.2)	43.1 (6.3)	.0018
E (cm/s)	77.5 (12.2)	73.9 (21.0)	.4159
A (cm/s)	59.2 (15.6)	61.8 (32.2)	.6845
E/A	1.4 (0.5)	1.4 (0.7)	.9797
Em (cm/s)	12.7 (2.8)	8.1 (2.6)	<.0001
E/Em	6.1 (1.1)	9.6 (2.7)	<.0001

LVMi calculated in relation to body surface area. IVS indicates left ventricular diastolic thickness of interventricular septum; PWT, left ventricular diastolic thickness of posterior wall; LVDd, left ventricular diastolic diameter; LA, left atrial diameter; *E*, early diastolic transmitral inflow velocity; *A*, late diastolic filling wave due to atrial contraction; Em, average of early diastolic mitral annular velocities calculated at the septal and lateral corners (Em = [Em septal + Em lateral]/2); *E*/Em, ratio of transmitral flow velocity to early diastolic velocity of the mitral annulus.

Conclusions.—Extended-length ECG can be considered an effective, low-cost, and low time-consuming clinical tool for distinguishing between PLVH and HCM (Table 2).

▶ The diagnosis of hypertrophic cardiomyopathy is often made erroneously, causing an athlete to withdraw from training unnecessarily to increase cardiac risk because of a drastic reduction in habitual physical activity, and possibly to develop a cardiac neurosis. There is growing acceptance that a resting electrocardiogram (ECG) provides a fallible tool to distinguish those that have a pathological abnormality.[1] However, there have recently been claims that an extended ECG record that uses a computer to look at QRS duration, heart rate variability, the signal-averaged ECG, QT interval dispersion, and T-wave complexity allows a more reliable diagnosis of pathology.[2] This article tested this hypothesis by comparing ECG patterns in small samples of athletes with physiological left ventricular hypertrophy and those thought to have hypertrophic myocardiopathy on the basis of 2-dimensional echocardiography showing a thickening of the left ventricular wall in the presence of a nondilated left ventricular chamber. There were relatively clear-cut differences between the 2 groups of subjects, but the weakness in the proof is that there was quite a large difference in ventricular mass between the 2 groups of individuals (Table 2). The crucial question is whether the test is effective when there is an equally massive physiological left ventricular hypertrophy and the comparison group has a histologically and/or genetically proven hypertrophic cardiomyopathy.

R. J. Shephard, MD (Lond), PhD, DPE

References

1. Pelliccia A, Maron BJ, Culasso F, et al. Clinical significance of abnormal electrocardiographic patterns in trained athletes. *Circulation.* 2000;102:278.
2. Barletta G, Lazzeri C, Franchi F, Del Bene R, Michelucci A. Hypertrophic cardiomyopathy: electrical abnormalities detected by the extended-length ECG and their relation to syncope. *Int J Cardiol.* 2004;97:43.

Aetiology of sudden cardiac death in athletes in the United Kingdom: a pathological study

de Noronha SV, Sharma S, Papadakis M, et al (Natl Heart and Lung Inst, London, UK; King's College Hosp and Univ Hosp Lewisham, London, UK; et al)
Heart 95:1409-1414, 2009

Objective.—To characterise the demographics and aetiology of sudden cardiac death (SCD) in athletes referred to a tertiary cardiac pathology centre in the UK.

Design.—Retrospective non-case controlled analysis.

Setting.—Cardiac pathology centre at the National Heart and Lung Institute and Royal Brompton Hospital.

Subjects.—Between 1996 and 2008, the hearts of 118 athletes were referred for pathological assessment to ascertain the precise aetiology of SCD.

Results.—The majority of athletes (n = 113; 96%) were male and most (107; 91%) were amateurs participating predominantly in football, rugby and running. The mean (SD) age of death was 28 (12) years (range 7–59); 75% athletes were aged ≤35 years. Most deaths (81%) occurred during or immediately after exercise. Antecedent symptoms of cardiac disease were reported in 21 (18%) subjects, and 20 (17%) had a family history of premature cardiovascular disease and/or SCD. 25 (21%) athletes had relevant past medical history which included a known history of cardiac disease. Cardiomyopathy was the commonest cause of death and accounted for 62% of all the SCDs. A significantly high proportion of athletes (23%) exhibited a morphologically normal heart. Atherosclerotic coronary disease accounted for only 3% of cases and was confined to athletes aged >35 years.

Conclusions.—SCD in sport is largely due to clinically silent cardiomyopathies or primary electrical disorders (morphologically normal heart). Antecedent symptoms and family history are absent in over 80% of cases, and therefore clinical screening with health questionnaires will fail to identify most athletes with potentially sinister cardiac disorders.

▶ The sudden death of an athlete is a rare event (incidence of 1:50 000-1:200 000).[1] Most sudden cardiac deaths in young athletes are due to hereditary or congenital cardiac anomalies, in particular, hypertrophic cardiomyopathy.[2] In contrast, the vast majority of sudden cardiac deaths in older athletes are secondary to atherosclerotic coronary artery disease. In this study based in the United Kingdom, cardiomyopathies were the most prevalent underlying pathology in sudden cardiac deaths related to athletic activity, consistent with previous studies in other parts of the world. Soccer and running were the sports most commonly associated with sudden cardiac deaths. Of the sudden cardiac death cases, 91% were amateur sportsmen and included 7 subjects who had participated in 2 to 23 marathons. The remaining 11 cases consisted of 7 athletes at a professional or semiprofessional level and 4 athletes who had previously participated in intensive physical training in the armed forces. Sudden death is often the first clinical manifestation of underlying heart disease in young athletes. The authors support the use of preparticipation cardiovascular screening in young athletes, using 12-lead ECG as a screening tool, and claim that this would probably have detected the underlying cardiac abnormality in a significant number of the victims.

D. C. Nieman, DrPH

References

1. Corrado D, Basso C, Rizzoli G, Schiavon M, Thiene G. Does sports activity enhance the risk of sudden death in adolescents and young adults? *J Am Coll Cardiol.* 2003;42:1959-1963.
2. Maron BJ, Thompson PD, Ackerman MJ, et al. Recommendations and considerations related to preparticipation screening for cardiovascular abnormalities in competitive athletes: 2007 update: a scientific statement from the American Heart Association Council on Nutrition, Physical Activity, and Metabolism: endorsed by the American College of Cardiology Foundation. *Circulation.* 2007; 115:1643-1655.

Physical Activity and All-cause Mortality: An Updated Meta-analysis with Different Intensity Categories

Löllgen H, Böckenhoff A, Knapp G (Ruhr-Univ, Remscheid, Germany; Univ of Essen/Duisburg, Germany; Technological Univ Dortmund, Germany)

Int J Sports Med 30:213-224, 2009

In a meta-analysis we investigated the effect of physical activity with different intensity categories on all-cause mortality. Many studies have reported positive effects of regular physical activity on primary prevention. This recent meta-analysis analyzed all-cause mortality with special reference to intensity categories. A computerized systematic literature search was performed in EMBASE, PUBMED, and MEDLINE data bases (1990–2006) for prospective cohort studies on physical leisure activity. Thirty-eight studies were identified and evaluated. The presentation refers to studies with 3 or 4 different intensities of regular physical activity according to a standard questionnaire. There was a significant association of lower all-cause mortality for active individuals compared with sedentary persons. For studies with three activity categories (mildly, moderately, and highly active) and multivariate-adjusted models, highly active men had a 22% lower risk of all-cause mortality (RR = 0.78; 95% CI: 0.72 to 0.84) compared to mildly active men. For women, the relative risk

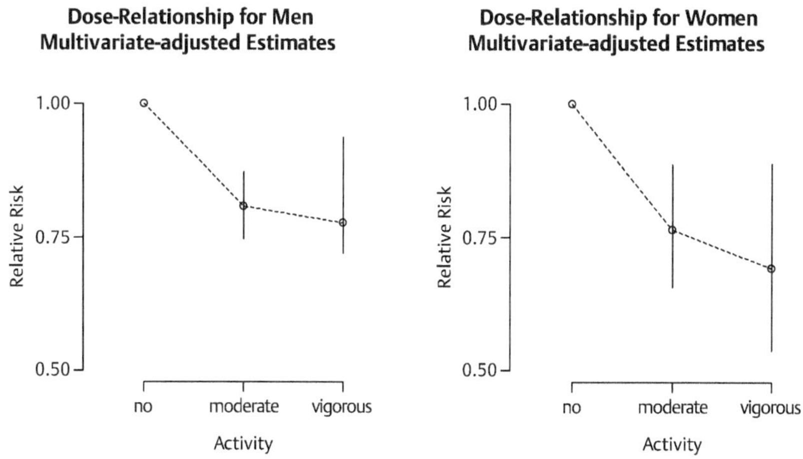

FIGURE 6.—Dose-response relationship based on meta-analytical results of multivariate-adjusted estimates for men (left) and women (right) in studies with three levels of activities (estimates plus 95% confidence intervals). (Reprinted from Löllgen H, Böckenhoff A, Knapp G. Physical activity and all-cause mortality: an updated meta-analysis with different intensity categories. *Int J Sports Med.* 2009;30:213-224.)

was 0.69 (95% CI: 0.53 to 0.90). We observed similar results in moderately active persons compared to mildly active individuals (RR = 0.81 for men and RR = 0.76 for women). This association of activity to all-cause mortality was similar and significant in older subjects. Regular physical activity over longer time is strongly associated with a reduction in all-cause mortality in active subjects compared to sedentary persons. There is a dose-response curve especially from sedentary subjects to those with mild and moderate exercise with only a minor additional reduction with further increase in activity level (Fig 6).

▶ Several meta-analyses have shown fairly conclusively that regular physical activity reduces both all-cause and cardiac mortality.[1-4] A number of quite large individual studies from the United States, such as observations made at the Cooper Clinic, have further suggested that in terms of reducing risk, the largest benefit is obtained from a small increase of habitual physical activity, and that the additional benefits from more vigorous physical activity are quite modest. However, the samples have often been biased, and possibly had a low initial level of habitual activity. Moreover, other studies such as those of Morris in England have argued that for protection against cardiac disease quite vigorous activity is required.[5] Nevertheless, the present meta-analysis appears to confirm the United States view, at least for all-cause mortality (Fig 6). The current analysis has a number of strengths. It is based on a very large pool of subjects (38 prospective studies from many countries, involving more than 271 000 participants), and a multivariate analysis of risk was attempted. On the other hand, not all of the studies that were included sorted results by intensity of effort; even when this was done, estimates of intensity were based on questionnaire data, and the number of levels and the cut-points identified differed from one study to another, making it difficult to pool data. There may have been some bias to a publication of studies where benefit was observed. Further, intensity was usually confounded with volume of activity, which is probably the important variable from the viewpoint of preventing the metabolic syndrome, and the more active individuals probably also had a healthier overall lifestyle. Finally, the primary objective of increased physical activity is not to reduce all-cause mortality, but rather to extend a person's quality-adjusted life expectancy. Nevertheless, the findings suggest there is value in persuading patients to exercise, even if they can undertake only quite modest intensities of effort.

R. J. Shephard, MD (Lond), PhD, DPE

References

1. Powell KE, Thompson PD, Caspersen CJ, Kendrick JS. Physical activity and the incidence of coronary heart disease. *Annu Rev Public Health*. 1987;8:253-287.
2. Berlin JA, Colditz GA. A meta-analsys of physical activity in the prevention of coronary heart disease. *Am J Epidemiol*. 1990;132:612-628.
3. Williams PD. Physical fitness and activity as a separate risk factor: a meta-analysis. *Med Sci Sports Exerc*. 2001;33:754-761.
4. Blair SN, Cheng Y, Holder JS. Is physical fitness or physical activity more important in defining health benefits? *Med Sci Sports Exerc*. 2001;33:379-399.
5. Morris JN, Clayton DG, Everett MG, Semmence AM, Burgess EH. Exercise in leisure time. Coronary attack and death rates. *Br Heart J*. 1990;63:325-334.

B-Type Natriuretic Peptides for the Evaluation of Exercise Intolerance

Mueller C, Maeder MT, Christ A, et al (Univ Hosp Basel, Switzerland)
Am J Med 122:265-272, 2009

Background.—Cardiopulmonary exercise testing is the method of choice for the differentiation of exercise intolerance. This study sought to assess the utility of B-type natriuretic peptide (BNP) and N-terminal-pro-B-type natriuretic peptide (NT-proBNP) for the identification of a cardiocirculatory exercise limitation.

Methods.—In 162 patients undergoing cardiopulmonary exercise testing, rest and peak exercise BNP and NT-proBNP levels were measured. In 94 patients fulfilling criteria for appropriate effort and sufficient diagnostic certainty, the accuracy of BNP and NT-proBNP for the prediction of a cardiocirculatory limitation, as assessed based on clinical and exercise testing data, was determined.

Results.—A cardiocirculatory limitation was identified in 27 (29%) patients. Median (interquartile range) resting BNP [162 (45-415) vs 39 (19-94) vs 24 (15-46) pg/mL; $P < .001$] and NT-proBNP [506 (129-1167) vs 77 (35-237) vs 34 (19-77) pg/mL; $P < .001$] were higher in patients with cardiocirculatory as compared with those with pulmonary limitation ($n = 28$) and those without cardiocirculatory or pulmonary limitation ($n = 39$). The area under the receiver operator characteristics

TABLE 4.—B-type Natriuretic Peptide (BNP) and N-terminal-pro-B-type Natriuretic Peptide (NT-proBNP) Kinetics

	Reference Group (n = 39)	Pulmonary Limitation (n = 28)	Cardiocirculatory Limitation (n = 27)	P Value
BNP at rest (pg/mL)	24 (15-46)	39 (19-94)	162 (45-415)‡§	<.001
BNP at peak exercise (pg/mL)	33 (15-56)*	54 (24-109)*	219 (32-484)*‡§	<.001
Δ BNP (pg/mL)	4 (0-16)	11 (0-24)	20 (8-124)‡	.007
% Δ BNP (%)	10 (0-76)	22 (0-43)	18 (2-53)	.81
NT-proBNP at rest (pg/mL)	34 (19-77)	77 (35-237)†	506 (129-1167)‡§	<.001
NT-proBNP at peak exercise (pg/mL)	34 (27-85)*	81 (36-253)*†	608 (130-1204)*‡§	<.001
Δ NT-proBNP (pg/mL)	3 (0-6)	4 (1-18)	20 (2-93)‡	.006
% Δ NT-proBNP (%)	8 (0-17)	5 (2-8)	7 (1-10)	.29

Δ BNP/Δ NT-proBNP = absolute increase in BNP/NT-proBNP; % Δ BNP/% Δ NT-proBNP = relative increase in BNP/NT-proBNP.

Data are given as median (interquartile range).

**P* <.05 compared with values at rest within the same group.

Post hoc tests †*P* <.05 reference vs pulmonary limitation; ‡*P* <.05 reference vs cardiocirculatory limitation; §*P* <.05 for pulmonary vs cardiocirculatory limitation.

curve for BNP and NT-proBNP to identify a cardiocirculatory limitation was 0.79 and 0.84, respectively ($P = .15$ for comparison of the curves). Sensitivity and specificity of the optimal BNP cutoff of 85 pg/mL were 63% and 84%, respectively. Sensitivity and specificity of the optimal NT-proBNP cutoff of 223 pg/mL were 74% and 85%, respectively. Peak exercise biomarkers were not more accurate than resting levels.

Conclusions.—Among patients referred for cardiopulmonary exercise testing for evaluation of unexplained exercise intolerance, BNP and NT-proBNP were similarly useful to identify those with a cardiocirculatory limitation (Table 4).

▶ The direct treadmill measurement of peak oxygen intake has long been the standard method of laboratory assessment of patients with pulmonary and cardiac disease. However, in many patients, caution on the part of the examiner or the person being tested leads to a low level of effort and, thus, rather equivocal peak oxygen intake values; in the present sample, patients with cardiac disease reached only 74 percent of their predicted maximal heart rate, with a final blood lactate concentration averaging less than 6 mM/L. There is thus continuing interest in finding a test that does not depend on the development of maximal effort by the patient.

Evidence is accumulating that increased levels of B-type natriuretic peptide (BNP) and its precursor peptide are helpful in distinguishing heart failure from other types pf dyspnea, although the underlying mechanism has yet to be determined.[1-4] The measurement of the resting BNP helps to distinguish a predominantly circulatory problem from a pulmonary limitation, which is important to the initiation of appropriate treatment. Significance can be attached to low values as indicators of normal cardiac function, although if values are high, further evaluation may be needed to determine the precise cardiac pathophysiology. The present data suggests that the peptide precursor tends to give a slightly better discrimination than BNP (although not significantly so), perhaps because of its longer half-life and, thus, lesser vulnerability to short-term changes in cardiac performance. Moreover, resting values are just as useful as those obtained during peak exercise (Table 4). Further evaluation of this test seems warranted.

R. J. Shephard, MD (Lond), PhD, DPE

References

1. Maisel AS, Krishnaswamy P, Nowak RM, et al. Rapid measurement of B-type natriuretic peptide in the emergency diagnosis of heart failure. *N Engl J Med.* 2002;347:161-167.
2. Mueller C, Scholer A, Laule-Kilian K, et al. Use of B-type natriuretic peptide in the evaluation and management of acute dyspnea. *N Engl J Med.* 2004;350:647-654.
3. Januzzi JL, vanKimmenade R, Lainchbury J, et al. NT-proBNP testing for diagnosis and short-term prognosis in acute destabilized heart failure: an international pooled analysis of 1256 patients: the International Collaborative of NT-proBNP Study. *Eur Heart J.* 2006;27:330-337.
4. Januzzi JL Jr, Camargo CA, Anwaruddin S, et al. The N-terminal Pro-BNP investigation of dyspnea in the emergency department (PRIDE) study. *Am J Cardiol.* 2005;95:948-954.

Relation of Vigorous Exercise to Risk of Atrial Fibrillation

Aizer A, Gaziano JM, Cook NR, et al (Brigham and Women's Hosp)
Am J Cardiol 103:1572-1577, 2009

Limited data suggest that athletes may have a higher risk of developing atrial fibrillation (AF); however, there has been no large prospective assessment of the relation between vigorous exercise and AF. Logistic regression analyses stratified by time were used to assess the association between frequency of vigorous exercise and risk of developing AF in 16,921 apparently healthy men in the Physicians' Health Study. During 12 years of follow-up, 1,661 men reported developing AF. With increasing frequency of vigorous exercise (0, 1, 1 to 2, 3 to 4, 5 to 7 days/week), multivariate relative risks for the full cohort were 1.0 (referent), 0.90, 1.09, 1.04, and 1.20 ($p = 0.04$). This risk was not significantly increased when exercise habits were updated or in models excluding variables that may be in the biological pathway through which exercise influences AF risk. In subgroup analyses, this increased risk was observed only in men <50 years of age (1.0, 0.94, 1.20, 1.05, 1.74, $p < 0.01$) and joggers (1.0, 0.91, 1.03, 1.30, 1.53, $p < 0.01$), where risks remained increased in all analyses. In conclusion, frequency of vigorous exercise was associated with an increased risk of developing AF in young men and joggers. This

TABLE 3.—Relative Risk of Atrial Fibrillation According to Frequency of Habitual Vigorous Exercise at Three Years, Stratified by Age Group

Variable: Frequency of Habitual Vigorous Exercise	Nonexercisers	<1 day/wk	1–2 days/wk	3–4 days/wk	5–7 days/wk	p Value for Trend
Age <50 yrs						
Age-adjusted (model 1)*						
RR (95% CI)	1.0	0.96 (0.56–1.63)	1.15 (0.84–1.57)	0.95 (0.71–1.28)	1.69 (1.22–2.33)	0.014
Multivariable model 2†						
RR (95% CI)	1.0	0.95 (0.55–1.66)	1.22 (0.88–1.68)	1.00 (0.73–1.36)	1.69 (1.21–2.37)	0.015
Multivariable model 3‡						
RR (95% CI)	1.0	0.94 (0.53–1.67)	1.20 (0.87–1.66)	1.05 (0.76–1.43)	1.74 (1.23–2.47)	<0.01
Age ≥50 yrs but <65 yrs						
Age-adjusted (model 1)*						
RR (95% CI)	1.0	0.87 (0.61–1.24)	1.01 (0.85–1.21)	0.97 (0.82–1.14)	1.09 (0.88–1.34)	0.57
Multivariable model 2†						
RR (95% CI)	1.0	0.88 (0.61–1.27)	1.02 (0.85–1.22)	0.97 (0.82–1.15)	1.07 (0.87–1.33)	0.65
Multivariable model 3‡						
RR (95% CI)	1.0	0.93 (0.65–1.35)	1.07 (0.89–1.29)	1.03 (0.86–1.22)	1.16 (0.93–1.44)	0.25
Age ≥65 yrs						
Age-adjusted (model 1)*						
RR (95% CI)	1.0	1.00 (0.51–1.95)	1.06 (0.77–1.46)	1.15 (0.88–1.49)	0.94 (0.67–1.31)	0.97
Multivariable model 2†						
RR (95% CI)	1.0	0.78 (0.37–1.64)	1.03 (0.75–1.43)	1.12 (0.86–1.47)	0.92 (0.66–1.29)	0.99
Multivariable model 3‡						
RR (95% CI)	1.0	0.81 (0.39–1.71)	1.10 (0.79–1.53)	1.12 (0.85–1.48)	0.97 (0.69–1.37)	0.86

*Model 1 controlled for age and treatment assignment (aspirin or placebo, β-carotene or placebo).

†Model 2 excluded possible physiologic intermediaries between exercise and AF. Model 2 controlled for age, treatment assignment (aspirin or placebo, β-carotene or placebo), parental history of premature myocardial infarction, alcohol intake, smoking habits, fish consumption, multivitamin intake, and vitamin C and E intakes.

‡Model 3 controlled for age, treatment assignment (aspirin or placebo, β-carotene or placebo), BMI, history of diabetes, history of hypertension, history of hyperlipidemia, parental history of premature myocardial infarction, alcohol intake, smoking habits, fish consumption, multivitamin intake, vitamin C intake, vitamin E intake, left ventricular hypertrophy, congestive heart failure, and evidence of cardiovascular disease.

risk decreased as the population aged and was offset by known beneficial effects of vigorous exercise on other AF risk factors (Table 3).

▶ Endurance athletes progressively increase their parasympathetic tone, and in some individuals the resting heart rate may drop below 30 beats/min. It has long been suspected that such low heart rates increase vulnerability to arrhythmias.[1-3] A second possible factor is atrial enlargement in endurance athletes.[4] The number of individuals with extreme bradycardia is small. Of greater importance to the practicing sports physician is the question whether participation in more moderate bouts of endurance activity also increases risks. The present report is based on a 12-year prospective study of some 16 000 physicians who were initially free of myocardial infarction, stroke, or ischemic attacks. There was a modest increase of risk of developing self-reported atrial fibrillation with increased frequency of vigorous exercise (arbitrarily defined as sufficient to break a sweat), but this was only significant after extensive statistical adjustments for other possible causes of atrial fibrillation; moreover, the effect was seen only in subjects < 50 years of age. Because 63% of the sample reported performing vigorous exercise for an average of 108 min/week, in many individuals the intensity is likely to have been moderate rather than very vigorous. In support of this view, the effect was seen only in the most committed exercisers who were active 5 to 7 times per week. The effect was also limited to joggers rather than participants in other sports (which may have had less of an endurance component). It remains unclear whether the decrease of risk with age (despite the development of structural changes predisposing to fibrillation) reflects a lesser intensity of activity or an age-related waning of parasympathetic tone. From the practical point of view, the many other benefits of exercise probably outweigh the risks of fibrillation even in younger individuals, although there may be merit in not pushing endurance training to its maximum.

For further reading on this subject I suggest an article by Kannael et al.[5]

R. J. Shephard, MD (Lond), PhD, DPE

References

1. Coelho A, Palileo E, Ashley W, et al. Tachyarrhythmias in young athletes. *J Am Coll Cardiol.* 1986;7:237-243.
2. Hood S, Northcote RJ. Cardiac assessment of veteran endurance athletes: a 12 year follow up study. *Br J Sports Med.* 1999;33:239-243.
3. Karjalainen J, Kujala UM, Kaprio J, Sarna S, Viitasalo M. Lone AF in vigorously exercising middle aged men: case-control study. *BMJ.* 1998;316:1784-1785.
4. Pelliccia A, Maron MJ, Di Paolo FM, et al. Prevalence and clinical significance of left atrial remodeling in competitive athletes. *J Am Coll Cardiol.* 2005;46: 690-696.
5. Kannel WB, Wolf PA, Benjamin EJ, Levy D. Prevalence, incidence, prognosis and predisposing conditions for atrial fibrillation: population-based estimates. *Am J Cardiol.* 1998;82:2N-9N.

Effect of cardiac rehabilitation on angiogenic cytokines in postinfarction patients

Lee B-C, Hsu H-C, Tseng W-YI, et al (Natl Taiwan Univ Hosp, Taipei; et al)
Heart 95:1012-1018, 2009

Objective.—To determine whether cardiac rehabilitation influences plasma levels of angiogenic cytokines and their correlation with myocardial blood flow (MBF).

Design.—Randomised controlled study.

Setting.—Tertiary cardiac centre.

Patients.—39 postinfarction patients randomised to either a 3-month training group (n = 20) or a non-training group (n = 19), and 19 normal controls.

Interventions.—Cardiac rehabilitation.

Main Outcome Measures.—MBF by cardiac magnetic resonance imaging, and plasma levels of stem cell factor (SCF), stromal-derived factor-1 (SDF-1), and vascular endothelial growth factor (VEGF) measured at enrolment and at 3 months after randomisation.

Results.—At baseline, when compared with the healthy subjects, postinfarction patients had a lower MBF in the infarcted myocardium during dipyridamole-induced stress (1.65 (0.58) vs 2.77 (0.78) ml/min/g, $p < 0.001$) but higher plasma levels of VEGF (3.65 (0.75) vs 2.77 (0.59) pg/ml, $p < 0.001$ expressed as the natural logarithm) and SDF-1 (2113 (345) vs 1869 (309) pg/ml, $p = 0.009$). Only SDF-1 was inversely associated with stress MBF in both remote ($r = -0.39$, $p = 0.03$) and infarcted myocardium ($r = -0.62$, $p < 0.001$). After 3 months, the training group's stress MBF had increased by 33% in the remote ($p < 0.001$) and 28% in infarcted myocardium ($p = 0.02$), while VEGF decreased by 9% ($p = 0.01$), and SDF-1 decreased by 11% ($p = 0.02$). The change in SDF-1 was inversely correlated with the change in stress MBF in both remote ($r = -0.40$, $p = 0.01$) and infarcted myocardium ($r = -0.50$, $p = 0.001$). In the non-training group, MBF and cytokines were unchanged.

Conclusion.—Cardiac rehabilitation improves stress MBF in postinfarction patients, with an inverse decrease in circulating angiogenic cytokines (Fig 2).

▶ Reports that cardiac rehabilitation increased myocardial vascularization were regarded with skepticism for a number of years. It was argued that other exercise-related factors such as an increase in maximal oxygen intake, an increase in muscle strength, and a decrease in exercise blood pressure reduced the oxygen cost of a given rate of working, and thus were adequate to explain the decrease in myocardial ischemia. However, recent research has underlined the potent effect of angiogenic cytokines in increasing the vascularization of ischemic areas of myocardium.[1] In this controlled study, maximal coronary blood flow was determined by dipyridamole infusion rather than by exercise, and coronary flow in response to this stimulus was plainly increased substantially in both infarcted and noninfarcted regions of the heart in response to 3 months of

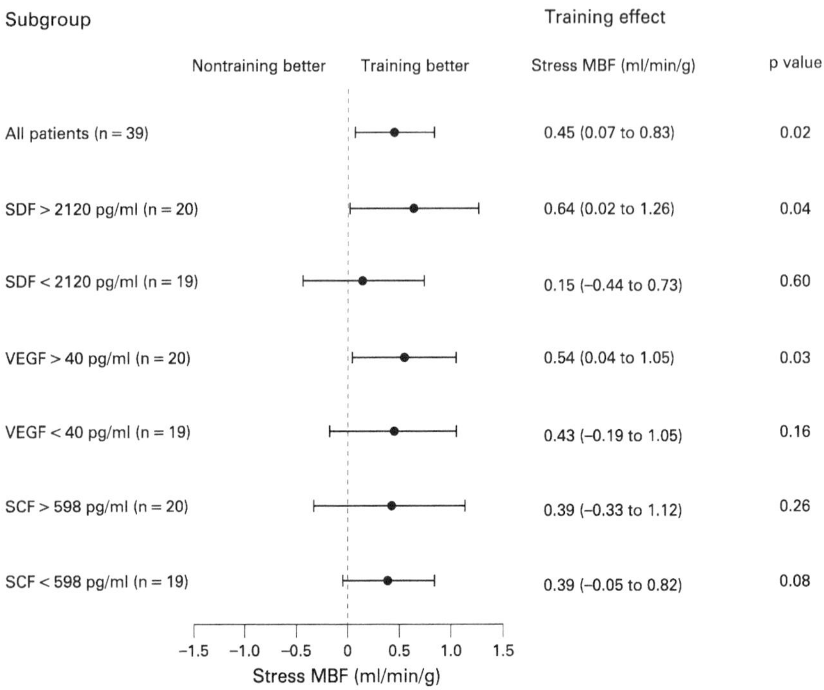

FIGURE 2.—Subgroup analyses of changes in stress myocardial blood flow (MBF) in the infarcted myocardium from baseline at 3-month follow-up. *Median values of the patient population were used to create subgroups of equal size. Oval dots show differences in least-squares means between groups; horizontal bars show the 95% confidence interval. SDF, stromal-derived factor-1; VEGF, vascular endothelial growth factor. (Reprinted from Lee B-C, Hsu H-C, Tseng W-YI, et al. Effect of cardiac rehabilitation on angiogenic cytokines in postinfarction patients. *Heart.* 2009;95:1012-1018, with permission from the BMJ Publishing Group.)

cycle ergometer training (20-minute sessions, 3 times per week, at 55%-70% of peak oxygen intake), and responses were correlated with stromal-derived factor-1 (SDF-1) cytokine levels (Fig 2). However, the concentration of the stimulating cytokines declined as a more adequate coronary flow was reestablished, suggesting the existence of a feedback loop. It would be interesting to learn the site of origin of the stimulating cytokines, and whether there would be virtue in prolonging the period of angiogenesis.

R. J. Shephard, MD (Lond), PhD, DPE

Reference

1. Wang Y, Johnsen HE, Mortensen S, et al. Changes in circulating mesenchymal stem cells, stem cell homing factor, and vascular growth factors in patients with acute ST elevation myocardial infarction treated with primary percutaneous coronary intervention. *Heart.* 2006;92:768-774.

Efficacy and Safety of Exercise Training in Patients With Chronic Heart Failure: HF-ACTION Randomized Controlled Trial

O'Connor CM, for the HF-ACTION Investigators (Duke Clinical Research Inst, Durham, NC; et al)

JAMA 301:1439-1450, 2009

Context.—Guidelines recommend that exercise training be considered for medically stable outpatients with heart failure. Previous studies have not had adequate statistical power to measure the effects of exercise training on clinical outcomes.

Objective.—To test the efficacy and safety of exercise training among patients with heart failure.

Design, Setting, and Patients.—Multicenter, randomized controlled trial of 2331 medically stable outpatients with heart failure and reduced ejection fraction. Participants in Heart Failure: A Controlled Trial Investigating Outcomes of Exercise Training (HF-ACTION) were randomized from April 2003 through February 2007 at 82 centers within the United States, Canada, and France; median follow-up was 30 months.

Interventions.—Usual care plus aerobic exercise training, consisting of 36 supervised sessions followed by home-based training, or usual care alone.

Main Outcome Measures.—Composite primary end point of all-cause mortality or hospitalization and prespecified secondary end points of all-cause mortality, cardiovascular mortality or cardiovascular hospitalization, and cardiovascular mortality or heart failure hospitalization.

Results.—The median age was 59 years, 28% were women, and 37% had New York Heart Association class III or IV symptoms. Heart failure etiology was ischemic in 51%, and median left ventricular ejection fraction was 25%. Exercise adherence decreased from a median of 95 minutes per week during months 4 through 6 of follow-up to 74 minutes per week during months 10 through 12. A total of 759 patients (65%) in the exercise training group died or were hospitalized compared with 796 patients (68%) in the usual care group (hazard ratio [HR], 0.93 [95% confidence interval {Cl}, 0.84-1.02]; *P* =.13). There were nonsignificant reductions in the exercise training group for mortality (189 patients [16%] in the exercise training group vs 198 patients [17%] in the usual care group; HR, 0.96 [95% Cl, 0.79-1.17]; *P* =.70), cardiovascular mortality or cardiovascular hospitalization (632 [55%] in the exercise training group vs 677 [58%] in the usual care group; HR, 0.92 [95% Cl, 0.83-1.03]; *P* =.14), and cardiovascular mortality or heart failure hospitalization (344 [30%] in the exercise training group vs 393 [34%] in the usual care group; HR, 0.87 [95% Cl, 0.75-1.00]; *P* =.06). In prespecified supplementary analyses adjusting for highly prognostic baseline characteristics, the HRs were 0.89 (95% Cl, 0.81-0.99; *P* =.03) for all-cause mortality or hospitalization, 0.91 (95% Cl, 0.82-1.01; *P* =.09) for cardiovascular mortality or cardiovascular hospitalization, and 0.85 (95% Cl, 0.74-0.99; *P* =.03) for

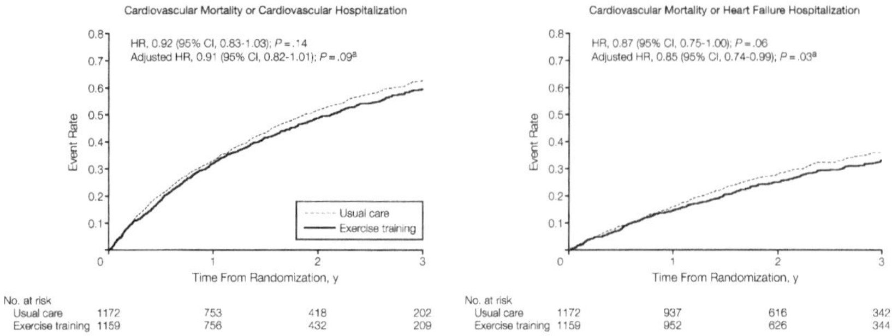

CI indicates confidence interval; HR, hazard ratio.
[a]Adjusted for key prognostic factors.

FIGURE 4.—Time to Cardiovascular Mortality or Cardiovascular Hospitalization and to Cardiovascular Mortality or Heart Failure Hospitalization. (Reprinted from O'Connor CM, for the HF-ACTION Investigators. Efficacy and safety of exercise training in patients with chronic heart failure: HF-ACTION randomized controlled trial. *JAMA*. 2009;301:1439-1450, with permission from American Medical Association. All rights reserved.)

cardiovascular mortality or heart failure hospitalization. Other adverse events were similar between the groups.

Conclusions.—In the protocol-specified primary analysis, exercise training resulted in nonsignificant reductions in the primary end point of all-cause mortality or hospitalization and in key secondary clinical end points. After adjustment for highly prognostic predictors of the primary end point, exercise training was associated with modest significant reductions for both all-cause mortality or hospitalization and cardiovascular mortality or heart failure hospitalization.

Trial Registration.—Clinicaltrials. gov Identifier: NCT00047437 (Fig 4).

▶ A very substantial trial is needed to assess the safety and efficacy of exercise training in terms of such outcomes as overall or cardiac mortality, and this is the first report that has attempted such an analysis for patients with congestive heart failure. It is encouraging to see that after adjustment for baseline characteristics, there was a small but statistically significant decrease of cardiac mortality for the patients enrolled in exercise programs (Fig 4). The authors do not comment on quality-adjusted life expectancy, but since there is also a significant enhancement in the quality of life, we can affirm that this also has been improved in response to exercise rehabilitation. The average 3-month gain of peak oxygen intake in the present study was small (< 5 percent) relative to the 10 to 15 percent gain seen in our study, and it would be interesting to know the effects on both mortality and quality-adjusted mortality of a more effective training program.

For further reading on this subject I suggest an article by Kavanagh et al.[1]

R. J. Shephard, MD (Lond), PhD, DPE

Reference

1. Kavanagh T, Myers MG, Baigrie RS, Mertens DJ, Sawyer P, Shephard RJ. Quality of life and cardiorespiratory function in chronic heart failure: effects of 12 months'; aerobic training. *Heart.* 1996;76:42-49.

Effects of Exercise Training on Health Status in Patients With Chronic Heart Failure: HF-ACTION Randomized Controlled Trial

Flynn KE, Piña IL, Whellan DJ, et al (Duke Univ School of Medicine, Durham, NC; Case Western Reserve Univ School of Medicine, Cleveland, OH; et al)
JAMA 301:1451-1459, 2009

Context.—Findings from previous studies of the effects of exercise training on patient reported health status have been inconsistent.

Objective.—To test the effects of exercise training on health status among patients with heart failure.

Design, Setting, and Patients.—Multicenter, randomized controlled trial among 2331 medically stable outpatients with heart failure with left ventricular ejection fraction of 35% or less. Patients were randomized from April 2003 through February 2007.

Interventions.—Usual care plus aerobic exercise training (n = 1172), consisting of 36 supervised sessions followed by home-based training, vs usual care alone (n = 1159). Randomization was stratified by heart failure etiology, which was a covariate in all models.

Main Outcome Measures.—Kansas City Cardiomyopathy Questionnaire (KCCQ) overall summary scale and key subscales at baseline, every 3 months for 12 months, and annually thereafter for up to 4 years. The KCCQ is scored from 0 to 100 with higher scores corresponding to better health status. Treatment group effects were estimated using linear mixed models according to the intention-to-treat principle.

Results.—Median follow-up was 2.5 years. At3 months, usual care plus exercise training led to greater improvement in the KCCQ overall summary score (mean, 5.21; 95% confidence interval, 4.42 to 6.00) compared with usual care alone (3.28; 95% confidence interval, 2.48 to 4.09). The additional 1.93-point increase (95% confidence interval, 0.84 to 3.01) in the exercise training group was statistically significant ($P < .001$). After 3 months, there were no further significant changes in KCCQ score for either group ($P = .85$ for the difference between slopes), resulting in a sustained, greater improvement overall for the exercise group ($P < .001$). Results were similar on the KCCQ subscales, and no subgroup interactions were detected.

Conclusions.—Exercise training conferred modest but statistically significant improvements in self-reported health status compared with usual care without training. Improvements occurred early and persisted over time.

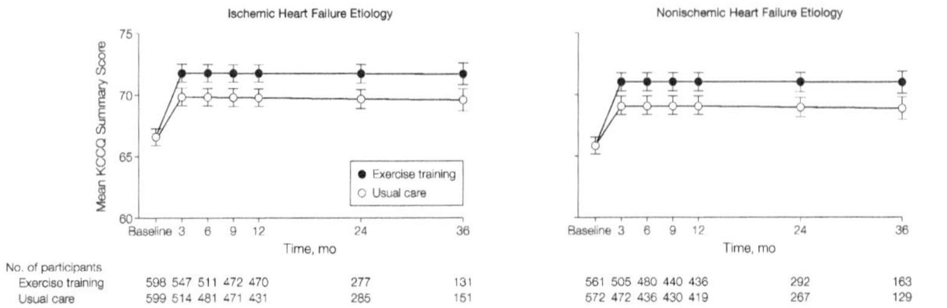

P = .001 for treatment effect for both ischemic and nonischemic heart failure. Error bars indicate standard errors at each time point.

FIGURE 2.—Predicted Mean Health Status Trajectories by Treatment Group. *P* = .001 for treatment effect for both ischemic and nonischemic heart failure. Error bars indicate standard errors at each time point. (Reprinted from Flynn KE, Piña IL, Whellan DJ, et al. Effects of exercise training on health status in patients with chronic heart failure HF-ACTION randomized controlled trial. *JAMA*. 2009;301:1451-1459, with permission from the American Medical Association.)

Trail Registration.—Clinicaltrials.gov Identifier: NCT00047437 (Fig 2).

▶ There is a general consensus that progressive exercise training is helpful in patients with stable congestive heart failure.[1] Research from our laboratory has shown a substantial gain of peak oxygen intake in response to 16 to 20 weeks of training, with associated gains in objective measurements of the quality of life;[2] continuation of observations to 52 weeks showed that gains were maintained but not increased with a longer period of training. Flynn and associates seem unaware of this previous work, but, nevertheless, it is useful to have our findings on quality of life (QOL) confirmed in a large-scale controlled trial (Fig 2). Given that some authors have found a dissociation between gains of peak oxygen intake and QOL score,[3,4] it is unfortunate that Flynn et al did not test correlations between these 2 variables. In the absence of such an association, the increase of QOL could reflect social support as much as physiological gains. The authors also speculate that the plateauing of response could reflect poor compliance with home-based training initiated at 3 months. However, in our study, plateauing was seen although supervised training was continued for a much longer period (52 weeks).

R. J. Shephard, MD (Lond), PhD, DPE

References

1. Shephard RJ. Exercise for patients with congestive heart failure. *Sports Medicine.* 1997;23:75-92.
2. Kavanagh T, Myers MG, Baigrie RS, et al. Quality of life and cardiorespiratory function in chronic heart failure: effects of 12 months'; aerobic training. *Heart.* 1996;76:42-49.
3. Keteyian SJ, Brawner CA, Schairer JR, Mertens DJ, Sawyer P, Shephard RJ. Effects of exercise training on chronotropic incompetence in patients with heart failure. *Am Heart J.* 1999;138:233-240.
4. Keteyian SJ, Levine AB, Brawner CA, et al. Exercise training in patients with heart failure: a randomized, controlled trial. *Ann Intern Med.* 1996;124:1051-1057.

Reduction in Circulating Testosterone Relates to Exercise Capacity in Men With Chronic Heart Failure

Jankowska EA, Filippatos G, Ponikowska B, et al (Military Hosp, Wroclaw, Poland; Athens Univ Hosp Attikon, Greece; Wroclaw Med Univ, Poland; et al)
J Cardiac Fail 15:442-450, 2009

Background.—We investigated whether anabolic deficiency was linked to exercise intolerance in men with chronic heart failure (CHF). Anabolic hormones (testosterone, dehydroepiandrosterone sulfate, insulin-like growth factor 1 [IGF1]) contribute to exercise capacity in healthy men. This issue remains unclear in CHF.

Methods and Results.—We studied 205 men with CHF (age 60 ± 11 years, New York Heart Association [NYHA] Class I/II/III/IV: 37/95/65/8; LVEF [left ventricular ejection fraction]: 31 ± 8%). Exercise capacity was expressed as peak oxygen consumption (peak VO_2), peak O_2 pulse, and ventilatory response to exercise (VE-VCO_2 slope). In multivariable models, reduced peak VO_2 (and reduced peak O_2 pulse) was associated with diminished serum total testosterone (TT) ($P < .01$) and free testosterone (eFT; estimated from TT and sex hormone globulin levels) ($P < .01$), which was independent of NYHA Class, plasma N-terminal pro-brain natriuretic peptide, and age. These associations remained significant even after adjustment for an amount of leg lean tissue. In multivariable models, high VE-VCO_2 slope was related to reduced serum IGF1 ($P < .05$), advanced NYHA Class ($P < .05$), increased plasma NT-proBNP ($P < .0001$), and borderline low LVEF ($P = .07$). In 44 men, reassessed after 2.3 ± 0.4 years, a reduction in peak VO_2 (and peak O_2 pulse) was accompanied by a decrease in TT ($P < .01$) and eFT ($P \leq .01$). Increase in VE-VCO_2 slope was related only to an increase in plasma NT-proBNP ($P < .05$).

Conclusions.—In men with CHF, low circulating testosterone independently relates to exercise intolerance. The greater the reduction of serum TT in the course of disease, the more severe the progression of exercise intolerance. Whether testosterone supplementation would improve exercise capacity in hypogonadal men with CHF requires further studies (Table 2).

▶ It has been recognized for a number of years that impaired muscle function makes a significant contribution to exercise intolerance in congestive heart failure.[1,2] The cause of this dysfunction has been less clear, although tissue hypoxia has been one common suggestion. Given the link between muscle weakness and a deficient production of anabolic steroids in the elderly,[3-6] a suppression of the anabolic axis is another possibility. The present cross-sectional study of a substantial sample of men with moderate congestive heart failure (average ejection fraction 31%) supports this suggestion (Table 2), particularly as the drop in testosterone concentration increases on follow-up of those with worsening cardiorespiratory function. Examination of the anabolic axis may be helpful in evaluating the prognosis of patients, as it

TABLE 2.—Associations between Clinical and Hormonal Variables and Exercise Capacity in 205 Men with CHF (Single Predictor Models)

Determinants	Peak VO_2 (mL ·min ·kg)	Peak VO_2 (% of Age-, Sex-, and Weight-Matched Predicted Values)	Peak O_2 Pulse (mL/beat)	VE-VCO_2 Slope
Age, year	$r = -0.34$ ($P < .0001$)	$r = 0.12$ ($P = .008$)	$r = -0.33$ ($P < .0001$)	$r = 0.02$ ($P = .83$)
LVEF, % (ln)	$r = 0.10$ ($P = .14$)	$r = 0.27$ ($P < .0001$)	$r = 0.16$ ($P = .02$)	$r = -0.27$ ($P < .0001$)
CHF etiology, ischemic vs. nonischemic	$t = -2.65$ ($P = .009$)	$t = 0.33$ ($P = .74$)	$t = -2.24$ ($P = .0.03$)	$t = 0.96$ ($P = .0.34$)
NYHA Class, I/II/III/IV	$r = -0.54$ ($P < .0001$)	$r = -0.34$ ($P < .0001$)	$r = -0.42$ ($P < .0001$)	$r = 0.21$ ($P = .002$)
Plasma NT-proBNP, pg/mL (ln)	$r = -0.30$ ($P < .0001$)	$r = -0.36$ ($P < .0001$)	$r = -0.27$ ($P < .0001$)	$r = 0.41$ ($P < .0001$)
Diabetes mellitus, yes vs. no	$t = -3.78$ ($P = .0002$)	$t = -0.63$ ($P = .53$)	$t = -1.51$ ($P = .13$)	$t = 0.28$ ($P = .78$)
Hemoglobin, g/dL	$r = 0.16$ ($P = .03$)	$r = 0.11$ ($P = .11$)	$r = 0.23$ ($P = .001$)	$r = -0.04$ ($P = .55$)
eGFR, mL min 1.73 m^2	$r = 0.16$ ($P = .03$)	$r = 0.06$ ($P = .43$)	$r = 0.15$ ($P = .03$)	$r = -0.04$ ($P = .56$)
Serum TT, ng/mL (ln)	$r = 0.30$ ($P < .0001$)	$r = 0.18$ ($P = .01$)	$r = 0.28$ ($P < .0001$)	$r = 0.08$ ($P = .27$)
Serum eFT, pg/mL (ln)	$r = 0.30$ ($P < .0001$)	$r = 0.16$ ($P = .02$)	$r = 0.25$ ($P < .0001$)	$r = -0.004$ ($P = .96$)
Serum DHEAS, ng/mL (ln)	$r = 0.36$ ($P < .0001$)	$r = 0.12$ ($P = .09$)	$r = 0.21$ ($P = .03$)	$r = -0.06$ ($P = .43$)
Serum IGF1, ng/mL (ln)	$r = -0.06$ ($P = .43$)	$r = -0.03$ ($P = .69$)	$r = -0.01$ ($P = 0.94$)	$r = -0.11$ ($P = .10$)

CHF, chronic heart failure; NYHA, New York Heart Association; LVEF, left ventricular ejection fraction; NT-proBNP, N-terminal pro-B-type natriuretic peptide; eGFR, estimated glomerular filtration rate; TT, total testosterone; eFT, estimated free testosterone; DHEAS, dehydroepiandrosterone sulfate; IGF1, insulin-like growth factor 1; VO_2, minute oxygen consumption; VCO_2, minute carbon dioxide production; VE, minute ventilation. Values are presented as correlatory coefficients, or *t*-value of the Student test, where appropriate with *P* values.

seems linked to mortality,[7] although the correlations are probably rather weak to be used in making predictions for individual patients. There would also seem some merit in adding anabolic steroids to the treatment of congestive heart failure patients when they enter a cardiac rehabilitation program,[8] particularly as endurance exercise alone can lead to some suppression of anabolic hormone secretion.

R. J. Shephard, MD (Lond), PhD, DPE

References

1. Coats AJ, Clark AAL, Piepoli M, Volterrani M, Poole-Wilson PA. Symptoms and quality of life in heart failure: the muscle hypothesis. *Br Heart J*. 1994;72:S36-S39.
2. Drexler H, Coats AJ. Explaining fatigue in congestive heart failure. *Annu Rev Med*. 1996;47:241-256.
3. Pitteloud N, Mootha VK, Dwyer AA, et al. Relationship between testosterone levels, insulin sensitivity, and mitochondrial function in men. *Diabetes Care*. 2005;28:1636-1642.
4. Izquierdo M, Häkkinen K, Antón A, et al. Maximal strength and power, endurance performance, and serum hormones in middle-aged and elderly men. *Med Sci Sports Exerc*. 2001;33:1577-1587.
5. Haydar ZR, Blackman MR, Tobin JD, Wright JG, Fleg JL. The relationship between aerobic exercise capacity and circulating IGF1 levels in healthy men and women. *J Am Geriatr Soc*. 2000;48:139-145.
6. Abbasi A, Duthie EH Jr, Sheldahl L, et al. Association of dehydroepiandrosterone sulfate, body composition, and physical fitness in independent community-dwelling older men and women. *J Am Geriatr Soc*. 1998;46:263-273.
7. Jankowska EA, Biel B, Majda J, et al. Anabolic deficiency in men with chronic heart failure: prevalence and detrimental impact on survival. *Circulation*. 2006; 114:1829-1837.
8. Malkin CJ, Pugh PJ, West JN, van Beek EJ, Jones TH, Channer KS. Testosterone therapy in men with moderate severity heart failure: a double-blind randomized placebo controlled trial. *Eur Heart J*. 2006;27:57-64.

Does Peak Oxygen Pulse Complement Peak Oxygen Uptake in Risk Stratifying Patients With Heart Failure?

Oliveira RB, Myers J, Araújo CGS, et al (Gama Filho Univ, Rio de Janeiro, Brazil; Stanford Univ, Palo Alto, CA; et al)
Am J Cardiol 104:554-558, 2009

There is scarce information regarding the prognostic utility of peak exercise oxygen pulse (peak O_2 pulse), a surrogate for stroke volume, in patients with heart failure (HF). From May 1994 to November 2007, 998 patients with HF underwent cardiopulmonary exercise testing. The ability of peak oxygen uptake (VO_2) and peak O_2 pulse to predict cardiac events was examined. Peak O_2 pulse was calculated by dividing peak VO_2 by heart rate at the time peak VO_2 was achieved and was expressed in both milliliters per beat and as a percentage achieved of the age-predicted value. There were 212 cardiac events (176 deaths, 26 transplantations, and 10 left ventricular assist device implantations) over a mean of 28 ± 26 months of follow-up. Peak VO_2 and age-predicted peak O_2 pulse were demonstrated by univariate and multivariate Cox regression analyses to be independent predictors of mortality ($p < 0.001$). The optimal cut points for peak VO_2 and age-predicted peak O_2 pulse (<14.3 and ≥14.3 [$mL/kg^{-1}/min^{-1}$] and < 85% and ≥85%, respectively) were established by areas under the receiver-operating characteristic curves. Patients exhibiting abnormalities for both responses had 4.8-fold (95% confidence interval 2.7 to 8.5) and 6.7-fold (95% confidence interval 4.1 to 11.1) higher risks for mortality and cardiac events, respectively, than those whose responses were normal. Age-predicted peak O2 pulse also predicted mortality in patients in the intermediate range of peak VO_2 (10 to 14 ($mL/kg^{-1}/min^{-1}$)). The 3-year mortality rate for patients in this range who had age-predicted peak O_2 pulse values < 85% was even slightly higher than those with peak VO_2 <10.1 ($mL/kg^{-1}/min^{-1}$). In conclusion, age-predicted peak O_2 pulse was a strong and independent predictor of cardiac mortality and complemented peak VO_2 in predicting risk in patients with HF.

▶ It is now well established that peak oxygen intake provides a useful index of prognosis in congestive heart failure; it reflects a combination of peak cardiac output and peripheral oxygen extraction. However, the dominant problem in most patients with congestive failure is a poor ejection fraction and thus a poor stroke volume. It thus seems logical to assess the predictive value of peak oxygen pulse, a relatively easily measured surrogate of peak stroke volume.[1-3] Previous assessments of the peak oxygen pulse have yielded conflicting results.[4,5]The follow-up period in this retrospective study of Oliveira et al was relatively short (an average of 28 months), but nevertheless yielded

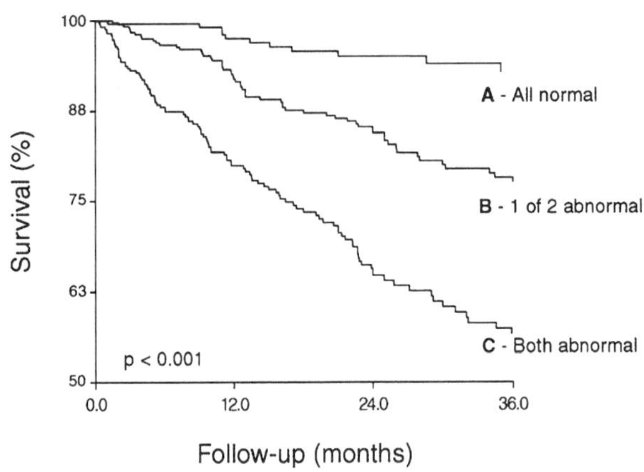

FIGURE 1.—Kaplan-Meier analyses for 3-year major cardiac events with normal and abnormal peak VO_2 and age-predicted peak O_2 pulse responses and their combination. Group A: peak $VO_2 \geq 14.3$ $mL/kg^{-1}/min^{-1}$ and age-predicted peak O_2 pulse ≥ 85%; group B: peak $VO_2 < 14.3$ $mL/kg^{-1}/min^{-1}$ or age-predicted peak O_2 pulse <85%; group C: peak VO_2 <14.3 $mL/kg^{-1}/min^{-1}$ and age-predicted peak O_2 pulse <85%. (Reprinted from Oliveira RB, Myers J, Araújo CGS, et al. Does peak oxygen pulse complement peak oxygen uptake in risk stratifying patients with heart failure? *Am J Cardiol.* 2009;104:554-558, with permission from Elsevier.)

176 deaths, adequate for assessing the merits of the 2 tests of prognosis. Univariate analysis showed the oxygen pulse to be at least as effective a predictor as peak oxygen intake, but the combination of the 2 tests yielded a much clearer identification of those who would undergo major cardiac events within the follow-up period (Fig 1); the risk of mortality was increased 4-fold, and the risk of a major event 6-fold if both test scores were below the arbitrary cut-point. The use of combined indices may be particularly helpful in assessing patients who have a peak oxygen intake in the range of 10 to 14 mL/(kg.min), as peak oxygen intake alone does not distinguish such individuals very well. One area that the authors suggest merits further research is the determination of an appropriate age adjustment for the peak oxygen pulse. It is also desirable to evaluate the proposed cut-points for both peak oxygen intake and peak oxygen pulse in a prospective trial.

R. J. Shephard, MD (Lond), PhD, DPE

References

1. Munhoz EC, Hollanda R, Vargas JP, et al. Flattening of oxygen pulse during exercise may detect extensive myocardial ischemia. *Med Sci Sports Exerc.* 2007;39: 1221-1226.
2. Whipp BJ, Higgenbotham MB, Cobb FC. Estimating exercise stroke volume from asymptotic oxygen pulse in humans. *J Appl Physiol.* 1996;81:2674-2679.
3. Chaudhry S, Arena R, Wasserman K, et al. Exercise-induced myocardial ischemia detected by cardiopulmonary exercise testing. *Am J Cardiol.* 2009;103:615-619.
4. Cohen-Solal A, Barnier P, Pessione F, et al. Comparison of the long-term prognostic value of peak exercise oxygen pulse and peak oxygen uptake in_patients with chronic heart failure. *Heart.* 1997;78:572-576.
5. Lavie CJ, Milani RV, Mehra MR. Peak exercise oxygen pulse and_prognosis in chronic heart failure. *Am J Cardiol.* 2004;93:588-593.

Effects of exercise training in patients with idiopathic pulmonary arterial hypertension

de Man FS, Handoko ML, Groepenhoff H, et al (Univ Med Ctr, Amsterdam; et al)

Eur Respir J 34:669-675, 2009

We determined the physiological effects of exercise training on exercise capacity and quadriceps muscle function in patients with idiopathic pulmonary arterial hypertension (iPAH).

In total, 19 clinically stable iPAH patients (New York Heart Association II-III) underwent a supervised exercise training programme for the duration of 12 weeks. Maximal capacity, endurance capacity and quadriceps function were assessed at baseline and after 12 weeks. In 12 patients, serial quadriceps muscle biopsies were obtained.

6-min walk distance and peak exercise capacity did not change after training. However, endurance capacity improved significantly after training, demonstrated by a shift of the anaerobic threshold to a higher workload (from 32 ± 5 to 46 ± 6 W; $p = 0.003$) together with an increase in exercise endurance time ($p < 0.001$). Moreover, exercise training increased quadriceps strength by 13% ($p = 0.005$) and quadriceps endurance by 34% ($p = 0.001$).

Training enhanced aerobic capacity of the quadriceps, by increasing capillarisation (1.36 ± 0.10 to 1.78 ± 0.13 capillaries per muscle fibre; $p < 0.001$) and oxidative enzyme activity, especially of the type-I (slow) muscle fibres. No changes were found in cross-sectional area and fibre type distribution.

Exercise training in iPAH improves exercise endurance and quadriceps muscle function, which is also reflected by structural changes of the quadriceps (Table 1).

▶ As in chronic obstructive pulmonary disease, patients with idiopathic pulmonary hypertension have a poor physical work capacity with impaired stroke volume, a tendency to lactic acidosis, and a deterioration of skeletal muscle function.[1,2] Enrollment in an exercise rehabilitation program thus seems desirable, but traditionally this has been avoided because of fears of provoking sudden cardiac death.[3] However, recent investigators have found exercise to be a practical form of therapy, and effective in improving the patient's quality of life.[4] The present report examined how far improvements in skeletal muscle function were responsible for the overall improvement in function. The exercise program included repeated bouts of aerobic training at 75% of peak oxygen intake for the second half of the 12-week program, but nevertheless there were no significant gains in walking distance or peak aerobic capacity (Table 1). However, the program of quadriceps strength and endurance exercises increased local capillarity and aerobic enzyme activity, with apparent increases in muscle performance (endurance > strength). One possible weakness in this conclusion is that the program may have increased patient

TABLE 1.—12-week Supervised Exercise Training Protocol

Week	Intensity	Exercise	Rest Time Min	Sets
Cycling				
1–3	50% $V'O_2$,max	2 min	2	10
4–6	50% $V'O_2$,max	3 min	2	7
7–9	75% $V'O_2$,max	4 min	2	6
10–12	75% $V'O_2$,max	5 min	2	5
Quadriceps strength				
1–3	50% ORM	12 rep	1	3
4–6	50% ORM	13 rep	1	3
7–9	75% ORM	14 rep	1	3
10–12	75% ORM	15 rep	1	3
Quadriceps endurance				
1–3	30% ORM	30 rep	1	3
4–6	30% ORM	40 rep	1	4
7–9	40% ORM	50 rep	1	5
10–12	40% ORM	60 rep	1	6

$V'O_2$,max: maximal oxygen uptake determined during cardiopulmonary exercise testing; ORM: one repetition maximum; rep: repetition. The exercise training consisted of cycle training (based on $V'O_2$,max assessed at baseline measurements) and quadriceps training (based on ORM assessed on the first day of training).

motivation; a more conclusive proof would have been obtained by electrical stimulation of the muscles before and after training. The sample size was also small, and there was some suggestion that not everyone responded to training; further studies on a larger sample are desirable to determine the characteristics of responders and nonresponders.

R. J. Shephard, MD (Lond), PhD, DPE

References

1. Deboeck G, Niset G, Lamotte M, Vachiéry JL, Naeije R. Exercise testing in pulmonary arterial hypertension and in chronic heart failure. *Eur Respir J.* 2004;23: 747-751.
2. Yasunobu Y, Oudiz RJ, Sun XG, Hansen JE, Wasserman K. End-tidal PCO2 abnormality and exercise limitation in patients with primary pulmonary hypertension. *Chest.* 2005;127:1637-1646.
3. Desai SA, Channick RN. Exercise in patients with pulmonary arterial hypertension. *J Cardiopulm Rehabil Prev.* 2008;28:12-16.
4. Mereles D, Ehlken N, Kreuscher S, et al. Exercise and respiratory training improve exercise capacity and quality of life in patients with severe chronic pulmonary hypertension. *Circulation.* 2006;114:1482-1489.

Physical activity and subclinical MRI cerebral infarcts: The ARIC Study

Dubbert PM, Penman AD, Evenson KR, et al (G.V. Sonny Montgomery Veterans Affairs Med Ctr, Jackson, MS; Univ of Mississippi Med Ctr, Jackson; Univ of North Carolina, Chapel Hill)

J Neurol Sci 284:135-139, 2009

Background.—We hypothesized that physical activity (PA), which is often associated with reduced risk of ischemic stroke, may also be associated with reduced risk of subclinical cerebral infarcts.

Objectives.—We studied the cross-sectional association between PA and subclinical cerebral infarcts among African-Americans in the Atherosclerosis Risk in Communities (ARIC) Study.

Methods.—PA self-reported at baseline and images from cerebral MRI examination obtained 6 years later were evaluated for presence and location of subclinical infarcts $\geq$ 3 mm in size. After exclusions, 944 participants were eligible for study.

Results.—The results suggested an inverse relationship between odds of having a subclinical cerebral infarct and level of PA on several measures, although the multivariable adjusted odds ratios (OR) were statistically significant only for the sport score. A 1-unit increase in the sport score, indicating more leisure PA, was associated with an adjusted OR for having a subclinical cerebral infarct of 0.62 (0.44–0.87), with a statistically significant monotonic trend across quartiles of the score ($P = 0.01$). There was no association of work scores with subclinical infarcts.

TABLE 3.—Adjusted Odds Ratios (95% CI) for Having a Subclinical Cerebral Infarct by Measures of PA

	Odds Ratio (95% CI) & P value				
	Model 1 Adjusted for Age and Sex	Model 2 Adjusted for Age, Sex, Center, Education, Smoking	Model 3A Adjusted for Age, Sex, Center, Education, Smoking and Hypertension	Model 3B Adjusted for Age, Sex, Center, Education, Smoking and Diabetes	Model 3C Adjusted for Age, Sex, Center, Education, Smoking and Fibrinogen
Sport (per 1-unit increase in score)	0.61 (0.45, 0.84) 0.003	0.62 (0.44, 0.86) 0.004	0.64 (0.46, 0.89) 0.01	0.60 (0.43, 0.84) 0.003	0.62 (0.44, 0.87) 0.01
Leisure (per 1-unit increase in score)	0.73 (0.53, 0.99) 0.04	0.77 (0.56, 1.05) 0.09	0.76 (0.56, 1.04) 0.09	0.79 (0.57, 1.08) 0.13	0.77 (0.56, 1.06) 0.11
Work (per 1-unit increase in score)	0.98 (0.81–1.19) 0.86	0.97 (0.80, 1.17) 0.76	0.99 (0.82, 1.20) 0.93	1.01 (0.84, 1.23) 0.90	0.99 (0.82, 1.20) 0.93
Regular activity (yes vs. no)	0.63 (0.40, 1.01) 0.05	0.69 (0.43, 1.11) 0.12	0.73 (0.45, 1.17) 0.19	0.68 (0.42, 1.10) 0.12	0.69 (0.42, 1.13) 0.14
Vigorous activity (yes vs. no)	0.64 (0.22, 1.84) 0.40	0.72 (0.25, 2.09) 0.55	0.84 (0.29, 2.45) 0.75	0.75 (0.26, 2.21) 0.61	0.77 (0.26, 2.23) 0.62
Walking (frequent vs. infrequent)	0.56 (0.32, 0.97) 0.04	0.59 (0.33, 1.03) 0.07	0.56 (0.31, 0.99) 0.05	0.62 (0.35, 1.09) 0.10	0.56 (0.31, 1.02) 0.06

Conclusions.—In African-Americans, sport PA was inversely related to subclinical MRI-detected cerebral infarcts assessed six years later.

► There is growing evidence of the value of regular physical activity in protecting against ischemic stroke.[1-3] However, much of the progressive loss of cerebral function seen in the elderly is attributable to subclinical lesions rather than an overt stroke,[4-6] and it is thus of considerable interest to examine whether regular physical activity has similar efficacy in preventing subclinical lesions. This prospective study obtained good MRI evidence of such lesions 6 years after an assessment of physical activity (although unfortunately not at entry to the study). One important limitation is reliance on the self-reported physical activity. The Baecke scale was used for this purpose. This instrument assesses physical activity on three 5-point scales—sport, leisure, and occupational activities. Differences of Baecke score between those with and without evidence of subclinical infarction were small, although because of a large sample size they were statistically significant for 1 of the 3 indices (sport, Table 3). Depending on the choice of covariates, there was also a suggestion of benefit in those subjects reporting frequent walking. Because the MRIs were only obtained at the end of the study, there remains at least a theoretical possibility that the subclinical lesions predisposed to a low level of physical activity, rather than the reverse. Thus, there remains a need for further observations, making objective and quantitative measurements of physical activity, and obtaining MRIs before and after the period of observation.

R. J. Shephard, MD (Lond), PhD, DPE

References

1. Evenson KR, Rosamond WD, Cai J, et al. Physical activity and ischemic stroke risk. The atherosclerosis risk in communities study. *Stroke.* 1999;30:1333-1339.
2. Oguma Y, Shinoda-Tagawa T. Physical activity decreases cardiovascular disease risk in women: review and meta-analysis. *Am J Prev Med.* 2004;26:407-418.
3. Lee I-M, Hennekens CH, Berger K, Buring JE, Manson JE. Exercise and risk of stroke in male physicians. *Stroke.* 1999;30:1-6.
4. Bokura H, Kobayashi S, Yamaguchi S, et al. Silent brain infarction and subcortical white matter lesions increase the risk of stroke and mortality: a prospective cohort study. *J Stroke Cerebrovas Dis.* 2006;15:57-63.
5. Longstreth WT Jr, Bernick C, Manolio TA, Bryan N, Jungreis CA, Price TR. Lacunar infarcts defined by magnetic resonance imaging of 3660 elderly people: the Cardiovascular Health Study. *Arch Neurol.* 1998;55:1217-1225.
6. Vermeer SE, Koudstaal PJ, Oudkerk M, Hofman A, Breteler MM. Prevalence and risk factors of silent brain infarcts in the population-based Rotterdam Scan study. *Stroke.* 2002;33:21-25.

A Self-Administered Graded Repetitive Arm Supplementary Program (GRASP) Improves Arm Function During Inpatient Stroke Rehabilitation: A Multi-Site Randomized Controlled Trial

Harris JE, Eng JJ, Miller WC, et al (Univ of British Columbia, Vancouver, Canada)

Stroke 40:2123-2128, 2009

Background and Purpose.—More than 70% of individuals who have a stroke experience upper limb deficits that impact daily activities. Increased amount of upper limb therapy has positive effects; however, practical and inexpensive methods of therapy are needed to deliver this increase in therapy.

Methods.—This was a multi-site single blind randomized controlled trial to determine the effectiveness of a 4-week self-administered graded repetitive upper limb supplementary program (GRASP) on arm recovery in stroke. 103 inpatients with stroke were randomized to the experimental group (GRASP group, n = 53) or the control group (education protocol, n = 50). The primary outcome measure was the Chedoke Arm and Hand Activity Inventory (CAHAI), a measure of upper limb function in activities of daily living. Secondary measures were used to evaluate grip strength and paretic upper limb use outside of therapy time. Intention-to-treat analysis was performed. Group differences were tested using analysis of covariance.

Results.—At the end of the 4-week intervention (approximately 7 weeks poststroke), the GRASP group showed greater improvement in upper limb function (CAHAI) compared to the control group (mean difference 6.2; 95% CI: 3.4 to 9.0; $P<0.001$). The GRASP group maintained this significant gain at 5 months poststroke. Significant differences were also found in favor of the GRASP protocol for grip strength and paretic upper limb use. No serious adverse effects were experienced.

Conclusion.—A self-administered homework exercise program provides a cost-, time-, and treatment-effective delivery model for improving upper limb recovery in subacute stroke.

▶ This well-designed, randomized controlled trial provides evidence that the addition of a 4-week monitored, self-administered, homework-based exercise program to a regular in-patient rehabilitation program, improves upper extremity function. The authors use valid outcome measures and show gains at 7 weeks and 5 months post-stroke. The implications are that monitored homework based programs may be an effective way to gain function. It would be interesting to apply these types of programs to persons with other types of impairments and functional deficits.

D. E. Feldman, PT, PhD

Brain Activity Changes Associated With Treadmill Training: After Stroke

Enzinger C, Dawes H, Johansen-Berg H, et al (Med Univ of Graz, Austria; Univ of Oxford, UK; Oxford Brookes Univ, UK; et al)

Stroke 40:2460-2467, 2009

Background and Purpose.—The mechanisms underlying motor recovery after stroke are not fully understood. Several studies used functional MRI longitudinally to relate brain activity changes with performance gains of the upper limb after therapy, but research into training-induced recovery of lower limb function has been relatively neglected thus far.

Methods.—We investigated functional reorganization after 4 weeks of treadmill training with partial body weight support in 18 chronic patients (mean age, 59.9 ± 13.5 years) with mild to moderate paresis (Motricity Index affected leg: 77.7 ± 10.5; range, 9 to 99) and gait impairment (Functional Ambulation Category: 4.4 ± 0.6; range, 3 to 5) due to a single subcortical ischemic stroke using repeated 3.0-T functional MRI and an ankle-dorsiflexion paradigm.

Results.—Walking endurance improved after training (2-minute timed walking distance: 121.5 ± 39.0 versus pre: 105.1 ± 38.1 m; $P = 0.0001$). For active movement of the paretic foot versus rest, greater walking endurance correlated with increased brain activity in the bilateral primary sensorimotor cortices, the cingulate motor areas, and the caudate nuclei bilaterally and in the thalamus of the affected hemisphere.

Conclusions.—Despite the strong subcortical contributions to gait control, rehabilitation-associated walking improvements are associated with cortical activation changes. This is similar to findings in upper limb rehabilitation with some differences in the involved cortical areas. We observed bihemispheric activation increases with greater recovery both in cortical and subcortical regions with movement of the paretic foot. However, although the dorsal premotor cortex appears to play an important role in recovery of hand movements, evidence for the involvement of this region in lower extremity recovery was not found (Table 2).

▶ A greater understanding of the central neurological processes associated with recovery from stroke would plainly be of value in the design of rehabilitation programs and in the triage of patients based on their recovery prospects.

TABLE 2.—Mobility Data Before and After Treadmill Training

Measure	Before Treadmill Training Mean ± 1 SD	Before Treadmill Training Median (IQR)	After Treadmill Training Mean ± 1 SD	After Treadmill Training Median (IQR)	P*
10-m timed walk, seconds	15.9 ± 20.3	9.4 (8.6–13.7)	12.1 ± 9.6	8.5 (7.9–11.7)	0.001
2-minute walk, meters	103.6 ± 38.1	114.6 (78.9–140.4)	119.7 ± 39.0	134.5 (97.1–152.1)	0.0001

IQR indicates interquartile range.
*Paired nonparametric Wilcoxon-test.

Previous studies of this question have been based mainly on patients with lesions affecting use of the arms, probably because it is easier to obtain MRI images on such individuals. Such investigations have demonstrated increased activity of the contralesional sensorimotor cortex with movement of the impaired limb soon after a stroke.[1,2] However, as recovery proceeds, the electrical activity shifts progressively to the ipsilateral sensorimotor cortex, this change being most obvious in those patients with the best prognosis for recovery of voluntary movement.[3,4] This study extends these observations to a small sample of patients with mild to moderate subcortical ischemic lesions affecting use of the lower limbs, as the group underwent 4 weeks of treadmill training with partial weight support (Table 2). Improved walking was associated with increased sensorimotor cortex activity on both sides of the brain, as might be expected from the establishment of altered cortical circuitry.[5] One difference from earlier studies of those with hand lesions was the absence of any involvement of the premotor cortex. It is necessary to underline several limitations to the study. In particular, lesions were not severe and did not involve the cortex. Moreover, there was no control group to examine what happens in the absence of formal supervised training.

R. J. Shephard, MD (Lond), PhD, DPE

References

1. Ward NS, Brown MM, Thompson AJ, Frackowiak RSJ. Neural correlates of outcome after stroke: a cross-sectional fMRI study. *Brain*. 2003;126:1430-1448.
2. Ward NS, Brown MM, Thompson AJ, Frackowiak RS. The influence of time after stroke on brain activations during a motor task. *Ann Neurol*. 2004;55:829-834.
3. Cramer SC, Parrish TB, Levy RM, et al. Predicting functional gains in a stroke trial. *Stroke*. 2007;38:2108-2114.
4. Loubinoux I, Dechaumont-Palacin S, Castel-Lacanal E, et al. Prognostic value of fMRI in recovery of hand function in subcortical stroke patients. *Cereb Cortex*. 2007;17:2980-2987.
5. Luft AR, Macko RF, Forrester LW, et al. Treadmill exercise activates subcortical neural networks and improves walking after stroke: a randomized controlled trial. *Stroke*. 2008;39:3341-3350.

Reduction in Incident Stroke Risk With Vigorous Physical Activity: Evidence From 7.7-Year Follow-Up of the National Runners' Health Study

Williams PT (Donner Laboratory, Berkeley, CA)
Stroke 40:1921-1923, 2009

Background and Purpose.—The purpose of this study was to assess the dose–response relationship between vigorous physical activity (running distance, km/d) and the participant-reported physician-diagnosed stroke.

Methods.—Age-adjusted survival analysis of 29 279 men and 12 123 women followed prospectively for 7.7 years.

Results.—One hundred men and 19 women reported incident strokes. Per km/d run, the age-and smoking-adjusted risk for stroke decreased

TABLE 3.—Risk Ratios for Categories of Daily Running Distance Relative to Current Physical Activity Guideline Levels (<2 km/day) From Cox-Proportional Hazard Model

	Males Only	Males and Females, Sex Adjusted
<2 km/day	1.00†	1.00*
2–3.9 km/day	0.76‡ (0.44, 1.37) *P*=0.35	0.82‡ (0.49, 1.42) *P*=0.47
4 to 5.9 km/day	0.48 (0.27, 0.90) *P*=0.02	0.55 (0.32, 0.99) *P*=0.04
6 to 7.9 km/day	0.59 (0.28, 1.21) *P*=0.15	0.54 (0.26, 1.10) *P*=0.09
≥8 km/day	0.29 (0.13, 0.64) *P*=0.002	0.40 (0.19, 0.79) *P*=0.009

All results are adjusted for age (age and age^2) and baseline smoking. Ranges within parentheses are the 95% confidence intervals. Significance of difference from all greater running distances are coded.
*P=0.05.
†P=0.03.
‡P=0.02.

12% in men ($P = 0.0007$), and 11% in men and women combined ($P = 0.001$), which remained significant when further adjusted for baseline diabetes, hypercholesterolemia, hypertension, and BMI (8% and 7% reduction per km/d run, respectively, $P = 0.03$). Men and women who ran ≥2 km/d (ie, exceeded the recommended AHA/CDC and NIH guideline activity level) had significantly lower risk than those who ran less ($P = 0.05$), and those who ran ≥4 km/d had significantly lower risk than those who ran 2 to 3.9 km/d ($P = 0.02$). Men and women who ran ≥8 km/d were at 60% lower risk than those who ran <2 km/d ($P = 0.002$).

Conclusions.—The risk for incident stroke is substantially reduced in those who exceed the guideline physical activity level, which cannot be attributed to less hypertension, diabetes, hypercholesterolemia, or body weight (Table 3).

▶ There is growing evidence of the value of regular physical activity in the prevention of ischemic stroke. The present large-scale cross-sectional study of runners is important both in showing substantial benefits that are independent of any effects from age, smoking, blood pressure, cholesterol levels, obesity, or diabetes, and in exploring the merits of exceeding currently recommended exercise guidelines for middle-aged adults. The data show a clear dose gradient for physician-diagnosed stroke (Table 3), and it seems that there is value in running at least 8 km/d, more than 4 times the currently recommended dose of exercise. However, the obvious weakness in such a cross-sectional analysis is that those who choose to engage in 4 times the recommended minimum of physical activity are unlikely to be representative of the general population. As in most exercise/health studies, there is an urgent need for prospective data.

For further reading on this subject I suggest an article by Goldstein et al.[1]

R. J. Shephard, MD (Lond), PhD, DPE

Reference

1. Goldstein LB, Adams R, Alberts MJ, et al. Primary prevention of ischemic stroke: a guideline from the American Heart Association/American Stroke Association Stroke Council. *Circulation.* 2006;113:e873-e923.

Upper Respiratory Tract Infection Symptoms in Ultramarathon Runners Not Related to Immunoglobulin Status

Peters EM, Shaik J, Kleinveldt N (Univ of KwaZulu-Natal, Durban, South Africa)

Clin J Sport Med 20:39-46, 2010

Objective.—To determine the association between variation in exercise load, immunoglobulin (Ig) status, and self-reported symptoms of upper respiratory tract infection (URTI) in ultramarathon runners.

Design.—Longitudinal observational field study.

Setting.—Four weeks before and 2 weeks after an 86.5-km Comrades Marathon, South Africa.

Participants.—Fourteen randomly selected, amateur, male, ultramarathon runners.

Main Outcome Measures.—Daily record of training and URTI symptom incidence. Salivary IgA and IgM at 28 days, 14 days, and 1 day (01PRE) before the race, immediately post race (IPR) and 1 (01 PR), 3, and 14 days post race. Serum cortisol, IgG, IgM, and IgA concentrations at 01PRE, IPR, and 01PR.

Results.—Mean weekly training distance varied from 89.4 kilometers per week (28.9 kilometers per week) to 4.2 kilometers per week (6.7 kilometers per week). Absolute and relative mucosal IgA and IgM concentrations were unaffected by pre-race taper in training volume ($P > 0.05$). IgA and IgM secretion rates decreased post race ($P = 0.018$; 0.008), returning to baseline by 01PR. Blood leukocyte, serum cortisol, and serum IgG concentrations increased at IPR ($P < 0.001$, <0001) and 01PR ($P = 0.009$), respectively. Upper respiratory tract infection symptom incidence was highest at 28PRE and 7 to 14 days post race but not related to salivary IgA and IgM secretion rates. Eight subjects (57%) who reported URTI symptoms pre race also reported these during days 7 to 14 post race.

Conclusions.—Upper respiratory tract infection symptom incidence was not associated with secretory Ig concentrations. Reactivation of pre-race viruses during the 2 weeks post race and exercise-induced inflammatory

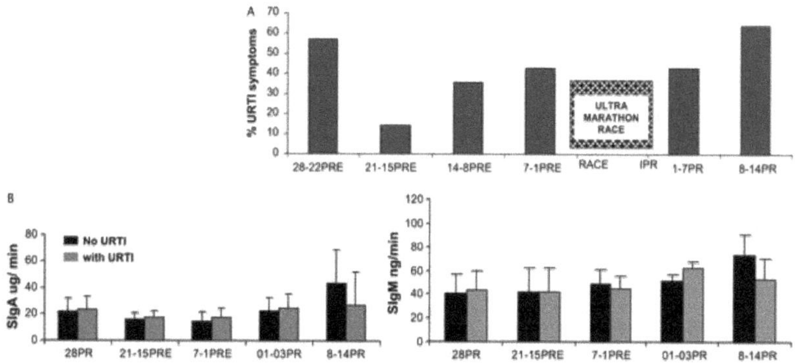

FIGURE 8.—A, Percentage of self-reported URTI symptoms (n = 14) at 4 time points preceding and 3 time points post participation in the Comrades Marathon. B, Mean ± SD salivary IgA (left, μg/min) and IgM (right, ng/min) secretion rates of subjects (n = 14) who reported URTI symptoms (n = 10) and those who did not (n = 4) at 2 time points preceding and 2 time points after participation in the Comrades Marathon. (Reprinted from Peters EM, Shaik J, Kleinveldt N. Upper respiratory tract infection symptoms in ultramarathon runners not related to immunoglobulin status. *Clin J Sport Med.* 2010;20:39-46.)

response are proposed as causes of the elevated URTI incidence at 28PRE and 7 to 14 days post race (Fig 8).

▶ Edith Peters has been one of the pioneers in relating upper respiratory symptoms to participation in ultramarathon events. One of the criticisms of her earlier work was that it was based on symptoms rather than clearly defined upper respiratory infections. Perhaps in consequence, the proportion of competitors affected was suspiciously high. As she appears to concede, this study seems beset by the same problem, with almost 60% of runners reporting upper respiratory symptoms 22 to 28 days before an ultramarathon run (Fig 8). This may explain the lack of relationship between secretory immunoglobulin concentrations and respiratory symptoms. The number of subjects (14) is also low for examining relationships between symptoms and immunoglobulin levels. Finally, the subjects examined did not show any depression of immunoglobulin levels (although this has been described in a substantial proportion of other reports,[1-8]). Nevertheless, Peters advances at least one alternative hypothesis that may merit further exploration—a reactivation of cold viruses by an ultraendurance run.[9-11]

R. J. Shephard, MD (Lond), PhD, DPE

References

1. MacKinnon LT, Chick TW, Van As A, Tomasi TB. Decreased secretory immunoglobulins following intense endurance exercise. *Sports Train Med Rehabil.* 1989; 1:209-218.
2. Gleeson M, McDonald WA, Pyne DB, et al. Salivary IgA levels and infection risk in elite swimmers. *Med Sci Sports Exerc.* 1999;31:67-73.
3. Gleeson M, McDonald WA, Pyne DB, et al. Immune status and respiratory illness for elite swimmers during a 12-week training cycle. *Int J Sports Med.* 2000;21: 1-6.

4. Nieman DC, Henson DA, Faoaga OR, et al. Change in salivary IgA following a competitive marathon race. *Int J Sports Med.* 2002;23:69-75.
5. Koch AJ, Smith AE, Fulmer CM, et al. Seasonal trends in salivary immunoglobulin A (IgA) and upper respiratory infections in NCAA Division II collegiate swimmers. *Med Sci Sports Exerc.* 2006;38:S412.
6. Tiollier E, Gomez-Merino D, Burnat P, et al. Intense training: mucosal immunity and incidence of respiratory infections. *Eur J Appl Physiol.* 2005;93:421-428.
7. Gomez-Merino D, Drogou C, Chennaoui M, Tiollier E, Mathieu J, Guezennec CY. Effects of combined stress during intense training on cellular immunity, hormones and respiratory infections. *Neuroimmunomodulation.* 2005;12:164-172.
8. Nieman DC, Tan SA, Lee JW, Berk LS. Complement and immunoglobulin levels in athletes and sedentary controls. *Int J Sports Med.* 1989;10:124-128.
9. Ekblom B, Ekblom O, Malm C. Infectious episodes before and after a marathon race. *Scand J Med Sci Sports.* 2006;16:287-293.
10. Gleeson M. Immune function in sport and exercise. *J Appl Physiol.* 2007;103: 693-699.
11. Pacque PFJ, Booth CK, Ball MJ, Dwyer DB. The effect of an ultra-endurance running race on mucosal and humoral immune function. *J Sports Med Phys Fitness.* 2007;47:496-501.

Cardiovascular Exercise Training Extends Influenza Vaccine Seroprotection in Sedentary Older Adults: The Immune Function Intervention Trial

Woods JA, Keylock KT, Lowder T, et al (Univ of Illinois, Urbana-Champaign)
J Am Geriatr Soc 57:2183-2191, 2009

Objectives.—To determine whether cardiovascular exercise training resulted in improved antibody responses to influenza vaccination in sedentary elderly people who exhibited poor vaccine responses.

Design.—Single-site randomized parallel-arm 10-month controlled trial.

Setting.—University of Illinois at Urbana-Champaign.

Participants.—One hundred forty-four sedentary, healthy older (69.9 ± 0.4) adults.

Interventions.—Moderate (60–70% maximal oxygen uptake) cardiovascular exercise was compared with flexibility and balance training.

Measurements.—The primary outcome was influenza vaccine response, as measured according to hemagglutination inhibition (HI) anti-influenza antibody titer and seroprotective responses (HI titer ≥40). Secondary measures included cardiovascular fitness and body composition.

Results.—Of the 160 participants enrolled, 144 (90%) completed the 10-month intervention with excellent compliance (~ 83%). Cardiovascular, but not flexibility, exercise intervention resulted in improvements in indices of cardiovascular fitness, including maximal oxygen uptake. Although not affecting peak (e.g., 3 and 6 weeks) postvaccine anti-influenza HI titers, cardiovascular exercise resulted in a significant increase in seroprotection 24 weeks after vaccination (30–100% dependent on vaccine variant), whereas flexibility training did not.

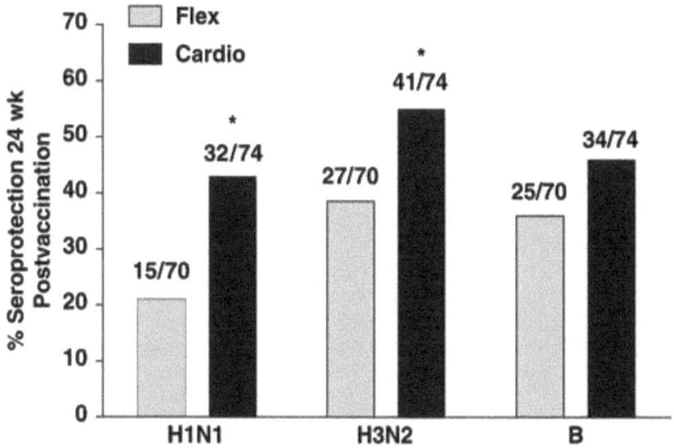

FIGURE 2.—Cardiovascular, but not flexibility, exercise intervention increased the percentage of study participants who achieved seroprotection (hemagglutination inhibition titer ≥40) 24 weeks after influenza vaccination. *Significant treatment difference ($P < .05$). (Reprinted from Woods JA, Keylock KT, Lowder T, et al. Cardiovascular exercise training extends influenza vaccine seroprotection in sedentary older adults: the immune function intervention trial. *J Am Geriatr Soc.* 2009;57:2183-2191, with permission from The American Geriatrics Society.)

Conclusion.—Participants randomized to cardiovascular exercise experienced improvements in influenza seroprotection throughout the entire influenza season, whereas those in the balance and flexibility intervention did not. Although there were no differences in reported respiratory tract infections, the exercise group exhibited reduced overall illness severity and sleep disturbance. These data support the hypothesis that regular endurance exercise improves influenza vaccine responses (Fig 2).

► Over the past 20 years there has been much research on the changes of immune function induced by various levels of habitual physical activity, but relatively few reports have examined the critical issue of resulting changes in resistance to viral and/or bacterial infection. Resistance to influenza infection is particularly important in the elderly, given that a fatal outcome to infection is not uncommon, and one important problem is the progressive waning of protection from vaccines over the influenza season; this seems to occur more rapidly in those who are elderly than in younger members of the population.[1,2] The present randomized controlled trial of an elderly population shows that regular cardiovascular exercise (thrice weekly aerobic activity at doses increasing to 45 to 60 min/session at 60% to 70% of the individual's maximal oxygen intake) does not change the immediate vaccine titer but substantially augments the likelihood of finding a protective titer at 24 weeks, relative to control subjects receiving simply flexibility and balance training (Fig 2). The findings support earlier cross-sectional comparisons[3,4] and one small longitudinal study[5] suggesting that vigorous aerobic activity enhances the response to vaccines. However, further research is needed to clarify whether there is an increased production of or a decreased loss of antibodies in subjects who are physically active.

R. J. Shephard, MD (Lond), PhD, DPE

References

1. Burns EA, Lum LG, L'Hommedieu G, Goodwin JS. Specific humoral immunity in the elderly: in vivo and in vitro response to vaccination. *J Gerontol Biol Sci*. 1993; 48:B231-B236.
2. McElhaney JE, Gravenstein S, Upshaw CM, Hooton JW, Krause P, Drinka P. Immune response to influenza vaccination in institutionalized elderly: effect on different T-cell subsets. *Vaccine*. 1998;16:403-409.
3. Keylock KT, Lowder T, Leifheit K, et al. Higher antibody, but not cell-mediated, responses to vaccination in high physically fit elderly. *J Appl Physiol*. 2007;102: 1090-1098.
4. Kohut ML, Cooper MM, Nickolaus MS, Russell DR, Cunnick JE. Exercise and psychosocial factors modulate immunity to influenza vaccine in elderly individuals. *J Gerontol A Biol Med Sci*. 2002;57A:M557-M562.
5. Kohut ML, Arntson BA, Lee W, et al. Moderate exercise improves antibody response to influenza immunization in older adults. *Vaccine*. 2004;22:2298-2306.

Are asthma-like symptoms in elite athletes associated with classical features of asthma?

Lund TK, Pedersen L, Anderson SD, et al (Copenhagen Univ Hosp, Denmark; Royal Prince Alfred Hosp, New South Wales, Australia)
Br J Sports Med 43:1131-1135, 2009

Background.—Asthma is frequent in elite athletes and clinical studies in athletes have found increased airway inflammation.

Objective.—To investigate asthma-like symptoms, airway inflammation, airway reactivity (AR) to mannitol and use of asthma medication in Danish elite athletes.

Methods.—The study group consisted of 54 elite athletes (19 with doctor-diagnosed asthma), 22 non-athletes with doctor-diagnosed asthma (steroid naive for 4 weeks before the examination) and 35 non-athletes without asthma; all aged 18–35 years. Examinations (1 day): questionnaires, exhaled nitric oxide (eNO) in parts per billion, spirometry, skin prick test, AR to mannitol and blood samples. Induced sputum was done in subjects with asthma.

Results.—No significant difference was found in values for eNO, AR and atopy between 42 elite athletes with and 12 without asthma-like symptoms. Elite athletes with doctor-diagnosed asthma had less AR (response dose ratio 0.02 (0.004) vs 0.08 (0.018) $p < 0.01$) and fewer sputum eosinophils (0.8% (0–4.8) vs 6.0% (0–18.5), $p < 0.01$) than non-athletes with doctor-diagnosed asthma. Use of inhaled corticosteroids was similar in the two groups (not significant). In all, 42 elite athletes had asthma-like symptoms but only 12 had evidence of current asthma.

Elite athletes without asthma had asthma-like symptoms more frequently than non-athletes without asthma (68.6% vs 25.7%, $p < 0.001$).

Conclusion.—Asthma-like symptoms in elite athletes are not necessarily associated with classic features of asthma and alone should not give a diagnosis of asthma. More studies are needed to further investigate if and how the asthma phenotype of elite athletes differs from that of classical asthma.

▶ Asthma, exercise-induced asthma (EIA), exercise-induced bronchospasm (EIB), and asthma-like symptoms in elite athletes are all hot topics in the current sports medicine literature. In part, this is because of the ever-changing regulations of the International Olympic Committee (IOC) and other antidoping agencies for the approval and documentation of use of medications such as short- and long-acting bronchodilators (beta-agonists) and inhaled corticosteroids (ICS). Other questions revolve around the concept of reactive bronchospasm, airway inflammation, and/or airway injury. It has been postulated that asthma in elite athletes, particularly in some sports where there is a high minute ventilation during exercise (eg, cross-country skiing) may be a different entity than the more classic asthma associated with allergy and atopy. This cross-sectional study examines Danish elite athletes and controls with and without doctor-diagnosed asthma. The only real difference in the groups was that the elite athletes currently receiving treatment for asthma were unable to discontinue their ICS prior to testing as the controls did, due to the demands of ongoing training and competition.

The findings are very interesting: exercise-related asthma-like symptoms are poor predictors of asthma in elite athletes, and the role of these self-reported symptoms in athletes is unclear. The differential diagnosis of vocal cord dysfunction (VCD) is not included, but detection of this frequently under-diagnosed condition is discussed elsewhere. This study also suggests that the asthma phenotype of elite athletes may differ from that of classic asthma, in that the analyses of induced sputum in this group demonstrated more neutrophils (suggesting injury and inflammation) than eosinophils (more indicative of allergy). Further research is obviously necessary to help elucidate a clearer understanding of the etiology and treatment of these entities.

C. Lebrun, MD

Are asthma-like symptoms in elite athletes associated with classical features of asthma?

Lund TK, Pedersen L, Anderson SD, et al (Copenhagen Univ Hosp, Denmark; Royal Prince Alfred Hosp, Camperdown, New South Wales, Australia)

Br J Sports Med 43:1131-1135, 2009

Background.—Asthma is frequent in elite athletes and clinical studies in athletes have found increased airway inflammation.

TABLE 3.—Clinical Characteristics for Elite Athletes and Non-athletes

	Elite Athletes		Non-athletes			
	Asthma (n = 19)	Non-asthma (n = 35)	Asthma (n = 22)	Non-asthma (n = 35)	p Value*	p Value†
eNO, ppb	25.2 (3.84)	21.3 (2.47)	43.4 (7.85)	14.7 (1.34)	NS (0.056)	<0.05
Atopy, n (%)	11 (57.9)	18 (51.4)	22 (100)	10 (28.6)	<0.01	0.051
Mannitol test, n (%)‡	4 (21.1)	1 (2.9)	18 (81.8)	2 (5.7)	<0.001	NS
RDR	0.018 (0.004)	0.007 (0.001)	0.083 (0.018)	0.011 (0.004)	<0.01	NS
B eosinophils, 10^9/litre	0.17 (0.02)	0.12 (0.01)	0.29 (0.04)	0.12 (0.02)	<0.02	NS
ACQ	3.7 (1.0)	0.5 (0.2)	7.4 (1.3)	0.2 (0.2)	<0.05	NS
Symptoms, n (%)§	18 (94.7)	24 (68.6)	21 (95.5)	9 (25.7)	NS	<0.001
Current asthma, n (%)	11 (57.9)	1 (2.9)	18 (81.8)	0 (0)	NS	NS
Treatment, n (%)¶	15 (78.9)	0 (0)	21 (95.5)	0 (0)	NS	NS

Asthma=subjects with doctor-diagnosed asthma before entering the study. One athlete with "non-asthma" had a positive mannitol challenge test and asthma-like symptoms and was classified as having current asthma.

ACQ, asthma control questionnaire (mean score); eNO, exhaled nitric oxide (parts per billion); RDR, response dose ratio.

*Between elite and non-elite patients with asthma;

†between elite and non-elite patients without asthma;

‡a positive mannitol challenge test;

§all asthma-like symptoms (rest+exercise);

¶use of any asthma medication.

Objective.—To investigate asthma-like symptoms, airway inflammation, airway reactivity (AR) to mannitol and use of asthma medication in Danish elite athletes.

Methods.—The study group consisted of 54 elite athletes (19 with doctor-diagnosed asthma), 22 non-athletes with doctor-diagnosed asthma (steroid naive for 4 weeks before the examination) and 35 non-athletes without asthma; all aged 18–35 years. Examinations (1 day): questionnaires, exhaled nitric oxide (eNO) in parts per billion, spirometry, skin prick test, AR to mannitol and blood samples. Induced sputum was done in subjects with asthma.

Results.—No significant difference was found in values for eNO, AR and atopy between 42 elite athletes with and 12 without asthma-like symptoms. Elite athletes with doctor-diagnosed asthma had less AR (response dose ratio 0.02 (0.004) vs 0.08 (0.018) p<0.01) and fewer sputum eosinophils (0.8% (0–4.8) vs 6.0% (0–18.5), p<0.01) than non-athletes with doctor-diagnosed asthma. Use of inhaled corticosteroids was similar in the two groups (not significant). In all, 42 elite athletes had asthma-like symptoms but only 12 had evidence of current asthma. Elite athletes without asthma had asthma-like symptoms more frequently than non-athletes without asthma (68.6% vs 25.7%, p<0.001).

Conclusion.—Asthma-like symptoms in elite athletes are not necessarily associated with classic features of asthma and alone should not give a diagnosis of asthma. More studies are needed to further investigate if and how the asthma phenotype of elite athletes differs from that of classical asthma (Table 3).

► There is a suspicion that some athletes have claimed symptoms of asthma in the belief that this will allow them access to bronchodilators that will enhance their performance. Certainly, the reported incidence of asthma is much higher in elite athletes than in the general population,[1,2] and the diagnosis is a poor predictor of exercise-induced bronchoconstriction.[3,4] This study shows little difference of such critical diagnostic measures as exhaled nitrous oxide, airway reactivity, and atopy between athletes with physician-diagnosed asthma and those who did not have asthma (Table 3). However, there is evidence of chronic airway inflammation in athletes with increased neutrophil counts.[5,6] Possibly, the direct inhalation of large volumes of cold, dry, and polluted air into the bronchi is causing a chronic inflammatory response. Symptoms may result, but these do not necessarily indicate asthma, and an athlete should not be treated for asthma on the basis of symptoms alone. The present findings would help to explain the poor response to asthmatic medication in many athletes with supposed asthma.[7,8]

R. J. Shephard, MD (Lond), PhD, DPE

References

1. Helenius IJ, Tikkanen HO, Sarna S, Haahtela T. Asthma and increased bronchial responsiveness in elite athletes: atopy and sport event as risk factors. *J Allergy Clin Immunol.* 1998;101:646-652.
2. Lumme A, Haahtela T, Ounap J, et al. Airway inflammation, bronchial hyperresponsiveness and asthma in elite ice hockey players. Eur Respir J2003;22:113–117.
3. Holzer K, Anderson SD, Douglass J. Exercise in elite summer athletes: challenges for diagnosis. *J Allergy Clin Immunol.* 2002;110:374-380.
4. Rundell KW, Im J, Mayers LB, Wilber RL, Szmedra L, Schmitz HR. Self-reported symptoms and exercise-induced asthma in the elite athlete. *Med Sci Sports Exerc.* 2001;33:208-213.
5. Bonsignore MR, Morici G, Vignola AM, et al. Increased airway inflammatory cells in endurance athletes: what do they mean? *Clin Exp Allergy.* 2003;33:14-21.
6. Boulet LP, Turcotte H, Langdeau JB, Bernier MC. Lower airway inflammatory responses to high-intensity training in athletes. *Clin Invest Med.* 2005;28:15-22.
7. Helenius I, Lumme A, Ounap J, et al. No effect of montelukast on asthma-like symptoms in elite ice hockey players. *Allergy.* 2004;59:39-44.
8. Sue-Chu M, Karjalainen EM, Laitinen A, Larsson L, Laitinen LA, Bjermer L. Placebo-controlled study of inhaled budesonide on indices of airway inflammation in bronchoalveolar lavage fluid and bronchial biopsies in cross-country skiers. *Respiration.* 2000;67:417-425.

Effects of chlorine and exercise on the unified airway in adolescent elite Scottish swimmers

Clearie KL, Vaidyanathan S, Williamson PA, et al (Univ of Dundee, UK)

Allergy 65:269-273, 2010

Background.—Chlorine metabolites and high training load may produce exercise-induced bronchospasm (EIB) in elite swimmers. The aim of this study was to assess the combined effects of chlorine and exercise on the unified airway of adolescent elite swimmers.

Methods.—The Scottish Midlands District squad were assessed during an indoor pool session at the National Swimming Academy. Athletes trained at least 8 h per week. Subjects underwent tidal (T_{NO}) and nasal (N_{NO}) exhaled NO and peak nasal inspiratory flow (PNIF) pre and post a 2 h session. A physiological exercise challenge assessed EIB in $n = 36$ swimmers (>10% fall in forced expiratory volume in 1 s (FEV_1)).

Results.—Combined and free chlorine levels (mg/l) were 1.66 and 0.3 respectively. $n = 36$ swimmers (mean age 13.3 years) were assessed: $n = 8$ (22%) had known asthma; $n = 13$ (36%) had a positive physiological challenge; 18 (50%) complained of symptoms suggestive of EIB. $n = 10/28$ (36%) who did not have asthma were found to have a positive exercise challenge. There was no significant association between reported exercise symptoms and positive exercise test. There was no significant change in T_{NO} or N_{NO} for pre *vs* postexposure, irrespective of asthma diagnosis or AHR. $n = 15$ (42%) swimmers complained of worsening nasal symptoms postexposure, but only $n = 7$ (14%) had a demonstrable fall in PNIF (mean 33 l/min). No significant association was found between PNIF and symptoms.

Conclusions.—Combined exposure to chlorine and exercise did not affect surrogate markers of inflammation in the unified airway. There was a high prevalence of undiagnosed EIB.

▶ Research that produces surprising findings always stimulates a number of questions: is the study valid? If so, does it indicate that we have been misled regarding certain questions? Or was there something unique about this particular group of subjects to produce certain results? In the case of this report, at least to this reviewer's way of looking at it, 3 findings raise eyebrows. First, chlorine in the pool had no effect on bronchial reactivity of the swimmers. Remembering my personal reactions to sophomore chemistry class, this is surprising. A large percentage of the swimmers had positive physiological tests for asthma that they did not know they had (10 of 28). This has been shown before, but this seems like a very large number. And, finally, half of the swimmers had symptoms "suggestive of exercise-induced bronchospasm (EIB)" but had negative tests. I suppose if such a symptom was shortness of breath, that might make sense. Overall, this study reminds us that it can be difficult to distinguish EIB and exertional breathlessness in highly competitve athletes.

T. Rowland, MD

7 Other Medical Conditions

A Prospective Study of Cardiorespiratory Fitness and Breast Cancer Mortality

Peel JB, Sui X, Adams SA, et al (Univ of South Carolina, Columbia; et al)

Med Sci Sports Exerc 41:742-748, 2009

Purpose.—Physical activity may protect against breast cancer. Few prospective studies have evaluated breast cancer mortality in relation to cardiorespiratory fitness (CRF), an objective marker of physiologic response to physical activity habits.

Methods.—We examined the association between CRF and risk of death from breast cancer in the Aerobics Center Longitudinal Study. Women ($N = 14{,}811$), aged 20 to 83 yr with no prior breast cancer history, received a preventive medical examination at the Cooper Clinic in Dallas, Texas, between 1970 and 2001. Mortality surveillance was completed through December 31, 2003. CRF was quantified as maximal treadmill exercise test duration and was categorized for analysis as low (lowest 20% of exercise duration), moderate (middle 40%), and high (upper 40%). At baseline, all participants were able to complete the exercise test to at least 85% of their age-predicted maximal heart rate.

Results.—A total of 68 breast cancer deaths occurred during follow-up (mean = 16 yr). Age-adjusted breast cancer mortality rates per 10,000 woman-years were 4.4, 3.2, and 1.8 for low, moderate, and high CRF groups, respectively (trend $P = 0.008$). After further controlling for body mass index, smoking, drinking, chronic conditions, abnormal exercise ECG responses, family history of breast cancer, oral contraceptive use, and estrogen use, hazard ratios (95% CI) for breast cancer mortality across incremental CRF categories were 1.00 (referent), 0.67 (0.35–1.26), and 0.45 (0.22–0.95) (trend $P = 0.04$).

Conclusions.—These results indicate that CRF is associated with a reduced risk of dying from breast cancer in women (Table 2).

▶ There is general agreement that regular physical activity is beneficial in the prevention of breast cancer.[1-4] What is unusual about the present large prospective study is the magnitude of the difference in risk between sedentary women and those judged to have a high level of cardiorespiratory fitness (as assessed from a simple rating of treadmill slope and speed). Blair and his

TABLE 2.—Rates and HR for Breast Cancer Mortality by Cardiorespiratory Fitness (CRF) Groups in 14,811 Women

	Low CRF	Moderate CRF	High CRF	*P* Value for Trend
No. of deaths	20	31	17	
No. of woman-years	42,488	96,714	103,554	
Rate*	4.4	3.2	1.8	0.008
Age-adjusted HR (95% CI)	1.00	0.72 (0.41–1.27)	0.42 (0.22–0.80)	0.008
Multivariate HR (95% CI)†	1.00	0.67 (0.35–1.26)	0.45 (0.22–0.95)	0.04

HR, hazard ratio; CI, confidence interval; CRF, cardiorespiratory fitness.
*Rate is expressed as per 10,000 woman-years and adjusted for age.
†Adjusted for age, BMI (kg·m−2), current smoking (yes or not), alcohol intake (≥5 drinks per week, or not), chronic conditions (hypertension, diabetes, or cardiovascular disease present or not for each), family history of breast cancer (present or not), abnormal exercise ECG responses (present or not), oral contraceptive use (yes or no), and estrogen use (yes or no).

associates are inclined to attribute the magnitude of the demonstrated benefit to the more accurate picture of habitual activity obtained from fitness measurements versus questionnaire assessments. One other potential factor influencing outcome is that the report is based on mortality rates; it is thus conceivable that those who engaged regularly in physical activity also engaged in other health practices such as regular self-examination of the breast, leading to earlier diagnosis, and treatment of any lesions; however, the sample tested (wealthy patrons of the Cooper Clinic) were all thought to be receiving regular breast examinations. The fitter individuals may also have been less prone to smoke, abuse alcohol, and develop excess weight, but the benefits of a high fitness level persisted after statistical control for these factors (Table 2). Further study is warranted to assess the relative importance of hormone suppression and the control of obesity to these major exercise effects.

R. J. Shephard, MD (Lond), PhD, DPE

References

1. Dallal CM, Sullivan-Halley J, Ross RK, et al. Long-term recreational physical activity and risk of invasive and in situ breast cancer: the California teachers study. *Arch Intern Med.* 2007;167:408-415.
2. Sesso HD, Paffenbarger RS Jr, Lee IM. Physical activity and breast cancer risk in the College Alumni Health Study (United States). *Cancer Causes Control.* 1998;9: 433-439.
3. Slattery ML, Edwards S, Murtaugh MA, et al. Physical activity and breast cancer risk among women in the southwestern United States. *Ann Epidemiol.* 2007;17: 342-353.
4. Thune I, Brenn T, Lund E, Gaard M. Physical activity and the risk of breast cancer. *N Engl J Med.* 1997;336:1269-1275.

Weight Lifting in Women with Breast-Cancer–Related Lymphedema

Schmitz KH, Ahmed RL, Troxel A, et al (Univ of Pennsylvania School of Medicine and Abramson Cancer Ctr, Philadelphia; Univ of Minnesota Med School, Minneapolis; et al)

N Engl J Med 361:664-673, 2009

Background.—Weight lifting has generally been proscribed for women with breast-cancer–related lymphedema, preventing them from obtaining the well-established health benefits of weight lifting, including increases in bone density.

Methods.—We performed a randomized, controlled trial of twice-weekly progressive weight lifting involving 141 breast-cancer survivors with stable lymphedema of the arm. The primary outcome was the change in arm and hand swelling at 1 year, as measured through displaced water volume of the affected and unaffected limbs. Secondary outcomes included the incidence of exacerbations of lymphedema, number and severity of lymphedema symptoms, and muscle strength. Participants were required to wear a well-fitted compression garment while weight lifting.

Results.—The proportion of women who had an increase of 5% or more in limb swelling was similar in the weight-lifting group (11%) and the control group (12%) (cumulative incidence ratio, 1.00; 95% confidence interval, 0.88 to 1.13). As compared with the control group, the weight-lifting group had greater improvements in self-reported severity of lymphedema symptoms ($P = 0.03$) and upper- and lower-body strength ($P < 0.001$ for both comparisons) and a lower incidence of lymphedema exacerbations as assessed by a certified lymphedema specialist (14% vs. 29%, $P = 0.04$). There were no serious adverse events related to the intervention.

Conclusions.—In breast-cancer survivors with lymphedema, slowly progressive weight lifting had no significant effect on limb swelling and resulted in a decreased incidence of exacerbations of lymphedema, reduced symptoms, and increased strength. (ClinicalTrials.gov number, NCT00194363.) (Table 3).

▶ Lymphedema is one of the most important complications following radical surgery for breast cancer. It has been considered a chronic condition, progressive, and incurable,[1] often with considerable resulting impairment of arm function.[2] Some Web sites have suggested that the problem is worsened by lifting children or heavy bags. However, the present small-scale but well-matched randomized controlled trial suggests that carefully graded weight-lifting exercises (90 minute group sessions twice per week, with a compression garment) are possible without harm (Table 4), enhancing muscle strength and functional capacity, controlling body fat content, and protecting against osteoporosis without increase of lymphedema.

For further reading on this subject I suggest articles from the American Cancer Society,[3] and Susan G. Komen for the Cure.[4]

R. J. Shephard, MD (Lond), PhD, DPE

TABLE 3.—Lymphedema Outcomes at 12 Months, According to Study Group.*

Variable	Weight Lifting No. of Patients With Data	Weight Lifting Value	Control No. of Patients With Data	Control Value	Cumulative Incidence Ratio or Mean Difference (95% CI)†	P Value‡
Change in interlimb volume difference						
≥5% increase — no. (%)	70	8 (11)	69	8 (12)	1.00 (0.88 to 1.13)	1.00
≥5% decrease — no. (%)	70	13 (19)	69	15 (22)	0.96 (0.81 to 1.14)	0.68
Mean interlimb volume discrepancy between baseline and 12 mo (percentage points)	70	−0.69±5.87	69	−0.98±7.31	−0.29 (−1.94 to 2.51)	0.80
Exacerbation — no. (%)	65	9 (14)	65	19 (29)	0.47 (0.23 to 0.97)	0.04
Change in no. of symptoms reported between baseline and 12 mo§	70	−1.81±2.16	69	−1.17±1.94	−0.63 (−1.32 to 0.06)	0.07
Change in severity of symptoms between baseline and 12 mo§	70	−0.51±0.80	69	−0.22±0.71	−0.29 (−0.54 to −0.03)	0.03

*Plus–minus values are means ±SD.

†The mean difference is given for the weight-lifting group as compared with the control group for the difference in interlimb volume discrepancies (the interarm difference over time) and changes in number and severity of symptoms. The cumulative incidence ratio is given for the weight-lifting group as compared with the control group for differences in percentages.

‡P values were calculated with the use of Fisher's exact test for between-group comparisons of percentages and the Wilcoxon rank-sum test for between-group comparisons of the difference in interlimb volume discrepancies and changes in number and severity of symptoms.

§Data were reported by patients regarding 14 symptoms: rings too tight, watch too tight, bracelets too tight, clothing too tight, puffiness, knuckles not visible, veins not visible, skin feels leathery, arm feels tired, pain, pitting, swelling after exercise, difficulty writing, or other. The change in severity of symptoms is the mean of the changes in severity for all 14 symptoms, with the possible severity score for each ranging from 0 (no symptom) to 4 (very severe).

References

1. Hayes SC, Janda M, Cornish B, et al. Lymphedema after breast cancer: incidence, risk factors, and effect on upper body function. *J Clin Oncol.* 2008;26:3536-3542.
2. Warren AG, Brorson H, Borud LJ, et al. Lymphedema: a comprehensive review. *Ann Plast Surg.* 2007;59:464-472.
3. *Lymphedema: what every woman with breast cancer should know.* Atlanta: American Cancer Society; 2009. http://www.cancer.org/docroot/%20MIT/content/MIT_7_2x_Lymphedema_and_Breast_Cancer.asp. Accessed July 20, 2009.
4. *Understanding breast cancer: after treatment: life issues: lymphedema.* Dallas: Susan G. Komen for the Cure; 2009. http://ww5.%20komen.org/BreastCancer/Lymphedema.%20html. Accessed July 20, 2009.

Prospective cohort study of lifetime physical activity and breast cancer survival

Friedenreich CM, Gregory J, Kopciuk KA, et al (Alberta Cancer Board, Calgary, Canada; et al)

Int J Cancer 124:1954-1962, 2009

Few studies have examined the association between physical activity and disease outcomes in breast cancer survivors. Here, we report the association between lifetime total physical activity performed prior to diagnosis and disease outcomes in a population-based sample of breast cancer survivors. A cohort of 1,231 women diagnosed with breast cancer between 1995 and 1997 was followed for a minimum of 8.3 years for any cancer progressions, recurrences and new primaries; and a minimum of 10.3 years for deaths. All treatment and follow-up care received was abstracted from medical records. Data on physical activity including type (occupational, household, recreational) and dose (frequency, intensity and duration) performed during the entire lifetime until diagnosis were examined in Cox proportional hazards models as well as with cumulative incidence curves. An average of 126 MET-hr/week were reported for total physical activity (of which 13.9, 46.9 and 65.3 MET-hr/week were, respectively, for recreational, occupational and household activity). A decreased risk of breast cancer death and all deaths was observed among women in the highest versus the lowest quartiles of recreational activity (MET-hr/week/year) (HR = 0.54, 95% CI = 0.36–0.79). Both moderate (0.56, 95% CI = 0.38–0.82) and vigorous intensity recreational activity (0.74, 95% CI = 0.56–0.98) decreased the risk of breast cancer death. Moderate intensity recreational activity decreased the risk of a recurrence, progression or new primary cancer (0.66, 95% CI = 0.48–0.91). No other association with breast cancer survival was observed for other types of physical activity. Prediagnosis recreational activity conferred a benefit

TABLE 1.—Selected Characteristics of Study Participants by Outcome after Breast Cancer, Alberta, Canada, 1995–2008 ($N = 1{,}225$)

Characteristics	M0 population All subjects	M0 population First Recurrences/ Progressions/New Primaries	Total population All Subjects	Total population Breast Cancer Deaths	Total population All Deaths
Total (*N*)	1,183	327	1,225	223	341
Lifetime physical activity (MET-hr/wk) [mean (SD)]					
Total	126.2 (43.4)	125.3 (43.6)	126.0 (43.2)	124.3 (43.7)	129.6 (46.3)
Recreational	14.0 (12.7)	13.9 (13.1)	13.9 (12.6)	13.3 (13.1)	13.2 (12.3)
Occupational	47.0 (28.7)	47.8 (27.3)	46.9 (25.8)	46.3 (25.7)	44.7 (27.8)
Household	65.2 (40.0)	63.7 (40.5)	65.3 (40.0)	64.7 (39.9)	71.7 (42.8)
Age at diagnosis (years) [mean (SD)]	56 (12.1)	54 (12.5)	56 (12.1)	55 (12.6)	59 (13.4)
BMI (kg/m^2) [mean (SD)]	27.5 (5.7)	28.2 (6.2)	27.4 (5.7)	27.7 (5.7)	27.5 (6.2)
Ever married (%)	95.9	94.2	96.1	93.7	95.3
Educational level (%)					
None	27.1	23.2	27.6	27.8	35.2
High school	16.7	19.9	16.6	18.8	17.6
Trade certificate	17.6	16.8	17.8	17.9	15.0
Other nonuniversity	22.8	23.2	22.4	20.2	20.2
University	15.8	16.8	15.6	15.2	12.0
Tumor stage (%)					
0	9.3	5.8	9.0	10.5	3.8
I	43.8	33.6	42.3	48.6	25.2
II	41.2	49.5	39.8	36.5	49.0
III+[1]	5.6	10.4	8.8	4.3	21.7
Missing	0.2	0.6	0.2	0.1	0.3
ER status (% positive)	69.2	66.7	68.2	57.8	63.3
PR status (% positive)	63.9	60.6	62.7	49.8	56.0
SBR grade (%)					
1	26.6	20.8	25.9	9.0	15.0
2	32.9	34.9	32.7	30.9	33.1
3	24.7	33.0	25.1	45.7	38.1
Unknown/Stage 0	15.8	11.3	16.3	14.3	13.8
Treatment[2] (%)					
Chemotherapy	34.5	45.9	35.6	61.4	44.9
Hormonal therapy	38.4	36.7	38.6	42.2	44.0
Radiation therapy	55.5	56.6	54.7	52.5	49.0
Postmenopausal (%)	62.3	57.5	62.4	58.7	69.8
Other comorbidities[2] (%)	47.1	51.7	47.3	49.8	56.6
Ever oral contraceptives use (%)	64.4	65.4	64.2	61.4	51.9
Ever HRT use (%)	34.7	30.6	34.0	22.9	28.7
Waist–hip ratio [mean (SD)]	0.79 (0.7)	0.80 (0.7)	0.79 (0.7)	0.81 (0.07)	0.81 (0.07)
First-degree family history of breast cancer (%)	18.8	18.3	18.4	14.3	16.1
Total pack-years of smoking for current and former smokers [mean (SD)]	9.4 (14.9)	9.5 (14.5)	9.6 (15.3)	10.0 (15.8)	12.1 (18.0)

[1]There were no Stage IV breast cancer cases in the M0 population.
[2]Excludes study subjects who had missing data on comorbidities ($n = 579$).

for survival after breast cancer. Moderate intensity recreational activity was particularly protective (Table 1).

▶ There is now good evidence that regular physical activity substantially reduces the risk of developing breast cancer.[1,2] However, this study demonstrates that a history of long-term physical activity also substantially improves prognosis after apparently successful treatment of such a cancer. There are a host of possible reasons for this, including a better control of body weight,[3,4] a lower prevalence of comorbidities,[5] an enhanced quality of life,[6,7] and specific changes in the inflammatory process,[8] immune function,[9,10] and insulin sensitivity.[11] The effect seems best with moderate rather than intensive recreational activity, and the difference in risk ratio for a recurrence (0.56) is quite impressive (Table 1).

R. J. Shephard, MD (Lond), PhD, DPE

References

1. Friedenreich CM. Physical activity and breast cancer risk: the effect of menopausal status. *Exerc Sport Sci Rev.* 2004;32:180-184.
2. Monninkhof EM, Elias SG, Vlems FA, et al. Physical activity and breast cancer: a systematic review. *Epidemiology.* 2007;18:137-157.
3. Rock CL, Demark-Wahnefried W. Can lifestyle modification increase survival in women diagnosed with breast cancer? *J Nutr.* 2002;132:3504S-3507S.
4. Ingram C, Courneya KS, Kingston D. The effects of exercise on body weight and composition in breast cancer survivors: an integrative systematic review. *Oncol Nurs Forum.* 2006;33:937-947.
5. Herman DR, Ganz PA, Petersen L, Greendale GA. Obesity and cardiovascular risk factors in younger breast cancer survivors: the Cancer and Menopause Study (CAMS). *Breast Cancer Res Treat.* 2005;93:13-23.
6. Hewitt JA, Mokbel K, van Someren KA, Jewell AP, Garrod R. Exercise for breast cancer survival: the effect on cancer risk and cancer-related fatigue (CRF). *Int J Fertil Womens Med.* 2005;50:231-249.
7. McNeely ML, Campbell KL, Rowe BH, Klassen TP, Mackey JR, Courneya KS. Effects of exercise on breast cancer patients and survivors: a systematic review and meta-analysis. *CMAJ.* 2006;175:34-41.
8. Fairey AS, Courneya KS, Field CJ, et al. Effect of exercise training on C-reactive protein in postmenopausal breast cancer survivors: a randomized controlled trial. *Brain Behav Immun.* 2005;19:381-388.
9. Fairey AS, Courneya KS, Field CJ, Bell GJ, Jones LW, Mackey JR. Randomized controlled trial of exercise and blood immune function in postmenopausal breast cancer survivors. *J Appl Physiol.* 2005;98:1534-1540.
10. Fairey AS, Courneya KS, Field CJ, Mackey JR. Physical exercise and immune system function in cancer survivors: a comprehensive review and future directions. *Cancer.* 2002;94:539-551.
11. Fairey AS, Courneya KS, Field CJ, Bell GJ, Jones LW, Mackey JR. Effects of exercise training on fasting insulin, insulin resistance, insulin-like growth factors, and insulin-like growth factor binding proteins in postmenopausal breast cancer survivors: a randomized controlled trial. *Cancer Epidemiol Biomarkers Prev.* 2003;12:721-727.

A prospective study of lifetime physical activity and prostate cancer incidence and mortality

Orsini N, Bellocco R, Bottai M, et al (Karolinska Institutet, Stockholm, Sweden; Univ of Milano-Bicocca, Milan, Italy; Univ of South Carolina, Columbia; et al)
Br J Cancer 101:1932-1938, 2009

Background.—The possible benefit of lifetime physical activity (PA) in reducing prostate cancer incidence and mortality is unclear.

Methods.—A prospective cohort of 45 887 men aged 45–79 years was followed up from January 1998 to December 2007 for prostate cancer incidence ($n = 2735$) and to December 2006 for its subtypes and for fatal ($n = 190$) prostate cancer.

Results.—We observed an inverse association between lifetime (average of age 30 and 50 years, and baseline age) total PA levels and prostate cancer risk. Multivariate-adjusted incidence in the top quartile of lifetime total PA decreased by 16% (95% confidence interval (CI) = 2–27%) compared with that in the bottom quartile. We also observed an inverse association between average lifetime work or occupational activity and walking or bicycling duration and prostate cancer risk. Compared with men who mostly sit during their main work or occupation, men who sit half of the time experienced a 20% lower risk (95% CI = 7–31%). The rate ratio linearly decreased by 7% (95% CI = 1–12%) for total, 8% (95% CI = 0–16%) for localised and 12% (95% CI = 2–20%) for

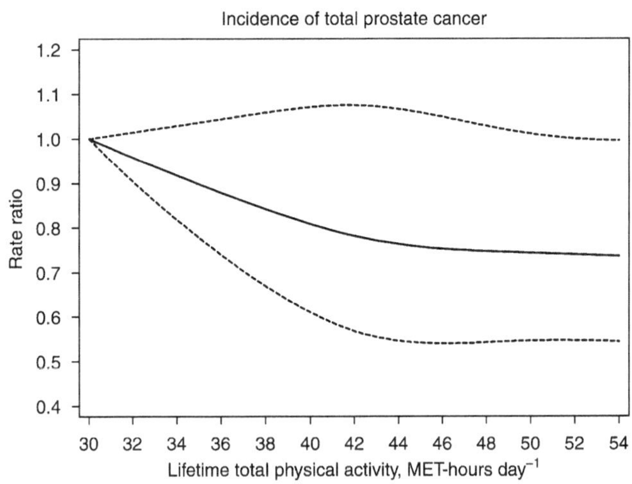

FIGURE 1.—Multivariate rate ratio for lifetime average total physical activity (average of age 30 and 50 years, and baseline age) as predictor of total incidence of prostate cancer rates. Data were fitted using a Cox regression model with restricted cubic splines. Data were adjusted for baseline age, waist–hip ratio, height, diabetes, alcohol consumption, smoking status, years of education, total energy intake, consumption of dairy product and red meat and parental history with respect to prostate cancer. Dotted lines represent 95% confidence limits. (Reprinted from Orsini N, Bellocco R, Bottai M, et al. A prospective study of lifetime physical activity and prostate cancer incidence and mortality. *Br J Cancer.* 2009;101:1932-1938.)

advanced prostate cancer for every 30 min per day increment of lifetime walking or bicycling in the range of 30 to 120 min per day.

Conclusions.—Our results suggest that not sitting for most of the time during work or occupational activity and walking or bicycling more than 30 min per day during adult life is associated with reduced incidence of prostate cancer (Fig 1).

▶ Investigators have reached varying conclusions regarding the efficacy of regular physical activity in the prevention of prostate cancer. This large and well-designed prospective trial from Sweden suggests a fairly small but statistically significant benefit (a 7% decrease of risk for each 30 minutes of walking per day) from what is described as lifelong physical activity (the average of levels reported at ages 30 and 50 years). Previous investigators have wondered whether lifelong relationships of this sort truly reflect a lifetime of physical activity or merely provide a better indication of activity because 2 assessments are made. However, given the slow onset of cancer, knowledge of physical activity over a long period is probably important to risk. It is important to underline that optimal level of protection requires more than the 30 minutes of daily activity found in some popular health recommendations. Mechanisms have yet to be clarified. Possibilities include a change in insulin resistance,[1] adiponectin levels,[2,3] insulin-like growth factors,[4] or testosterone.[5]

R. J. Shephard, MD (Lond), PhD, DPE

References

1. Goodyear LJ, Kahn BB. Exercise, glucose transport, and insulin sensitivity. *Annu Rev Med.* 1998;49:235-261.
2. Kelesidis I, Kelesidis T, Mantzoros CS. Adiponectin and cancer: a systematic review. *Br J Cancer.* 2006;94:1221-1225.
3. Bluher M, Brennan AM, Kelesidis T, et al. Total and high-molecular weight adiponectin in relation to metabolic variables at baseline and in response to an exercise treatment program: comparative evaluation of three assays. *Diabetes Care.* 2007; 30:280-285.
4. Chan JM, Stampfer MJ, Giovannucci E, et al. Plasma insulin-like growth factor-I and prostate cancer risk: a prospective study. *Science.* 1998;279:563-566.
5. Eaton NE, Reeves GK, Appleby PN, Key TJ. Endogenous sex hormones and prostate cancer: a quantitative review of prospective studies. *Br J Cancer.* 1999;80: 930-934.

Cardiorespiratory Fitness and Digestive Cancer Mortality: Findings from the Aerobics Center Longitudinal Study

Peel JB, Sui X, Matthews CE, et al (Univ of South Carolina, Columbia; Vanderbilt Univ Med Ctr, Nashville, TN; et al)

Cancer Epidemiol Biomarkers Prev 18:1111-1117, 2009

Although higher levels of physical activity are inversely associated with risk of colon cancer, few prospective studies have evaluated overall digestive system cancer mortality in relation to cardiorespiratory fitness (CRF).

The authors examined this association among 38,801 men ages 20 to 88 years who performed a maximal treadmill exercise test at baseline in the Aerobics Center Longitudinal Study (Dallas, TX) during 1974 to 2003. Mortality was assessed over 29 years of follow-up (1974-2003). Two hundred eightythree digestive system cancer deaths occurred during a mean 17 years of observation. Age-adjusted mortality rates per 10,000 person-years according to low, moderate, and high CRF groups were 6.8, 4.0, and 3.3 for digestive system cancer ($P_{trend} < 0.001$). After adjustment for age, examination year, body mass index, smoking, drinking, family history of cancer, personal history of diabetes, hazard ratios (95% confidence intervals) for overall digestive cancer deaths for those in the middle and upper 40% of the distribution of CRF relative to those in the lowest 20% were 0.66 (0.49-0.88) and 0.56 (0.40-0.80), respectively. Being fit (the upper 80% of CRF) was associated with a lower risk of mortality from colon [0.61 (0.37-1.00)], colorectal [0.58 (0.37-0.92)], and liver cancer [0.28 (0.11-0.72)] compared with being unfit (the lowest 20% of CRF). These findings support a protective role of CRF against total digestive tract, colorectal, and liver cancer deaths in men (Figure 3).

▶ The beneficial influence of regular physical activity upon the risk of colon cancer is well established, so it is not surprising to see that there is also an association between fitness and a decreased overall risk of digestive system cancers. However, the very large size of the initial sample and the long average period of follow-up also enabled the Cooper Clinic group to evaluate possible beneficial

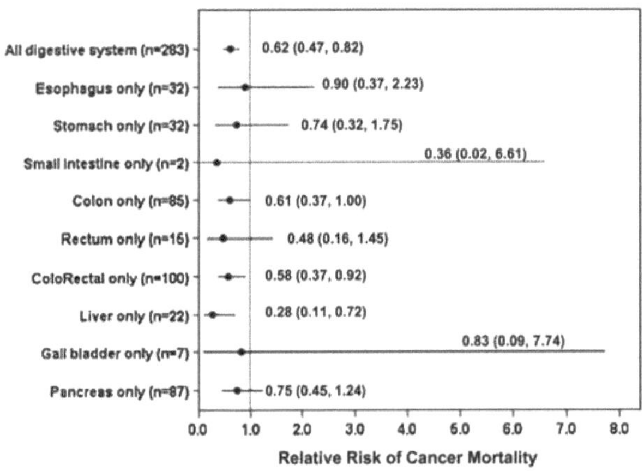

FIGURE 3.—Risk of site-specific digestive cancer mortality associated with being fit (the upper 80% of the distribution of CRF) as defined by achieving at least a moderate level of fitness during maximal exercise testing, ACLS, Dallas, TX, 1974-2003. The reference group was the unfit group (the lowest 20% of the distribution of CRF). We used Cox proportional hazards models to estimate the HR, which include age, examination year, smoking, alcohol intake, personal history of diabetes, family history of cancer, and BMI as covariates. *Bars*, 95% CI. (Reprinted from Peel JB, Sui X, Matthews CE, et al. Cardiorespiratory fitness and digestive cancer mortality: findings from the aerobics center longitudinal study. *Cancer Epidemiol Biomarkers Prev.* 2009;18:1111-1117.)

effects of fitness on the risk of death from hepatic cancer. The 95% confidence limits of benefit were quite broad, but the hazard ratio for the fit individuals (the upper 80% of the sample in terms of a treadmill endurance time) was 0.28, which is both noteworthy and statistically significant (Fig 3). Despite the sample size, positive trends for small intestine, pancreatic, and gall bladder cancers (where some authors have found benefit) were not proven. There remains scope both to explore these trends with even larger samples and to elucidate mechanisms, which may include changes in immune function,[1-3] as well as alterations in the speed of transit of the gastrointestinal contents. As with any epidemiological study, there are some caveats to the present findings. Baseline data allowed control for a number of potentially interfering factors, but it was not possible to control for the important questions of dietary fiber and fat intake, which may have differed in the more health conscious and fitter subjects. Also, the diagnostic end-point was death, so it is conceivable that part of the apparent benefit of a higher level of physical fitness came from a longer survival after diagnosis and any resultant surgery. Finally, as in all studies of Cooper Clinic patients, the study was limited to an elite "white" segment of United States society.

R. J. Shephard, MD (Lond), PhD, DPE

References

1. Lee IM. Exercise and physical health: cancer and immune function. *Res Q Exerc Sport.* 1995;66:286-291.
2. Shephard RJ, Shek PN. Associations between physical activity and susceptibility to cancer: possible mechanisms. *Sports Med.* 1998;26:293-315.
3. McTiernan A, Ulrich C, Slate S, Potter J. Physical activity and cancer etiology: associations and mechanisms. *Cancer Causes Control.* 1998;9:487-509.

Randomized Controlled Trial of the Effects of Aerobic Exercise on Physical Functioning and Quality of Life in Lymphoma Patients

Courneya KS, Sellar CM, Stevinson C, et al (Univ of Alberta, Canada; Cross Cancer Inst, Edmonton, AB, Canada; Alberta Cancer Board, Canada; et al)
J Clin Oncol 27:4605-4612, 2009

Purpose.—Lymphoma patients commonly experience declines in physical functioning and quality of life (QoL) that may be reversed with exercise training.

Patients and Methods.—We conducted a randomized controlled trial in Edmonton, Alberta, Canada, between 2005 and 2008 that stratified 122 lymphoma patients by major disease type and current treatment status and randomly assigned them to usual care (UC; n = 62) or 12 weeks of supervised aerobic exercise training (AET; n = 60). Our primary end point was patient-rated physical functioning assessed by the Trial Outcome Index-Anemia. Secondary end points were overall QoL, psychosocial functioning, cardiovascular fitness, and body composition.

Results.—Follow-up assessment for our primary end point was 96% (117 of 122) at postintervention and 90% (110 of 122) at 6-month follow-up. Median adherence to the supervised exercise program was 92%. At postintervention, AET was superior to UC for patient-rated physical functioning (mean group difference, +9.0; 95% CI, 2.0 to 16.0; $P = .012$), overall QoL ($P = .021$), fatigue ($P = .013$), happiness ($P = .004$), depression ($P = .005$), general health ($P < .001$), cardiovascular fitness ($P < .001$), and lean body mass ($P = .008$). Change in peak cardiovascular fitness mediated the change in patient-rated physical functioning. AET did not interfere with chemotherapy completion rate or treatment response. At 6-month follow-up, AET was still borderline or significantly superior to UC for overall QoL ($P = .054$), happiness ($P = .034$), and depression ($P = .009$) without an increased risk of disease recurrence/progression.

Conclusion.—AET significantly improved important patient-rated outcomes and objective physical functioning in lymphoma patients without interfering with medical treatments or response. Exercise training to improve cardiovascular fitness should be considered in the management of lymphoma patients.

▶ Previous trials have shown aerobic exercise to benefit patients with other types of cancer, including lesions of the breast[1] and prostate,[2] but this is the first systematic trial of aerobic conditioning in lymphomas. Given the differences in demographics, pathology, symptoms, treatment, and prognosis, Courneya and associates caution against assuming that the findings of exercise programs for other forms of carcinoma can necessarily be transferred to patients with lymphoma. The authors are to be commended for having assembled a substantial sample of subjects with lymphoma and to have persuaded most of the group to adhere to a stratified randomized controlled trial, although their initial sample comprised only 132 of 1416 patients contacted. One other weakness in the trial to date is plainly the duration of follow-up; it is a little rash to draw conclusions about the relative rates of recurrence in experimental and control groups after an interval of only 6 months, particularly as many of the control group subsequently began to exercise. A larger trial would also be required to draw conclusions about possible differences in response between Hodgkin's and other types of lymphoma. The dose of supervised aerobic exercise was substantial, rising 40 to 45 minutes at 75% of peak aerobic power 3 times per week. Many of the program-related gains were in patient-rated quality of life, but there was also a substantial gain in peak aerobic power (4-5 ml/[kg.min], or more than 20% over the initial values, Fig 4 in the original article) that appeared to mediate the gain in physical functioning. Given the complaints of fatigue associated with both the disease and its treatment, it seems important to expand upon this innovative study.

R. J. Shephard, MD (Lond), PhD, DPE

References

1. McNeely ML, Campbell KL, Rowe BH, Klassen TP, Mackey JR, Courneya KS. Effects of exercise on breast cancer patients and survivors: a systematic review and meta-analysis. *CMAJ*. 2006;175:34-41.
2. Thorsen L, Courneya KS, Stevinson C, Fosså SD. A systematic review of physical activity in prostate cancer survivors: outcomes, prevalence, and determinants. *Support Care Cancer*. 2008;16:987-997.

Incident Diverticular Disease Is Inversely Related to Vigorous Physical Activity

Williams PT (Donner Laboratory, Berkeley, CA)

Med Sci Sports Exerc 41:1042-1047, 2009

Purpose.—In 1995, the Health Professionals Follow-up Study published an isolated report of lower diverticular disease risk in physically active men, particularly among those who ran. The purpose of this article was to assess whether this finding can be verified among older men and women of the National Runners' Health Study.

Methods.—Survival analyses were applied to incident disease occurring during 7.7 yr of follow-up in 9072 men and 1664 women, representing 84% follow-up of the original ≥50-yr-old cohort. In addition to the usual running distance ($km \cdot d^{-1}$), 80% of the baseline respondents included 10-km footrace performance times (a measure of cardiorespiratory fitness). Results were adjusted for age, sex, and reported intakes of meat, fish, fruit, and alcohol.

Results.—A total of 127 men and 21 women reported clinically diagnosed diverticular disease since baseline. The risk for incident diverticular disease decreased 6.2% per $km \cdot d^{-1}$ run ($P = 0.04$). Relative to men and women who ran ≤ 2 $km \cdot d^{-1}$, those who ran an average of >8 $km \cdot d^{-1}$ had 48% lower risk ($P = 0.05$). Each meter-per-second increment in the 10-km performance was associated with a 68% risk reduction ($P = 0.04$). Men and women who ran >4 $m \cdot s^{-1}$ had 70% lower risk for diverticular disease than those who ran ≤ 2.8 $m \cdot s^{-1}$ ($P = 0.01$), which persisted when adjusted for baseline body mass index (69% risk reduction, $P = 0.02$) or usual running distance (36% risk reduction, $P = 0.03$).

Conclusion.—These results demonstrate an inverse association between vigorous physical activity and incident diverticular disease among older men and women but are limited by their reliance on self-reported physician diagnosis (Fig 2).

▶ Diverticulitis affects as many as a half of older North American adults, often with resultant colicky pain, altered bowel habits, or intestinal inflammation. However, diverticulitis is apparently not a common problem in developing societies. This difference has commonly been explained by the greater proportion of roughage in the traditional diet,[1] but it is also possible that the decline of habitual physical activity in modern society may play some role. This article

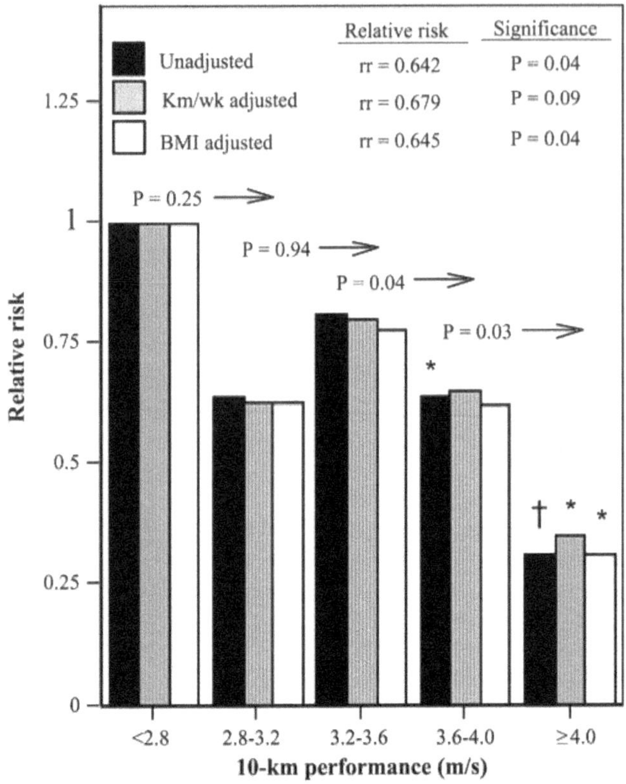

FIGURE 2.—Relative risk of self-reported physician-diagnosed diverticular disease by cardiorespiratory fitness (10-km race performance time) relative to the least-fit (slowest) runners, adjusted for age, sex, pack-years of cigarette consumption, and intake of meat, fish, fruit, and alcohol. Additional adjustment for usual running distance ($km \cdot d^{-1}$) and BMI where indicated. Significance levels relative to the least fit runners are coded: $^{*}P < 0.05$, $\dagger P < 0.01$. Significance levels relative to all faster men are presented above the *bars* and to the left of the *arrows* (e.g., men who ran faster than 3.6 $m \cdot s^{-1}$ were significantly less likely to report physician-diagnosed diverticular disease than those who ran 3.2–3.6 $m \cdot s^{-1}$, $P = 0.04$). Relative risks (rr) per meter-per-second increment in the 10-km performance (as a continuous variable) are presented at the top. (Reprinted from Williams PT. Incident diverticular disease is inversely related to vigorous physical activity. *Med Sci Sports Exerc*. 2009;41:1042-1047.)

tests the latter possibility using data from a 7-year follow-up of a large sample of older men and women participating in the United States National Runners' Study; the group were initially free of diverticular disease. The data, adjusted for diet and body mass index, show a substantial and negative association between the reported daily running distance and the patient-reported incidence of physician-diagnosed diverticulitis (Fig 2), although the threshold for benefit (running 2 km/d) exceeds many current national physical activity guidelines. The findings confirm results from one previous study of younger men,[2] and the present authors attribute benefit to an exercise-induced increase of colonic motility.

R. J. Shephard, MD (Lond), PhD, DPE

References

1. Painter NS, Burkitt DP. Diverticular disease of the colon, a 20th century problem. *Clin Gastroenterol.* 1975;4:3-21.
2. Aldoori WH, Giovannuvvi EL, Rimm EB, et al. Prospective study of physical activity and the risk of symptomatic diverticular disease in men. *Gut.* 1995;36: 276-282.

Relationship of Incident Glaucoma versus Physical Activity and Fitness in Male Runners

Williams PT (Lawrence Berkeley Laboratory, CA)

Med Sci Sports Exerc 41:1566-1572, 2009

Purpose.—To assess the dose–response relationship of vigorous physical activity (running distance, $km \cdot d^{-1}$) or cardiorespiratory fitness (meters-per-second pace during a 10-km footrace) to the risk for incident glaucoma.

Design.—Prospective epidemiologic cohort study.

Methods.—Participant-reported, physician-diagnosed incident glaucoma was compared with distance run per week and 10-km footrace performance in a cohort of 29,854 male runners without diabetes followed prospectively for 7.7 yr. The survival analyses were adjusted for age, hypertension, current and past cigarette use, and intakes of meat, fish, fruit, and alcohol.

Results.—Two hundred incident glaucoma cases were reported during follow-up. The risk for reported glaucoma decreased 37% per meter per second increment in a 10-km race performance ($P = 0.005$). Relative to the least fit men (i.e., slowest, $\leq 3.5\ m \cdot s^{-1}$), the risk for incident-reported glaucoma declined 29% in those who ran 3.6–4.0 $m \cdot s^{-1}$ ($P = 0.06$), 54% for those who ran 4.1–4.5 $m \cdot s^{-1}$ ($P = 0.001$), 51% for those who ran 4.6–5.0 $m \cdot s^{-1}$ ($P = 0.04$), and glaucoma was nonexistent among the 781 men who exceeded 5.0 $m \cdot s^{-1}$ ($P = 0.03$). The risk for incident, reported glaucoma decreased 5% per kilometer per day run at baseline ($P = 0.04$), which remained significant when adjusted for the 10-km race performance (5% reduction per kilometer per day, $P = 0.04$), and both body mass index and race performance ($P = 0.04$). Baseline hypertension was unrelated to the incident glaucoma.

Conclusions.—These data provide preliminary evidence that vigorous physical activity may reduce glaucoma risk, which, in the absence of medical record validation, could represent ocular hypertension in addition to frank glaucoma. Additional follow-up with validation is needed to identify the type of glaucoma affected.

▶ Glaucoma is a condition that ultimately affects up to 1% of the population, with progressive optic nerve neuropathy and visual field loss.[1,2] An acute bout of exercise is known to reduce intraocular pressure,[3,4] but given that hypertension is known to be one of the factors predisposing to glaucoma,

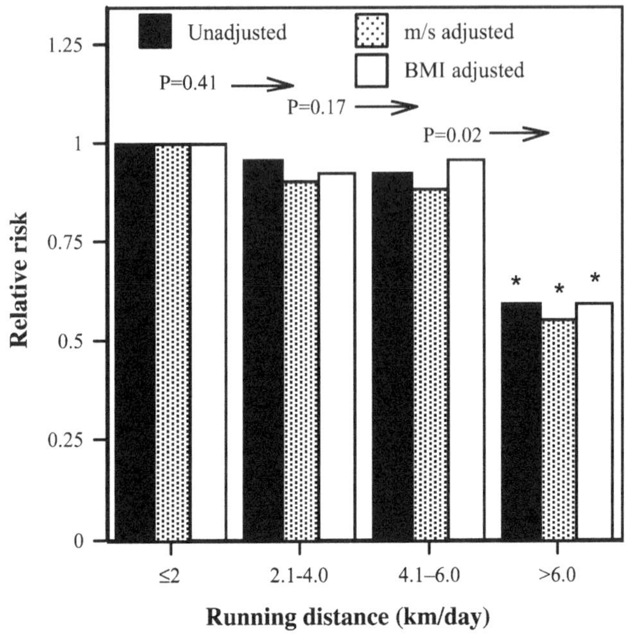

FIGURE 2.—Relative risk of incident glaucoma by running distance ($km \cdot d^{-1}$) relative to the men averaging $\leq 2\ km \cdot d^{-1}$, adjusted for age, education, hypertension medication use, current and past cigarette use, and intakes of meat, fish, fruit, and alcohol. Significance levels relative to all longer distanced runners are presented above the *bars* and to the left of the *arrows* (e.g., men who exceeded $6\ km \cdot d^{-1}$ had significantly lower risk for incident glaucoma than those who ran $4.1–6\ km \cdot d^{-1}$, at $P = 0.02$). *Asterisk* (*) signifies that men who exceeded $6\ km \cdot d^{-1}$ had significantly lower risk relative to men who ran $\leq 6\ km \cdot d^{-1}$ ($P \leq 0.02$) with or without adjustment for BMI or fitness. Additional adjustment for 10-km performance and baseline BMI where indicated. (Reprinted from Williams PT, Relationship of incident glaucoma versus physical activity and fitness in male runners. *Med Sci Sports and Exerc.* 2009;41:1566-1572, with permission from the American College of Sports Medicine.)

physical activity seems most likely to be of benefit through a progressive reduction of systemic blood pressure. The effect of regular exercise on blood pressure is small, and several previous studies from a group of Asian investigators have suggested the reduction in intraocular pressure is similarly quite limited, generally around 1 mm Hg.[5-7] However, observations on patients with established glaucoma found a larger effect,[8] a 4-6 mm Hg reduction in pressure. Paul Williams' study is based on a group of dedicated runners who typically cover long distances each week. Within this specialized population, benefit was seen both in those running more than 6 km/day (Fig 2) and the fittest members of the group (as judged by their speed over a 10 km race). Previous studies from the same author have suggested other ocular benefits from distance running in terms of the incidence of cataract and macular degeneration.[9,10] Two lessons emerge: firstly, one should consider the eyes when listing the benefits of regular physical activity to our patients, and secondly, in order to attain these benefits, it may be necessary to exceed most of the currently proposed exercise guidelines.

R. J. Shephard, MD (Lond), PhD, DPE

References

1. American Academy of Ophthalmology, Glaucoma Panel. *Primary Open-Angle Glaucoma. Preferred Practice Pattern Committee.* San Francisco, CA: American Academy of Ophthalmology; 2000: 1-36.
2. Collaborative Normal-Tension Glaucoma Study Group. Comparison of glaucomatous progression between untreated patients with normal-tension glaucoma and patients with therapeutically reduced intraocular pressures. *Am J Ophthalmol.* 1998;126:487-497.
3. Kiuchi Y, Mishima HK, Hotehama Y, Furumoto A, Hirota A, Onari K. Exercise intensity determines the magnitude of IOP decrease after running. *Jpn J Ophthalmol.* 1994;38:191-195.
4. Karabatakis VE, Natsis KI, Chatzibalis TE, et al. Correlating intraocular pressure, blood pressure, and heart rate changes after jogging. *Eur J Ophthalmol.* 2004;14:117-122.
5. Qureshi IA. Effects of exercise on intraocular pressure in physically fit subjects. *Clin Exp Pharmacol Physiol.* 1996;23:648-652.
6. Qureshi IA. Does physical fitness influence intraocular pressure? *J Pak Med Assoc.* 1997;47:81-84.
7. Qureshi IA, Xi XR, Wu XD, Zhang J, Shiarkar E. The effect of physical fitness on intraocular pressure in Chinese medical students. *Zhonghua Yi Xue Za Zhi (Taipei).* 1996;58:317-322.
8. Passo MS, Goldberg L, Elliot DL, Van Buskirk EM. Exercise training reduces intraocular pressure among subjects suspected of having glaucoma. *Arch Ophthalmol.* 1991;109:1096-1098.
9. Williams PT. Prospective study of incident age-related macular degeneration in relation to vigorous physical activity during 7-year follow-up. *Invest Ophthalmol Vis Sci.* 2009;50:101-106.
10. Williams PT. Independent effects of vigorous physical activity and fitness on incident cataract during 7.6-year follow-up. *Invest Ophthalmol Vis Sci.* 2009;50: 95-100.

Assessment of a Sixteen-Week Training Program on Strength, Pain, and Function in Rheumatoid Arthritis Patients

Flint-Wagner HG, Lisse J, Lohman TG, et al (Boise State Univ, ID; Arizona Arthritis Ctr, Tucson; Univ of Arizona, Tucson; et al)
J Clin Rheumatol 15:165-171, 2009

Objective.—To assess the effects of a 16-week progressive, individualized, high-intensity strength training program on muscle strength, pain, and function in patients with rheumatoid arthritis (RA).

Methods.—Twenty-four RA patients (men, n = 5; women, n = 19) receiving infliximab participated in a randomized controlled trial. The strength training (ST) group (n = 16) participated in a supervised program 3 times per week, and the control (C) group (n = 8) continued with standard of care as overseen by their rheumatologist. Assessments were completed at baseline and at weeks 8 and 16. Strength was measured by 3 repetition maximum (3RM), isometric hand dynamometer, and isokinetic dynamometer. A 100-mm visual analogue scale was used to assess pain. Functional performance was derived from a timed 50-foot walk and the Health Assessment Questionnaire Disability Index.

Results.—The mean percent increase in strength (3RM) for the ST group from baseline to week 16 was 46.1% ± 31.6% ($P < 0.01$) (mean of all three 3RM exercises: hammer curl, leg press, and incline dumbbell press), with mean gains in strength up to 4 times that of baseline values reported in all strength training exercises (upper and lower body) performed during exercise sessions. On average, right-hand grip strength increased by 2.9 ± 4.0 kg in the ST group, in comparison with a loss of 1.2 ± 3.0 kg in the C group over 16 weeks. The ST group had a 53% reduction in pain, in comparison with almost no change in the C group. The ST group had a significant improvement in 50-foot walk time, with a mean reduction of−1.2 ± 1.6 seconds, in comparison with the C group (mean increase of 0.8 ± 1.0 seconds; $P = 0.01$) over the 16 weeks. There was a clinically important difference (predefined as mean change ±0.25) in the Health Assessment Questionnaire Disability Index in the ST group (−0.4 ± 0.4) but not in the C group (−0.1 ± 0.4).

Conclusion.—High-intensity strength training in RA patients with varying levels of disease activity and joint damage had a large, significant effect on strength, and led to improvements in pain and function, with additive patient benefits beyond the effect of their infliximab use.

▶ The main message in this article is that high intensity strength training in patients with rheumatoid arthritis may be beneficial in terms of increasing strength and function, and it does not have any detrimental effects with respect to increasing disease activity. The sample is small, especially the control group (only 8 patients), and there are multiple comparisons done. Thus, the level of evidence is rather low. However, I believe that the important conclusion here is that high intensity strength training did no harm and has a potential benefit for these patients. Often patients with rheumatoid arthritis are not enrolled in high intensity strengthening programs, and the focus has traditionally been on improving range of motion and mobility. This pilot study indicates that patients with this condition may safely participate in an individualized, supervised, high-intensity strengthening program without adverse effects on their disease status. Further, they appear to benefit from this intervention, although there is a need for a larger sample to substantiate this conclusion.

D. E. Feldman, PT, PhD

Assessment of a Sixteen-Week Training Program on Strength, Pain, and Function in Rheumatoid Arthritis Patients

Flint-Wagner HG, Lisse J, Lohman TG, et al (Boise State Univ, ID; Arizona Arthritis Ctr, Tucson; Univ of Arizona, Tucson; et al)

J Clin Rheumatol 15:165-171, 2009

Objective.—To assess the effects of a 16-week progressive, individualized, high-intensity strength training program on muscle strength, pain, and function in patients with rheumatoid arthritis (RA).

Methods.—Twenty-four RA patients (men, n = 5; women, n = 19) receiving infliximab participated in a randomized controlled trial. The strength training (ST) group (n = 16) participated in a supervised program 3 times per week, and the control (C) group (n = 8) continued with standard of care as overseen by their rheumatologist. Assessments were completed at baseline and at weeks 8 and 16. Strength was measured by 3 repetition maximum (3RM), isometric hand dynamometer, and isokinetic dynamometer. A 100-mm visual analogue scale was used to assess pain. Functional performance was derived from a timed 50-foot walk and the Health Assessment Questionnaire Disability Index.

Results.—The mean percent increase in strength (3RM) for the ST group from baseline to week 16 was 46.1% ± 31.6% ($P < 0.01$) (mean of all three 3RM exercises: hammer curl, leg press, and incline dumbbell press), with mean gains in strength up to 4 times that of baseline values reported in all strength training exercises (upper and lower body) performed during exercise sessions. On average, right-hand grip strength increased by 2.9 ± 4.0 kg in the ST group, in comparison with a loss of 1.2 ± 3.0 kg in the C group over 16 weeks. The ST group had a 53% reduction in pain, in comparison with almost no change in the C group. The ST group had a significant improvement in 50-foot walk time, with a mean reduction of−1.2 ± 1.6 seconds, in comparison with the C group (mean increase of 0.8 ± 1.0 seconds; $P = 0.01$) over the 16 weeks. There was a clinically important difference (predefined as mean change ± 0.25) in the Health Assessment Questionnaire Disability Index in the ST group (−0.4 ± 0.4) but not in the C group (−0.1 ± 0.4).

Conclusion.—High-intensity strength training in RA patients with varying levels of disease activity and joint damage had a large, significant

TABLE 2.—Mean Strength Changes (%) (Mean ± SD) From 3RMs for Strength Training (ST) Group

Exercises	Baseline to Week 8 (n = 16)	*P*	Weeks 8–16 (n = 16)	*P*	Baseline to Week 16 (n = 16)	*P*
Leg press (%)	25.1 ± 22.4	0.001†	20.8 ± 14	0.000†	46.4 ± 35.2	0.000†
Hammer curl, right arm (%)	19.0 ± 20.3	0.0001†	15.4 + 23.7	0.005*	34.1 ± 20.6	0.000†
Hammer curl, left arm (%)	32.6 ± 46.5	0.0001†	12.1 ± 17.2	0.002*	43.1 ± 19.0	0.000†
Incline dumbbell press, right (%)	38.8 ± 22.7	0.0001†	16.0 ± 17.7	0.021*	55.6 ± 38.3	0.000†
Incline dumbbell press, left (%)	36.4 ± 25.6	0.005*	15.3 ± 20.7	0.059*	48.1 ± 32.7	0.000†
Total mean strength change (%)	28.9 ± 18.9	0.000†	21 ± 11	0.000†	46.1 ± 31.6	0.000†

*Significant at $P \leq 0.005$.
†Significant at $P \leq 0.0002$.

effect on strength, and led to improvements in pain and function, with additive patient benefits beyond the effect of their infliximab use (Table 2).

▶ Rheumatoid arthritis is one of the most common problems in older women, but there have been relatively few trials of exercise programs for this condition. The general consensus has been that, provided the patient is not suffering from an acute exacerbation, it is helpful to encourage an increase of physical activity.[1-8] This study is based on a small controlled trial, and it confirms current wisdom, showing gains in both strength and physical performance and a reduction of pain in response to a supervised strength training program (Table 2). Because of supervision, patients were able to continue some exercise, even during flare-ups of their disorder. Nevertheless, the conclusion is a little suspect because 6 of the 16 patients in the experimental group ceased exercising. Moreover, reported gains of isometric strength (40%-50%) were much larger than the change in walking speed (9%) or isokinetic strength, suggesting that scores for the isometric strength test may have been influenced by practice of the required movements. Also, the improvement in symptom score has not been found in all previous studies. Plainly, there remains scope for larger controlled trials and, in view of the drop-outs, a comparison of results based on intention to treat.

R. J. Shephard, MD (Lond), PhD, DPE

References

1. Hakkinen A, Sokka T, Kotaniemi A, Hannonen P. A randomized two-year study of the effects of dynamic strength training on muscle strength, disease activity, functional capacity, and bone mineral density in early rheumatoid arthritis. *Arthritis Rheum.* 2001;44:515-522.
2. Hakkinen A, Sokka T, Kotaniemi A, et al. Muscle strength characteristics and central bone mineral density in women with recent onset rheumatoid arthritis compared with healthy controls. *Scand J Rheumatol.* 1999;28:145-151.
3. Rall LC, Meydani SN, Kehayias JJ, Dawson-Hughes B, Roubenoff R. The effect of progressive resistance training in rheumatoid arthritis. *Arthritis Rheum.* 1996;39: 415-426.
4. Hakkinen A. Effectiveness and safety of strength training in rheumatoid arthritis. *Curr Opin Rheumatol.* 2004;16:132-137.
5. Van Den Ende CHM, Breedveld F, le Cessie S, Dijkmans BA, de Mug AW, Hazes JM. Effect of intensive exercise on patients with active rheumatoid arthritis: a randomized clinical trial. *Ann Rheum Dis.* 2000;59:615-621.
6. Van Den Ende CHM, Hazes JMW, le Cessie S, et al. Comparison of high and low intensity training in well controlled rheumatoid arthritis. results of a randomised clinical trial. *Ann Rheum Dis.* 1996;55:798-805.
7. Komatireddy GR, Leitch RW, Cella K, Browning G, Minor M. Efficacy of low load resistive muscle training in patients with rheumatoid arthritis functional class II and III. *J Rheumatol.* 1997;24:1531-1539.
8. Stenstrom CH, Minor MA. Evidence for the benefit of aerobic and strengthening exercise in rheumatoid arthritis. *Arthritis Rheum.* 2003;49:428-434.

Differences in gait parameters between healthy subjects and persons with moderate and severe knee osteoarthritis: A result of altered walking speed?

Zeni JA Jr, Higginson JS (Univ of Delaware, Newark)

Clin Biomech 24:372-378, 2009

Background.—While knee osteoarthritis has been shown to affect a multitude of kinematic, kinetic and temporo-spatial gait parameters, few investigations have examined the effect of increasing levels of radiographic osteoarthritis severity on these gait parameters. Fewer still have investigated the effect of walking speed on gait variables in persons with knee osteoarthritis. The objective of this study was to investigate the influence of walking speed on biomechanical variables associated with joint loading in persons with varying severities of medial compartment knee osteoarthritis.

Methods.—Twenty-one persons with moderate osteoarthritis (Kellgren–Lawrence score 2–3) and 13 persons with severe osteoarthritis (Kellgren–Lawrence score of 4) participated. Twenty-two persons without knee pain or radiographic evidence of arthritis comprised a healthy control group. Sagittal plane kinetics, knee adduction moment, sagittal plane knee excursion, ground reaction forces and knee joint reaction forces were calculated from three-dimensional motion analysis at 1.0 m/s, self-selected and fastest tolerable walking speeds. Differences were analyzed using multivariate analysis of variance and multivariate analysis of covariance with speed as a covariate.

Findings.—Persons with knee osteoarthritis showed significantly lower knee and ankle joint moments, ground reaction forces, knee reaction force and knee excursion when walking at freely chosen speeds. When differences in walking speed were accounted for in the analysis, the only difference found at all conditions was decreased knee joint excursion.

Interpretation.—Compared to a healthy control group, persons with knee OA demonstrate differences in joint kinetics and kinematics. Except for knee excursion, these differences in gait parameters appear to be a result of slower freely chosen walking speeds rather than a result of disease progression.

▶ Patients with knee osteoarthritis (OA) have been shown to present with temporal-spatial, kinematic, and kinetic changes during a clinical gait analysis compared with healthy subjects. However, few investigators have examined the association between increasing knee OA severity (as assessed using radiographic evidence), walking speed, and changes in the clinical gait analysis values. In this study, 34 patients with moderate and severe knee OA and 22 healthy individuals underwent clinical gait assessments at 3 walking speeds. Although many kinematic and kinetic differences were noted between the OA and healthy groups and between the 2 OA groups, the authors' found that most of the gait differences could be attributed to a change in walking speed—patients with knee OA walked slower thereby modulating most of the other gait values. Only the knee range of motion change was independent of gait speed. The authors conclude that a change in the knee range of motion, which is independent of walking speed, may be the defining kinematic characteristic of persons with knee OA. As such, the more practical kinematic knee examination during gait may provide valuable information to the clinician regarding the severity of knee OA.

M. R. Pierrynowski, PhD

Incidence of severe knee and hip osteoarthritis in relation to different measures of body mass: a population-based prospective cohort study

Lohmander LS, de Verdier MG, Rollof J, et al (Lund Univ, Sweden; AstraZeneca R&D, Lund, Sweden)

Ann Rheum Dis 68:490-496, 2009

Objective.—To determine in a prospective population-based cohort study relationships between different measures of body mass and the incidence of severe knee and hip osteoarthritis defined as arthroplasty of knee or hip due to osteoarthritis.

Materials and Methods.—Body mass index (BMI), waist circumference, waist–hip ratio (WHR), weight and percentage of body fat (BF%) were measured at baseline in 11 026 men and 16 934 women from the general population. The incidence of osteoarthritis over 11 years was monitored by linkage with the Swedish hospital discharge register.

Results.—471 individuals had knee osteoarthritis and 551 had hip osteoarthritis. After adjustment for age, sex, smoking and physical activity, the relative risks (RR) of knee osteoarthritis (fourth vs first quartile) were 8.1 (95% CI 5.3 to 12.4) for BMI, 6.7 (4.5 to 9.9) for waist circumference, 6.5 (4.6 to 9.43) for weight, 3.6 (2.6 to 5.0) for BF% and 2.2 (1.7 to 3.0) for WHR. Corresponding RR for hip osteoarthritis were 2.6 (2.0 to 3.4) for BMI, 3.0 (2.3 to 4.0) for weight, 2.5 (1.9 to 3.3) for waist, 1.3 (0.99 to 1.6) for WHR and 1.5 (1.2 to 2.0) for BF%.

Conclusion.—All measures of overweight were associated with the incidence of knee osteoarthritis, with the strongest relative risk gradient observed for BMI. The incidence of hip osteoarthritis showed smaller but significant differences between normal weight and obesity. Our results support a major link between overweight and biomechanics in increasing the risk of knee and hip osteoarthritis in men and women (Fig 1).

▶ This is the first study to compare the incidence of severe knee and hip osteoarthritis in men and women in relation to different measures of overweight. Results show that body mass index (BMI), weight, and waist circumference were major risk factors for knee arthroplasty or osteotomy as a result of osteoarthritis, with the highest relative risks (RR) for subjects with the highest BMI (Fig 1). BMI, weight, and waist were also important risk factors for osteoarthritis of the hip leading to arthroplasty (Fig 1). Both mechanical factors induced by high body weight and metabolic or inflammatory factors related

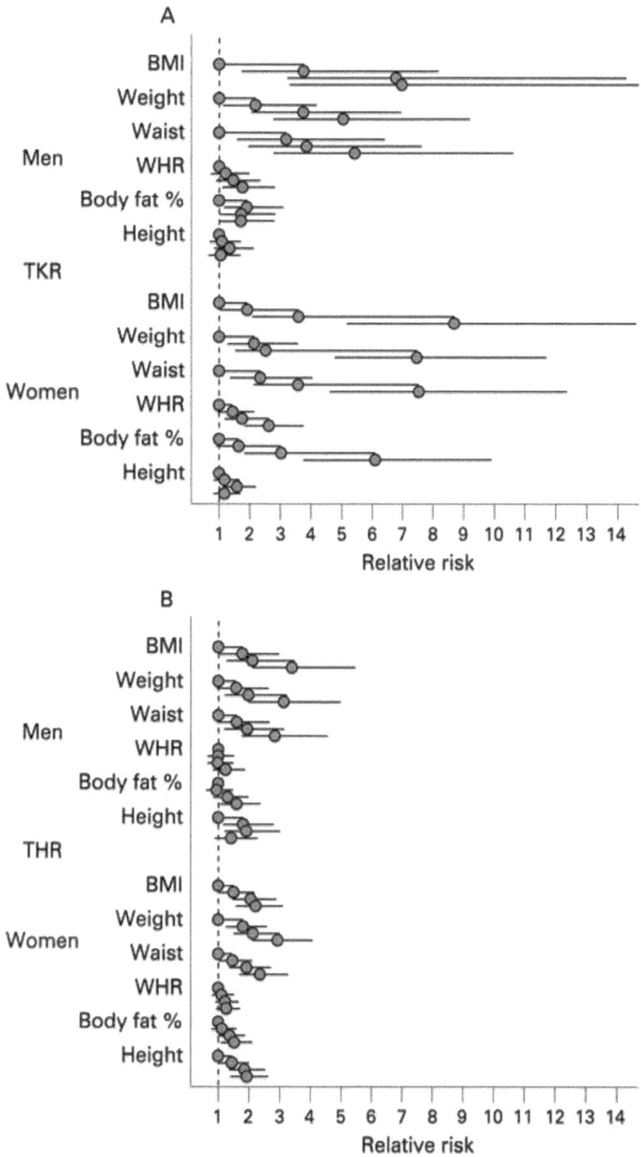

FIGURE 1.—Adjusted relative risks (RR) for men and women for total knee replacement (TKR) or osteotomy for severe knee osteoarthritis (top), or total hip replacement (THR) for severe hip osteoarthritis (bottom). Error bars show 95% CI for RR estimates; each group of four symbols represent quartiles 1 to 4. The dotted line corresponds to RR 1. BMI, body mass index; WHR, waist–hip ratio. (Reprinted from Lohmander LS, de Verdier MG, Rollof J, et al. Incidence of severe knee and hip osteoarthritis in relation to different measures of body mass: a population-based prospective cohort study. *Ann Rheum Dis.* 2009;68:490-496, with permission from the BMJ Publishing Group, Ltd.)

to obesity contribute to osteoarthritis.[1] This study found that BMI was associated more closely with knee and hip osteoarthritis than waist-hip ratio (WHR) or percentage of body fat (BF%). Mechanical factors associated with overweight are more strongly related to knee and hip osteoarthritis than metabolic or inflammatory factors. Many other factors, however, contribute to osteoarthritis, including age, joint malalignment, and traumatic joint injury.[2] Nonetheless, a high BMI is definitely one of the strongest risk factors for osteoarthritis. Research with twins indicates a 9% to 13% increase in risk of knee osteoarthritis for every kilogram gain in weight during mid-life.[3] Weight loss in individuals with osteoarthritis reduces force loads and inflammatory factors within the joint, improving the potential for slowing down the progress of osteoarthritis.[4]

D. C. Nieman, DrPH

References

1. Pottie P, Presle N, Terlain B, Netter P, Mainard D, Berenbaum F. Obesity and osteoarthritis: more complex than predicted! *Ann Rheum Dis.* 2006;65:1403-1405.
2. Blagojevic M, Jinks C, Jeffery A, Jordan KP. Risk factors for onset of osteoarthritis of the knee in older adults: a systematic review and meta-analysis. *Osteoarthritis Cartilage.* 2009 September 2 (Epub ahead of print).
3. Cicuttini FM, Baker JR, Spector TD. The association of obesity with osteoarthritis of the hand and knee in women: a twin study. *J Rheumatol.* 1996;23:1221-1226.
4. Messier SP, Gutekunst DJ, Davis C, DeVita P. Weight loss reduces knee-joint loads in overweight and obese older adults with knee osteoarthritis. *Arthritis Rheum.* 2005;52:2026-2032.

Early physical and occupational therapy in mechanically ventilated, critically ill patients: a randomised controlled trial

Schweickert WD, Pohlman MC, Pohlman AS, et al (Univ of Pennsylvania, Philadelphia; Univ of Chicago, IL; et al)

Lancet 373:1874-1882, 2009

Background.—Long-term complications of critical illness include intensive care unit (ICU)-acquired weakness and neuropsychiatric disease. Immobilisation secondary to sedation might potentiate these problems. We assessed the efficacy of combining daily interruption of sedation with physical and occupational therapy on functional outcomes in patients receiving mechanical ventilation in intensive care.

Methods.—Sedated adults (≥18 years of age) in the ICU who had been on mechanical ventilation for less than 72 h, were expected to continue for at least 24 h, and who met criteria for baseline functional independence were eligible for enrolment in this randomised controlled trial at two university hospitals. We randomly assigned 104 patients by computer-generated, permuted block randomisation to early exercise and mobilisation (physical and occupational therapy) during periods of daily interruption of sedation (intervention; n=49) or to daily interruption of sedation with therapy as ordered by the primary care team (control; n=55). The primary endpoint—the number of patients returning to independent functional status at hospital discharge—was defined as the ability to perform six activities of daily living and the ability to walk independently. Therapists who undertook patient assessments were blinded to treatment assignment. Secondary endpoints included duration of delirium and ventilator-free days during the first 28 days of hospital stay. Analysis was by intention to treat. This trial is registered with ClinicalTrials.gov, number NCT00322010.

Findings.—All 104 patients were included in the analysis. Return to independent functional status at hospital discharge occurred in 29 (59%) patients in the intervention group compared with 19 (35%) patients in the control group (p=0·02; odds ratio 2·7 [95% CI 1·2–6·1]). Patients in the intervention group had shorter duration of delirium (median 2·0 days, IQR 0·0–6·0 *vs* 4·0 days, 2·0–8·0; p = 0·02), and more ventilator-free days (23·5 days, 7·4–25·6 *vs* 21·1 days, 0·0–23·8; p=0·05) during the 28-day follow-up period than did controls. There was one serious adverse event in 498 therapy sessions (desaturation less than 80%). Discontinuation of therapy as a result of patient instability occurred in 19 (4%) of all sessions, most commonly for perceived patient-ventilator asynchrony.

Interpretation.—A strategy for whole-body rehabilitation—consisting of interruption of sedation and physical and occupational therapy in the earliest days of critical illness—was safe and well tolerated, and resulted in better functional outcomes at hospital discharge, a shorter duration of delirium, and more ventilator-free days compared with standard care.

▶ This is a very important article that provides strong evidence for the implementation of daily interruption of sedation combined with physical therapy for patients who are critically ill and on mechanical ventilation. The methods of this randomized controlled trial are sound, well-described, and support that physical or occupational therapy should be started in the intensive care unit. The intervention was safe and well-tolerated. Patients who received the early physical and occupational therapy treatment (along with interruption in sedation) improved with respect to functional status at discharge, shorter duration of ICU associated delirium, and longer time breathing without assistance.

Besides the findings that patients who received the intervention had a better functional outcome at discharge from hospital and a shorter duration of delirium, the study supports coordination of multidisciplinary care for critically ill persons. This article highlights the importance of maximizing outcomes in persons who are critically ill with respect to quality of life and functional outcomes.

D. E. Feldman, PT, PhD

Dose response and efficacy of spinal manipulation for chronic cervicogenic headache: a pilot randomized controlled trial

Haas M, Spegman A, Peterson D, et al (Western States Chiropractic College, Portland, OR; Geisinger Ctr for Health Res, Danville, PA; et al)

Spine J 10:117-128, 2010

Background Context.—Systematic reviews of randomized controlled trials suggest that spinal manipulative therapy (SMT) is efficacious for care of cervicogenic headache (CGH). The effect of SMT dose on outcomes has not been studied.

Purpose.—To compare the efficacy of two doses of SMT and two doses of light massage (LM) for CGH.

Patient Sample.—Eighty patients with chronic CGH.

Main Outcome Measures.—Modified Von Korff pain and disability scales for CGH and neck pain (minimum clinically important difference = 10 on 100-point scale), number of headaches in the last 4 weeks, and medication use. Data were collected every 4 weeks for 24 weeks. The primary outcome was the CGH pain scale.

Methods.—Participants were randomized to either 8 or 16 treatment sessions with either SMT or a minimal LM control. Patients were treated once or twice per week for 8 weeks. Adjusted mean differences (AMD) between groups were computed using generalized estimating equations for the longitudinal outcomes over all follow-up time points (profile) and using regression modeling for individual time points with baseline characteristics as covariates and with imputed missing data.

Results.—For the CGH pain scale, comparisons of 8 and 16 treatment sessions yielded small dose effects: $|AMD| \leq 5.6$. There was an advantage for SMT over the control: AMD = −8.1 (95% confidence interval = −13.3 to −2.8) for the profile, −10.3 (−18.5 to −2.1) at 12 weeks, and −9.8 (−18.7 to −1.0) at 24 weeks. For the higher dose patients, the advantage was greater: AMD = −11.9 (−19.3 to −4.6) for the profile, −14.2 (−25.8 to −2.6) at 12 weeks, and −14.4 (−26.9 to −2.0) at 24 weeks. Patients receiving SMT were also more likely to achieve a 50% improvement in pain scale: adjusted odds ratio = 3.6 (1.6 to 8.1) for the profile, 3.1 (0.9 to 9.8) at 12 weeks, and 3.1 (0.9 to 10.3) at 24 weeks. Secondary outcomes showed similar trends favoring SMT. For SMT patients, the mean number of CGH was reduced by half.

Conclusions.—Clinically important differences between SMT and a control intervention were observed favoring SMT. Dose effects tended to be small (Fig 2).

▶ This study is concerned with spinal manipulation treatment for cervicogenic headache (ie, headache associated with neck pain and dysfunction). The strengths of this study are the randomized trial design, the comparisons between an 8-week treatment course of spinal manipulation and a 16-week treatment course in addition to controls receiving light massage as the intervention, and the use of well-accepted outcome measures. At baseline, the 4 groups

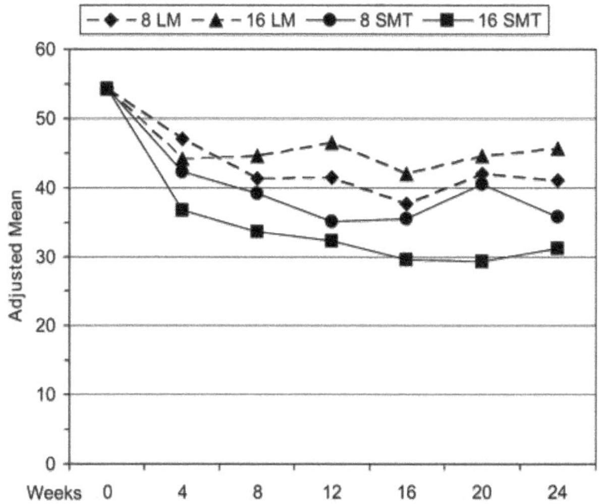

FIGURE 2.—Adjusted mean cervicogenic headache (CGH) pain. Predicted follow-up means were computed using simultaneous regression analysis adjusted for the baseline covariates. The analysis assumes that all groups start at the grand baseline mean pain (shown at Week 0). (Reprinted from Haas M, Spegman A, Peterson D, et al. Dose response and efficacy of spinal manipulation for chronic cervicogenic headache: a pilot randomized controlled trial. *Spine J*. 2010;10:117-128, with permission from Elsevier Inc.)

seemed quite similar except for neck functional disability, which was lower in the 16-visit group, possibly accounting for the lack of a difference in improvement between the 8- and 16-week groups. Although the sample was small (started out with 20 in each group), there is evidence that spinal manipulation for cervicogenic headache is more effective in reducing pain than a control intervention of light massage (Fig 2). However, there were no significant differences in patient outcomes between the 8- and 16-week spinal manipulation groups.

D. E. Feldman, PT, PhD

A Study to Evaluate the Feasibility of an Aerobic Exercise Program in Patients With Migraine

Varkey E, Cider Å, Carlsson J, et al (Cephalea Headache Centre, Gothenburg, Sweden; Göteborg Univ, Sweden)
Headache 49:563-570, 2009

Objectives.—The aim of this study was to develop and evaluate an exercise program to improve maximum oxygen uptake ($VO_{2\ max}$) in untrained patients with migraine without making their migraines worse.

Patients and Methods.—Twenty-six patients were studied at a headache clinic in Sweden. The exercise program, based on indoor cycling, was

TABLE 1.—Results from Migraine Specific Quality of Life Questionnaire (MSQoL), Maximal Oxygen (VO_{2max}), and Migraine Status

	MSQoL (points)†	VO_{2max} (mL/kg/minute)	Migraine Attacks/Month	Days with Migraine	Intensity of Pain (VAS in mm)†	Doses of Acute Medicine
Baseline	58 (37)	32.9 (9.8)	4.7 (2.0)	7.5 (3.6)	57 (36)	7.6 (3.7)
Treatment			3.9 (1.6) ns	6.4 (3.3) ns	42 (34) ns	6.6 (2.5) ns
Last month of treatment			3.6 (1.9) $P = .027$	5.4 (3.6) $P < .01$	47 (33) $P = .019$	5.8 (3.7) $P = .024$
After treatment	65 (25) $P < .01$	36.2 (8.1) $P = .044$				

Mean values with standard deviations (in parentheses).
ns = nonsignificant; VAS = visual analog scale.
†Median value with interquartile range (given within parentheses) significant change from baseline.

performed 3 times per week during 12 weeks. $VO_{2\ max}$, migraine status, side effects, and quality of life were evaluated.

Results.—$VO_{2\ max}$ increased from 32.9 mL/kg/minute to 36.2 mL/kg/minute ($P = .044$). Quality of life increased and significant improvements in migraine status (attack frequency, symptom intensity, and intake of medicine) were seen. During the 12 weeks of exercise, on one occasion one patient had a migraine attack, which started immediately after training. No other side effects were reported.

Conclusions.—The evaluated exercise program was well tolerated by the patients and improved their $VO_{2\ max}$ with no deterioration of migraine status (Table 1).

▶ Some previous reports have suggested that exercise can be a trigger for migraine attacks.[1] Perhaps because of this fear, patients with migraines tend to have less flexibility and a low maximal oxygen intake.[2] This study was not controlled, but it is reassuring that only 1 of the 26 patients triggered a migraine attack over 12 weeks of thrice weekly cycle ergometer training that increased the predicted maximal oxygen intake (Åstrand/Ryhming test) by some 10%. Individual training sessions began with a 10-minute warm-up, and then 20 minutes at a Rating of Perceived Exertion of 14 to 16 on the Borg Scale ("hard"), with a final 5-minute warm down. Most patients actually reported an improvement in their migraine (Table 1), although this would have been more convincing given a control group.

R. J. Shephard, MD (Lond), PhD, DPE

References

1. Kelman L. The triggers or precipitants of the acute migraine attack. *Cephalalgia.* 2007;27:394-402.
2. Neususs K, Neumann B, Steinhoff BJ, Thegeder H, Bauer A, Reimers D. Physical activity and fitness in patients with headache disorders. *Int J Sports Med.* 1997;18: 607-611.

Sleep Is Not Disrupted by Exercise in Patients with Chronic Fatigue Syndromes

Togo F, Natelson BH, Cherniack NS, et al (UMDNJ-New Jersey Med School, Newark; et al)

Med Sci Sports Exerc 42:16-22, 2010

Purpose.—Patients with chronic fatigue syndrome (CFS) report that exertion produces dramatic symptom worsening. We hypothesized this might be due to the exacerbation of an underlying sleep disorder, which we have previously demonstrated to exist.

Methods.—Female patients with CFS and matched healthy controls with no evidence of major depressive disorder were studied with overnight polysomnography on a baseline night and on a night after their performance of a maximal exercise test.

Results.—CFS patients as a group had evidence for disturbed sleep compared with controls. Although exercise improved sleep for healthy subjects, it did not do this for the group as a whole. When we stratified the sample on the basis of self-reported sleepiness after a night's sleep, the patient group with reduced morning sleepiness showed improvement in sleep structure, whereas those with increased morning sleepiness continued to show evidence for sleep disruption.

Conclusions.—Sleep is disturbed in CFS patients as a group, but exercise does not exacerbate this sleep disturbance. Approximately half the patients studied actually sleep better after exercise. Therefore, activity-related symptom worsening is not caused by worsened sleep (Fig 1).

► Opinions on the value of exercise in chronic fatigue syndrome (CFS) differ widely, in part because it is a rather poorly defined and diffuse syndrome. However, there are reports of a dramatic worsening of symptoms with even mild exertion[1] and other hand studies showing considerable benefit from exercise training.[2] One commonly reported manifestation of the syndrome is a disturbance of sleep,[3] and one might wonder whether this would be exacerbated by the arousing effect of exercise. In healthy people, the effect of exercise on subsequent sleep depends on timing; if exercise is taken early in the day, it helps a person to sleep well,[4] but it can have the opposite effect late at night. This study involved a relatively homogeneous population of women with CFS (as defined by the standard psychiatric diagnostic criteria) and healthy controls. Sleep after a single late afternoon bout of exercise (progressive maximal exercise on a cycle ergometer) was studied by both self-report and polysomnography. In the initial control period, sleep duration did not differ from that of control subjects, but the sleep was of poorer quality, with less deep sleep. The exercise bout shortened sleep latency in the healthy subjects. In the individuals with CFS, the good news is that sleep patterns were not worsened by the exercise bout; indeed, in about a half of the group, sleep was improved (Fig 1). The authors of this report suggest that patients helped by exercise could be distinguished by their initial absence of morning sleepiness. However, the extent of benefit was relatively small and was probably of

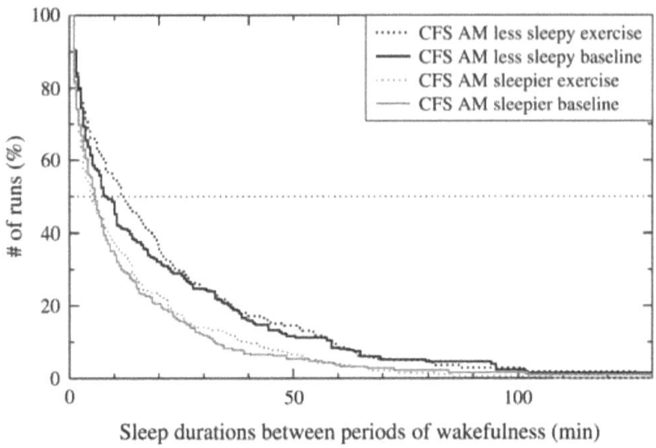

FIGURE 1.—Survival curves of every episode of sleep (i.e., a bout of sleep preceded and followed by periods of wakefulness) for patients in the AM less sleepy and in the AM sleepier groups for whole-night hypnograms on the baseline and postexercise nights stratified by the duration of the sleep episode. To compare sleep continuity between groups, all data from all subjects in each group were pooled, and a group survival curve was generated using standard statistical techniques (9). Patients in the AM less sleepy group showed a significant shift toward longer bouts of sleep on the postexercise night compared with the baseline night. (Reprinted from Togo F, Natelson BH, Cherniack NS, et al. Sleep is not disrupted by exercise in patients with chronic fatigue syndromes. *Med Sci Sports Exerc.* 2010;42:16-22.)

no great clinical significance. It would be interesting to repeat the experiment with exercise performed earlier during the day. From the present data, it looks as if any symptom that follows an exercise bout in patients with CFS cannot be attributed to a disturbance of sleep.

R. J. Shephard, MD (Lond), PhD, DPE

References

1. King C, Jason LA. Improving the diagnostic criteria and procedures for chronic fatigue syndrome. *Biol Psychol.* 2005;68:87-106.
2. Afari N, Buchwald D. Chronic fatigue syndrome: a review. *Am J Psychiatry.* 2003; 160:221-236.
3. Togo F, Natelson BH, Cherniack NS, FitzGibbons J, Garcon C, Rapoport DM. Sleep structure and sleepiness in chronic fatigue syndrome with or without coexisting fibromyalgia. *Arthritis Res Ther.* 2008;10:R56.
4. Youngstedt SD. Effects of exercise on sleep. *Clin Sports Med.* 2005;24:355-365.

Cystatin C a Marker for Renal Function after Exercise

Mingels A, Jacobs L, Kleijnen V, et al (Univ Hosp Maastricht, Netherlands)
Int J Sports Med 30:668-671, 2009

Renal impairment is common during and after severe exercise. In clinical practice, renal function is evaluated using serum creatinine, urine parameters, and equations to estimate the Glomular Filtration Rate (GFR). However, creatinine levels may be biased by skeletal muscle damage and the GFR equations, requiring age, gender and body weight, are shown to be inadequate in normals. In the present study, we show that serum cystatin C and creatinine concentrations were elevated after marathon running in 26% and 46% of the 70 recreational male runners, respectively, possibly because of reduction in renal blood flow. The mean cystatin C increase was twice as low as compared to creatinine (21% and 41%, respectively), suggesting that cystatin C is indeed less biased by muscle damage. Future research has to reveal whether training diminishes the elevation in renal markers. Overall, cystatin C seems a more reliable method to establish renal function during and after extensive exercise.

▶ Impairment of renal function, probably due in part to a reduction of renal blood flow and resulting tissue ischemia, is well recognized after a bout of prolonged endurance exercise such as a marathon run.[1] In some instances, it can progress to rhabdomyolysis and acute renal failure.[2,3] Assessment of such renal injury has typically been based on serum creatinine measurements—either an absolute increase >26.4≥ mol/L, or a 1.5-fold relative increase in serum concentration. However, there are 2 problems in applying the standard clinical technique in sports medicine, as underlined by the authors of this article: 1) Creatinine levels may be elevated not only by poor renal function but also by exercise-induced muscle injury. 2) Background creatinine levels depend in part on the individual's muscle mass, and in some groups of athletes muscle mass may be much above norms for the general population.[4,5] One potential alternative is to measure levels of serum cystatin C, a nonglycolysated cysteine protease inhibitor produced by all nucleated cells. Serum concentrations of this substance also reflect glomerular filtration, and are said to be less influenced by issues of age, gender, and muscle mass.[4] In the present trial, dehydration-corrected serum concentrations of cystatin C showed only half as large an increase as creatinine immediately following a marathon run (see Fig 1 in the original article). It is of some concern that both indicators showed a substantial proportion of marathoners with an acute depression of renal function, even though there was recovery within 24 hours. The proportion of runners showing a pathological change was smaller in terms of cystatin C data than as indicated by serum creatinine measurements, but comparison with some gold standard is needed before we can be really certain which of the 2 measurements is giving the correct assessment of risk.

R. J. Shephard, MD (Lond), PhD, DPE

References

1. Bellinghieri G, Savica V, Santoro D. Renal alterations during exercise. *J Ren Nutr.* 2008;18:158-164.
2. Clarkson PM. Exertional rhabdomyolysis and acute renal failure in marathon runners. *Sports Med.* 2007;37:361-363.
3. Le Meur Y, Paraf F, Szelag JC, Aldigier JC, Leroux-Robert C. Acute renal failure in a marathon runner" role of glomerular bleeding in tubular injury. *Am J Med.* 1998;105:251-262.

4. Vinge E, Lindergard B, Nilsson-Ehie P, Grubb A. Relationships among serum cytastatin C, serum creatinine. Lean tissue mass and glomerular filtration rate in healthy adults. *J Clin Lab Invest.* 1999;59:587-592.
5. Banfi G, Del Fabbro M, Lippi G. Relation between serum creatinine and body mass index in elite athletes of different sport disciplines. *Br J Sports Med.* 2006; 40:675-678.

Fiberoptic Videolaryngoscopy During Bicycle Ergometry: A Diagnostic Tool for Exercise-Induced Vocal Cord Dysfunction

Tervonen H, Niskanen MM, Sovijärvi AR, et al (Helsinki Univ Central Hosp, Finland)

Laryngoscope 119:1776-1780, 2009

Objectives/Hypothesis.—Exercise-induced vocal cord dysfunction is difficult to diagnose because the paradoxical vocal cord adduction should be observed during exercise. Our goal was to develop and validate a new diagnostic method for exercise-induced vocal cord dysfunction by combining continuous fiberoptic laryngoscopy with a bicycle ergometry test.

Methods.—Thirty consecutive patients referred to a laryngologist because of suspicion of exercise-induced vocal cord dysfunction and 15 healthy controls underwent the exercise test until dyspnea or exhaustion rated as 18–19/20 on the Borg scale. Laryngeal findings, electrocardiography, blood pressure, heart rate, and respiratory rate were monitored, and forced expiratory flow in the first second was measured before and after the exercise. The medical history was assessed by use of a structured questionnaire.

Results.—Among the 30 patients, 27 (90%) performed the test successfully, as did all controls. Diagnostic signs of inspiratory stridor, supraglottic collapse, and vocal cord adduction appeared in five (19%) patients but in none of the controls. Of the 30 patients referred, the laryngologist considered 25 to be suspect. Of them, 9 (36%) showed signs diagnostic or highly suspect for exercise-induced vocal cord dysfunction. Of the 15 patients whose dyspnea could be induced during the test, nine (60%) were suspected of having exercise-induced vocal cord dysfunction.

Conclusions.—Fiberoptic videolaryngoscopy during bicycle ergometry was a well-tolerated and relatively easily established diagnostic tool that could induce dyspnea in more than one half the patients examined. If the symptom of dyspnea appeared, the most frequent diagnosis was exercise- induced vocal cord dysfunction (Fig 1).

▶ While exercise-induced asthma (EIA) is a relatively common diagnosis in sport medicine, vocal cord dysfunction (VCD) can mimic this condition and/or co-exist with it. Proper diagnosis is essential to facilitate proper treatment and to avoid unnecessary administration of asthma medications, including high-dose corticosteroids with their potentially severe side effects. VCD or exercise-induced VCD (EIVCD) presents with inspiratory stridor and dyspnea

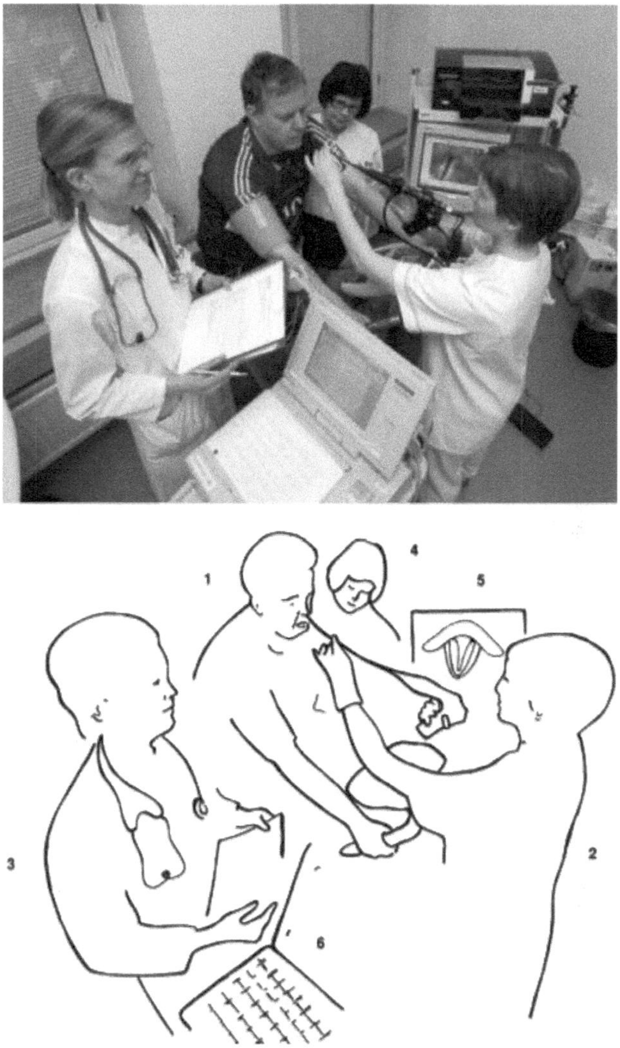

FIGURE 1.—A photo and a schematic presentation of the laryngeal team performing exercise test. 1 = patient; 2 = ear, nose, and throat specialist; 3 = anesthesiologist; 4 = nurse; 5 = computer-based videolaryngostroboscopy equipment; 6 = 12-lead electrocardiogram monitor. [Color figure can be viewed in the online issue, which is available at www.interscience.wiley.com.]. (Reprinted from Tervonen H, Niskanen MM, Sovijärvi AR, et al. Fiberoptic videolaryngoscopy during bicycle ergometry: a diagnostic tool for exercise-induced vocal cord dysfunction. *Laryngoscope*. 2009;119:1776-1780.)

during exercise. Dysphagia, dysphonia, and cough can be the typical symptoms, and patients are frequently taking antireflux medications in addition to bronchodilators and inhaled corticosteroids. EIVCD is caused by paradoxical closure of the vocal cords during the dyspneic attack, and the gold standard for diagnosis is therefore actual visualization of this phenomenon during exercise. Findings on direct laryngoscopy (transnasal fiberoptic scope) include supraglottic collapse of arytenoids and aryepiglottic folds toward the aditus of the larynx as well as vocal cord adduction. A negative provocation test does not preclude the diagnosis, and because EIVCD is an episodic symptom not always appearing in the same exercise surroundings, it can be difficult to detect.

Some authors have used a method based on continuous videolaryngoscopy during treadmill exercise,[1] but the space requirements and technical demands of running on a treadmill (especially for older patients or those with impaired physical condition) limit its practicality in crowded outpatient facilities. The technique described in this article uses a cycle ergometer and a progressive exercise load in combination with ECG and respiratory rate monitoring, and is suitable for a laryngeal outpatient department and for patients of various ages and physical conditions. A color figure of the set-up and a video of the procedure can be viewed in the online issue, which is available at http://www.interscience.wiley.com. It is important to consider the entity of EIVCD in patients with exercise-induced dyspnea, especially if screening for asthma or EIA is inconclusive and there is little or no response to the usual treatment regimens for these conditions. Referral to an ENT specialist for diagnostic testing may aid in the diagnosis.

C. Lebrun, MD

Reference

1. Heimdal J-H, Roksund O, Halvorsen T, Skadberg B, Olofson J. Continuous laryngoscopy exercise test: a method for visualizing laryngeal dysfunction during exercise. *Laryngoscope*. 2006;116:52-57.

8 Environment Factors

Determining a "Do Not Start" Temperature for a Marathon on the Basis of Adverse Outcomes

Roberts WO (Univ of Minnesota Med School, Minneapolis)

Med Sci Sports Exerc 42:226-232, 2010

Introduction.—Marathon races faced with unexpectedly hot conditions must make a decision to start or not to start. The current race cancellation parameters may not reflect the safety profile of an individual race, and a universal temperature may not work an individual race.

Methods.—A retrospective review of the number of starters, finishers, and finish line medical encounters was used to calculate the rate of "unsuccessful" marathon starters from race records, where unsuccessful is defined as medical encounters seen for any reason in the finish medical area plus marathon starters who did not finish. Unsuccessful marathon starters were plotted against the race start wet bulb globe temperature (WBGT), and the WBGT level at which a mass casualty incident (MCI) occurred was used to calculate a "do not start" WBGT.

Results.—A start WBGT of >21°C resulted in MCI or midrace cancellation in several races. Twin Cities Marathon data show a rapid increase in the rate of unsuccessful marathoner starters above a start WBGT of 13°C. The event experienced an area-wide MCI at a start WBGT of 21°C with an unsuccessful starter rate of 160 per 1000 finishers.

Conclusions.—Marathons in northern latitudes (>40°) held in "unexpectedly" hot conditions when the participants are not acclimatized and the start WBGT is >21°C often end in either race cancellation or an MCI. It would seem prudent not to start these races in similar conditions. The rate of unsuccessful marathon starters per 1000 marathon finishers plotted against start WBGT generates a curve that can be used to estimate a do not start level. The do not start WBGT for Twin Cities Marathon is 20.5°C on the basis of this model.

► Endurance runners frequently develop very high rectal temperatures over the course of a marathon event, particularly if the day is sunny. The question thus arises whether this is dangerous for participants. The figures observed are often much higher than the cut-off limits of 39.0°C to 39.5°C that Human Experimentation Committees set for laboratory investigations; the latter are based largely on experience with workers in the deep gold mines of South Africa, where a well-trained and heat-acclimated labor force engages in hard physical exercise for 8 hours per day under physically awkward and very humid conditions.

The cut-off temperature for endurance competition is commonly based not on rectal temperatures but rather on the wet bulb globe thermometer (WBGT) reading at the outset of an event. The figure that the American College of Sports Medicine (ACSM) recommended for cancellation of an endurance event in a 1996 "Position Stand" (a WBGT of 28°C) is based on studies of fit young marines.[1] A revised ACSM "Position Stand" published in 2007 was even more liberal, suggesting that if participants were acclimated, a race could continue to an initial WBGT as high as 30°C.[2] Given the large number of participants in most marathons, there is scope for epidemiological study of the validity of this position, and Dr Roberts has made a valuable contribution in this regard. Taking data from past Twin Cities marathons, he has shown a relationship between starting temperature and two indices of heat stress—the proportion of starters not completing a race and the proportion of incidents requiring medical attention (Fig 1 in the original article). The number of runners who failed to complete the event began to increase exponentially from a very low initial WBGT (13°C), and the initial WBGT threshold for medical incidents (corresponding to a situation where 10% of runners did not complete the event) was about 20.5°C. Findings might differ if the runners were younger, better trained, and heat acclimated, but, nevertheless, these data suggest an urgent need to revisit the current ACSM environmental temperature recommendations for races involving a broad spectrum of the general public.

R. J. Shephard, MD (Lond), PhD, DPE

References

1. Armstrong LE, Epstein Y, Greenleaf JE, et al. American College of Sports Medicine. position stand: heat and cold illnesses during long distance running. *Med Sci Sports Exerc.* 1996;28:i-x.
2. American College of Sports Medicine. Position Stand: exertional heat illness during training and competition. *Med Sci Sports Exerc.* 2007;30:556-572.

Effects of Environmental Heat Stress (35°C) with Simulated Air Movement on the Thermoregulatory Responses during a 4-km Cycling Time Trial

Altareki N, Drust B, Atkinson G, et al (Liverpool John Moores Univ, United Kingdom)
Int J Sports Med 30:9-15, 2009

The aim of the present investigation was to examine the influence of environmental heat stress (35°C) on 4-km cycling time trial performance using simulated environmental conditions and facing air velocities that closely reflect competitive situations. Nine competitive cyclists (age 34 ± 5 years, maximal oxygen uptake $61.7 \pm 8.6\ ml \cdot kg^{-1} \cdot min^{-1}$) completed a simulated 4-km cycling time trial in laboratory ambient temperatures (dry bulb temperatures) of 35°C and 13°C (relative humidity 60%, air velocity 5.6 m/s). Mean performance time was reduced in 35°C (390.1 ± 19.6 s) compared to 13°C (382.8 ± 18.2 s) (95% CI of difference = 4.0 to 10.6 s; $p < 0.01$). This was consistent with a decline in mean power output throughout the duration of exercise in 35°C compared with 13°C ($p < 0.01$). Mean skin temperature and mean body temperatures were elevated at rest and throughout the duration of exercise in 35°C ($p < 0.01$). A higher level of muscle temperature was also observed at the onset and cessation of exercise in 35°C ($p < 0.01$). The rate of heat storage (35°C, 413.6 ± 130.8 $W \cdot m^{-2}$; 13°C, 153.1 ± 112.5 $W \cdot m^{-2}$) representative of the entire 4-km time trial was greater in the heat ($p < 0.01$). When expressed per kilometre, however, difference in the rate of heat storage between conditions declined during the final kilometre of exercise ($p = 0.06$). We conclude that the current decrements in self-selected work-rate in the heat are mediated to some extent through afferent feedback arising from changes in heat storage at rest and during the early stages of exercise which serve to regulate the subsequent exercise intensity in attempt to preserve thermal homeostasis.

▶ Although performance of a brief period of exercise is increased under hot conditions,[1] the performance of prolonged exercise is reduced.[2,3] Noakes has argued that this is evidence that somewhere in our brains there is a "central governor" that restricts energy expenditure to protect the body against fatal heat stress.[4] However, the governor has never been demonstrated, and most investigators do not accept this hypothesis. The authors of this article suggest that the moderation of effort under the conditions of their study is based, at least in part, on a peripheral reflex, reflecting increased heat storage in skin and muscle, both at rest and in the early phases of an exercise bout in the heat (see Fig 4 in the original article); their data showed little cardiovascular or thermal strain, so these factors did not contribute to the moderation of effort. One strong point in this study was the provision of air movement equivalent to that encountered during a cycling competition; many trials on a treadmill or a laboratory cycle ergometer have exacerbated the effects of a given environmental temperature because there has been little air movement in the exercise laboratory. However, there was no simulation of radiant heating, which is often a further challenge in actual competition. Surprisingly, the rating of perceived exertion was no greater when the 4 km trial was run under hot conditions, so this was not a factor reducing exercise intensity.

For further reading on this subject I suggest an article by Tatterson et al.[5]

R. J. Shephard, MD (Lond), PhD, DPE

References

1. Ball D, Burrows C, Sargeant AJ. Human power output during repeated sprint cycle exercise: the influence of thermal stress. *Eur J Appl Physiol Occup Physiol.* 1999; 79:360-366.
2. Gonzalez-Alonso J, Teller C, Andersen SL, Jensen FB, Hyldig T, Nielsen B. Influence of body temperature on the development of fatigue during prolonged exercisein the heat. *J Appl Physiol.* 1999;86:1032-1039.
3. Parkin JM, Carey MF, Zhao S, Febbraio MA. Effect of ambient temperature on human skeletal muscle metabolism during fatiguing submaximal exercise. *J Appl Physiol.* 1999;86:902-908.

4. St Clair Gibson A, Noakes TD. Evidence for complex system integration and dynamic neural regulation of skeletal muscle recruitment during exercise in humans. *Br J Sports Med.* 2004;38:797-806.
5. Tatterson AJ, Hahn AG, Martin DT, Febbraio MA. Effects of heat stress on physiological responses and exercise performance in elite cyclists. *J Sci Med Sport.* 2000;3:186-193.

Sodium Balance During U.S. Football Training in the Heat: Cramp-Prone vs. Reference Players

Horswill CA, Stofan JR, Lacambra M, et al (Gatorade Sports Science Inst, Barrington, IL; et al)
Int J Sports Med 30:789-794, 2009

U.S. football players with a history of heat cramps were evaluated for the effect of physical training, sodium intake, and loss of sweat sodium on whole blood sodium concentration (BNa). Athletes ($n = 14$ males, 24 ± 1 y) were recruited and studied based on medical history, age, and position. The reference group (R, $n = 8$ without a cramping history) and cramp-prone group (C, $n = 6$, history of whole-body cramps associated with extensive sweat loss during exercise in the heat) were measured for body mass and BNa (ISTAT) before and after team training of 2.2 h in hot conditions (WBGT = 29–32°C). Intake and loss of fluid and sodium were also measured to determine respective acute balance. In R, BNa was stable pre- to post-training (138.9 ± 1.8 to 139.0 ± 2.0 mmol/L) while it tended to decline in C (137.8 ± 2.3 to 135.7 ± 4.9 mmol/L), and three subjects in C had BNa values below 135 mmol/L (131.7 ± 2.9 mmol/L). C consumed a greater percentage of total fluid as water ($p < 0.05$). Mean sweat sodium concentration was (52.6 ± 29.2 mmol/L for C and 38.3 ± 18.3 mmol/L for R ($p > 0.05$). Compared to R, C tended to experience a decline in BNa and greater acute sodium imbalance. These changes may place cramp-prone players at greater risks for developing acute sodium deficits during training.

▶ Cramps can be a very painful and debilitating experience for an athlete, and disruptive to well-planned tactics in a team sport. The problem was originally noted by industrial physiologists (miners' cramps in hot mines, and stokers' cramps on the old steamships). In such cases, the problem was thought to be an excessive loss of salt, and it could readily be treated by administration of additional salt. Large losses of fluid and salt have also been described in football players who are prone to cramps.[1-3] This small-scale study compared individuals who were prone to cramps with reference players during a bout of training in hot conditions. It found that while plasma sodium concentrations did not change in the reference group, those susceptible to cramps sustained a decrease in plasma sodium of some 2 mMol/L, perhaps caused by a combination of the ingestion of a greater volume of water (Fig 1 in the original article) and the excretion of sweat with a higher sodium ion content. One weakness in the study is that none of the subjects developed cramps during the period of observation. Further, no intergroup comparisons of urinary sodium losses were made. I now suffer from frequent nocturnal cramps, and I attribute this to declining renal function and a resultant increase in sodium loss. It is tempting to blame the athletes' cramps on salt depletion, but this does not always seem responsible for the muscle spasm. Maughan[4] found that 18% of marathon runners suffered from cramps, usually around the 35 km mark of a race, but the affected individuals had similar plasma electrolyte concentrations to their peers that were unaffected. Sustained abnormal spinal reflex activity secondary to fatigue was suggested as the cause in such situations.[5] Nevertheless, given the effectiveness of salt in treating stokers (and my own nocturnal cramps), it seems worthwhile trying salt administration as an initial treatment for athletes who are afflicted with repeated cramps.

R. J. Shephard, MD (Lond), PhD, DPE

References

1. Fowkes-Godek S, Bartolozzi AR, Godek JJ. Sweat rate and fluid turnover in American football platers compared to runners in a hot humid environment. *Br J Sports Med.* 2004;39:205-211.
2. Jacobson BH, Ranzone J, Vardiman P. Comparison of fluid weight loss between heat-related episodes and non-episodes in football players. *Int J Sports Med.* 2001;22:95-100.
3. Stofan JR, Zachwiecja JJ, Horswi CA, et al. Sweat and sopdium losses in NCAA football players; a precursor to cramps? *Int J Sports Nutr Exerc Metab.* 2005;15: 641-652.
4. Maughan RJ. Exercise-induced muscle cramps: a prospective study. *J Sport Sci.* 1986;4:31-34.
5. Schwellnus MP, Derman EW, Noakes TD. Aetiology of skeletal muscle cramps during exercise. A novel hyouthesis. *J Sport Sci.* 1997;15:277-285.

Effect of Preexercise Electrolyte Ingestion on Fluid Balance in Men and Women

Johannsen NM, Lind E, King DS, et al (Pennington Biomedical Res Ctr, Baton Rouge, LA; SUNY College at Oneonta, NY; Iowa State Univ, Ames)
Med Sci Sports Exerc 41:2017-2025, 2009

Purpose.—This article aimed to study the effect of preexercise ingestion of an electrolyte-containing beverage and meal on fluid balance during exercise in men and women.

Methods.—Twenty healthy, college-aged people (10 males, 10 females; mean ± SD = 51.2 ± 9.8 $mL \cdot kg^{-1} \cdot min^{-1}$) exercised at 58 ± 4% $\dot{V}O_{2peak}$ for 90 min, 45 min after ingesting 355 mL of chicken noodle soup (SOUP; 167 $mmol \cdot L^{-1} Na^+$), carbohydrate–electrolyte beverage (CE; 16 $mmol \cdot L^{-1} Na^+$), or water (WATER). After 90 min of exercise, participants completed a physical performance task (PPT) consisting of the calculated work that would be completed in 30 min at 60% $\dot{V}O_{2peak}$ ($n = 19$). Water was allowed *ad libitum* throughout all trials.

Results.—Fluid balance was improved in SOUP compared with WATER (-251 ± 418 vs -657 ± 593 g, respectively; $P = 0.002$) because of greater water intake and retention throughout the trial. Water intake was also greater in CE compared with WATER mostly because of an increase during the PPT. Plasma osmolality increased after ingestion of SOUP and remained elevated throughout exercise compared with both CE and WATER. Men and women had similar fluid balance results, with women having lower relative water intake and evaporative water losses compared with men. Physical performance was similar in all trials.

Conclusions.—SOUP ingested before exercise improves fluid balance because of increased *ad libitum* water intake and reduced proportional urinary water loss. The increase in water intake and, subsequently, the improved fluid balance may be because of a greater plasma osmolality before and throughout exercise (Fig 1).

▶ If an athlete is planning to exercise in the heat, it seems reasonable to preload with fluid and/or minerals; in one early study, we recommended the ingestion of 500 ml of fluid some 30 minutes before a marathon event, followed by an intake of 150 ml every 15 minutes while running. Some trials with water and/or glycerol have had mixed success, provoking a desire to urinate during the event. However, sodium ions should help retain the water within the body, at least on a short-term basis, and the American College of Sports Medicine position stand has promoted the taking of sodium-containing fluids or snacks to stimulate thirst and reduce the desire to urinate in those who plan to undertake prolonged exercise under warm conditions.[1] Previous studies have supported this suggestion. Looking at the very high salt content of many soups, a bowl of warm soup seems a very palatable way of combining salt and fluid preloading, and indeed we found soup a very effective way of getting both fluids and nutrients into an athlete who made a 5000 km cross-Canada run. The present

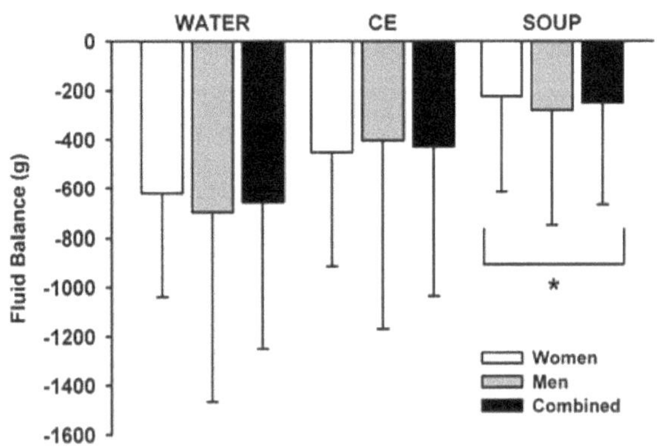

FIGURE 1.—Fluid balance after 90 min of steady-state exercise at 55% $\dot{V}O_{2peak}$ and subsequent PPT (mean ± SD). *Significantly different from WATER (treatment effect, $P < 0.05$). (Reprinted from Johannsen NM, Lind E, King DS, et al. Effect of preexercise electrolyte ingestion on fluid balance in men and women. *Med Sci Sports Exerc.* 2009;41:2017-2025, with permission from the American College of Sports Medicine.)

small-scale controlled trial of chicken-noodle soup versus a more traditional carbohydrate beverage versus water shows a substantial advantage of water retention to the soup drinkers (Fig 1). This reflected a greater water intake (water was provided ad libitum whole exercising) and a slightly reduced urinary water loss. Despite sex differences in fluid balance, the pattern of benefit was similar in male and female subjects. Plasma sodium levels were surprisingly similar in all 3 subject groups. The task was relatively modest (90 minutes of cycle ergometry at 55% of maximal oxygen intake and a wet bulb temperature of 16°C, presumably without any radiant heat load). The soup group had a net water loss of only about 300 ml. There remains a need for information on what happens when exercising under conditions where heavy sweating is likely. Finally, although fluid balance was improved by the soup, the study could not, of course, prove that its salt content was responsible—there may have been effects from other constituents; it would be interesting to repeat the experiment using a low-salt soup.

For further reading on this subject I suggest articles by Greenleaf et al,[2,3] and Sims et al.[4]

R. J. Shephard, MD (Lond), PhD, DPE

References

1. Sawka MN, Burke LM, Eichner ER, et al. American College of Sports Medicine position stand. Exercise and fluid replacement. *Med Sci Sports Exerc.* 2007;39: 377-390.
2. Greenleaf JE, Jackson CGR, Geelen G, Keil LC, Hinghofer-Szalkay H, Whittam JH. Plasma volume expansion with oral fluids in hypohydrated men at rest and during exercise. *Aviat Space Environ Med.* 1998;69:837-844.
3. Greenleaf JE, Looft-Wilson R, Wisherd JL, et al. Hypervolemia in men from fluid ingestion at rest and during exercise. *Aviat Space Environ Med.* 1998;69:374-386.
4. Sims ST, van Vilet L, Cotter JD, Rehrer NJ. Sodium loading aids fluid balance and reduces physiological strain of trained men exercising in the heat. *Med Sci Sports Exerc.* 2007;39:123-130.

Comparison of regional patch collection vs. whole body washdown for measuring sweat sodium and potassium loss during exercise

Baker LB, Stofan JR, Hamilton AA, et al (Gatorade Sports Science Inst, Barrington, IL)

J Appl Physiol 107:887-895, 2009

This study compared simultaneous whole body washdown (WBW) and regional skin surface (REG) sweat collections to generate regression equations to predict WBW sweat Na^+ concentration ($[Na^+]$) and K^+ concentration ($[K^+]$) from single- and five-site REG sweat patch collections. Athletes (10 men, 10 women) cycled in a plastic chamber for 90 min in the heat. Before exercise, the subject and bike were washed with deionized water. After the onset of sweating, sterile patches were attached to the forearm, back, chest, forehead, and thigh and removed on saturation. After exercise, the subject and bike were washed with ammonium sulfate solution to

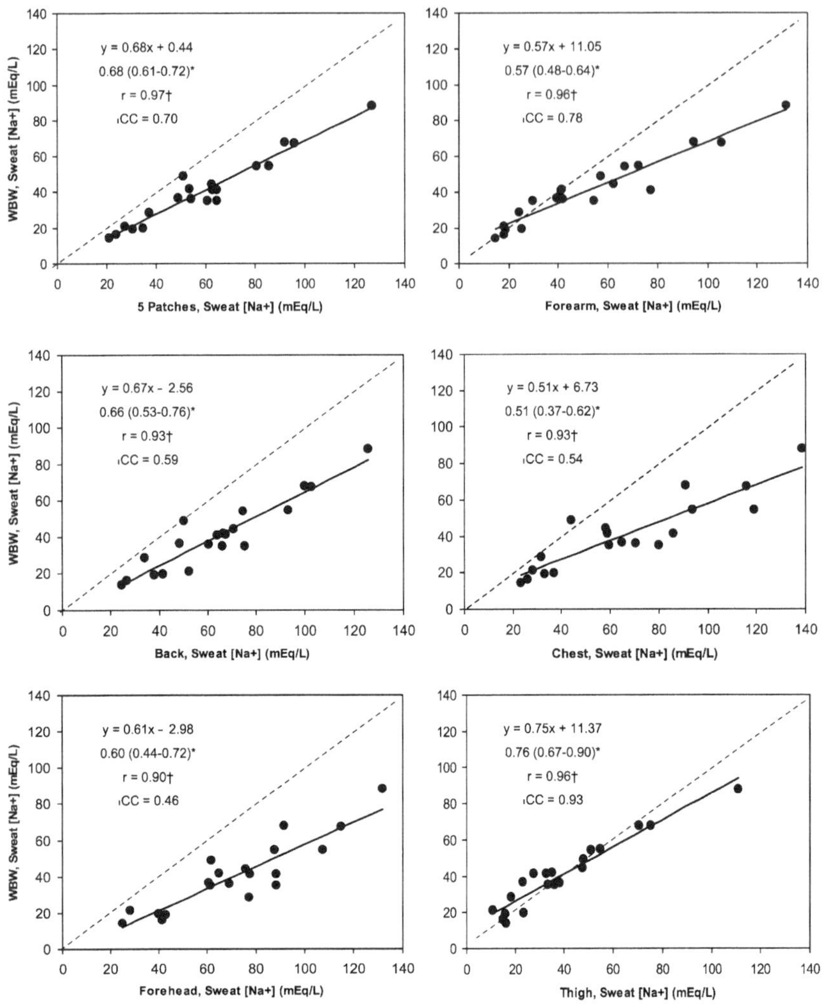

FIGURE 1.—Regression of 5-site and individual regional (REG) patch sweat Na^+ concentration ($[Na^+]$) on whole body washdown (WBW) sweat $[Na^+]$. Dashed line is line of identity. The 5-site REG sweat $[Na^+]$ was calculated from an equation weighted for local sweat rate and body surface area (35). ICC, intraclass correlation coefficient between WBW and each REG method (<0.40 indicates poor reliability, 0.40–0.75 indicates good reliability, >0.75 indicates excellent reliability; Ref. 32). Editor's note: Please check the original article for full reference. *Bootstrapped slopes with 95% confidence intervals (10,000 iterations); †$P < 0.05$ (Pearson correlation). (Reprinted from Baker LB, Stofan JR, Hamilton AA, et al. Comparison of regional patch collection vs. whole body washdown for measuring sweat sodium and potassium loss during exercise. *J Appl Physiol.* 2009;107:887-895, with permission from the American Physiological Society.)

collect all sweat electrolyte loss and determine the volume of unevaporated sweat. All individual patch sites and five-site REG (weighted for local sweat rate and body surface area) were significantly ($P = 0.000$) correlated with WBW sweat $[Na^+]$. The equation for predicting WBW sweat $[Na^+]$

from five-site REG was $y = 0.68x + 0.44$ [$r = 0.97$, intraclass correlation coefficient (ICC) = 0.70] and did not differ between sexes. There were sex differences in the regression results between five-site REG and WBW sweat [K^+] (men: $y = 0.74x + 0.30$, $r = 0.89$, ICC = 0.73; women: $y = 0.04x + 3.18$, $r = 0.03$, ICC = 0.00). Five-site REG sweat [Na^+] and [K^+] significantly overestimated that of WBW sweat (59 ± 27 vs. 41 ± 19 meq/l, $P = 0.000$ and 4.4 ± 0.7 vs. 3.6 ± 0.7 meq/l, $P = 0.000$, respectively). For both sexes, the best sites for predicting WBW sweat [Na^+] and [K^+] were the thigh (1 ± 8 meq/l < WBW, $P = 1.000$, $y = 0.75x + 11.37$, $r = 0.96$, ICC = 0.93) and chest (0.2 ± 0.3 meq/l > WBW, $P = 1.000$, $y = 0.76x + 0.55$, $r = 0.89$, ICC = 0.87), respectively. In conclusion, regression equations can be used to accurately and reliably predict WBW sweat [Na^+] and [K^+] from REG sweat collections when study conditions and techniques are similar to that of the present protocol (Fig 1).

▶ There are many good reasons for understanding sweat losses of mineral ions, from the prevention of muscle cramps and possibly even hyponatremia to the choice of appropriate replacement fluids.[1] It has generally been argued that collection of all of the sweat that has been secreted is important to accurate data; the use of regional sweat absorbing patches has been thought to exaggerate losses of sodium ions, and either to underestimate or overestimate potassium losses.[2,3] Problems arise from regional differences of sweat secretion, interactions between occlusive patches and sweat production, and possibly even electrolyte leaching from the stratum corneum. However, the procedure for collecting all of the secreted sweat is extremely cumbersome, as the present report makes clear, and interest thus continues in the possibility of collecting useful information from regional patches. The present small study seems to be one of the few that makes a direct comparison between the 2 techniques. It shows that the patches tend to overestimate sodium losses, but nevertheless can be used in equations that provide surprisingly good estimates (Fig 1). The closest predictions can be obtained from 5 patches, but a reasonable estimate can be based on data from any one of the 5 sites; the choice depends in part on restrictions imposed by a particular sport. The overall data underline the point we made many years ago that normally sweat is hypotonic, so the end-result of heat exposure is an increase of plasma sodium[1]; in most cases, hyponatremia will develop only if an excess of water is drunk, and plasma normality can usually be restored by a small increase of salt intake following an event.

R. J. Shephard, MD (Lond), PhD, DPE

References

1. Verde T, Shephard RJ, Corey P, Moore R. Sweat composition in exercise and in the heat. *J Appl Physiol.* 1982;53:1540-1545.
2. Patterson MJ, Galloway SDR, Nimmo MA. Variations in regional sweat composition in normal human males. *Exp Physiol.* 2000;85:869-875.
3. Shirreffs SM, Maughan RJ. Whole body sweat collection in humans: an improved method with preliminary data on electrolyte content. *J Appl Physiol.* 1997;82:336-341.

Urine dipstick testing to rule out rhabdomyolysis in patients with suspected heat injury

Young SE, Miller MA, Docherty M (Darnall Army Med Ctr, TX; et al)
Am J Emerg Med 27:875-877, 2009

Background.—Heat injury is a common, potentially life-threatening medical condition. In austere or mass-casualty conditions an easy to use, sensitive screening test could be a valuable tool to care providers and evacuation planners.

Objective.—The objective of the study was to determine if a simple urine dipstick test for blood is sensitive for detection of rhabdomyolysis in the suspected heat injury patient.

Material and Methods.—A convenience sample of patients presenting to a military community hospital Emergency Department during summer months with a presenting complaint consistent with suspected heat injury had urine dipstick testing performed for blood and compared with the results of formal urinalysis and serum creatine kinase.

Results.—60 patients were enrolled in the study, seven had creatine kinase levels greater than 1000U/L, 14 had levels greater than 500U/L, and 26 had levels greater than 250 U/L. Using 1000U/L, urine dipstick testing had a sensitivity of 14% and a specificity of 85%.

Conclusions.—Urine dipstick testing for blood is not a useful screening test for rhabdomyolysis in patients suspected to have significant heat injury (Table 1).

▶ Rhabdomyolysis is a feature of severe heat stress, and can progress to renal failure, arrhythmia, and death. The idea of using a simple urinary dipstick as a method of screening participants in an event where there have been a massive number of heat casualties is thus worth considering. The main objection to use of myoglobin levels as a clinical tool seems the relatively slow time course of muscle damage. The myoglobin concentration in the serum does not begin to rise until about 2 hours after the initiating event,[1] and does not peak till about 6 hours. Renal failure is not the only hazard of heat stress, and the idea of allowing a person to continue in competition or other physically demanding activity until myoglobin is detectable in the urine seems unwise. In my view, it would be better to specify rectal temperatures at which exercise should be halted and treatment

TABLE 1.—Performance of UD in the Evaluation of Patients with Suspected Heat Injury

	Serum CK (U/L)			
	≤500	>500	≤1000	>1000
UD				
Positive	7	2	8	1
Negative	39	12	45	6

begun. The authors of this report note that as judged from creatine kinase release, considerable muscle damage must occur before the dipstick gives a reliable indication of this problem (Table 1). The findings are also limited by the fact that some patients had received fluids before the dipstick tests were performed.

R. J. Shephard, MD (Lond), PhD, DPE

Reference

1. Penn AS. Myoglobinuria. In: Engel AG, Banker BQ, eds. *Myology.* New York: Mcgraw-Hill; 1986:1785-1805.

Efficacy of Field Treatments to Reduce Body Core Temperature in Hyperthermic Subjects

Sinclair WH, Rudzki SJ, Leicht AS, et al (James Cook Univ, Queensland, AUSTRALIA; Directorate of Occupational Health and Safety, Canberra, AUSTRALIA; et al)

Med Sci Sports Exerc 41:1984-1990, 2009

Purpose.—To contrast the effects of three postcooling techniques in reducing body core temperature (T_c) in exercise-induced hyperthermic participants on the cessation of exercise.

Methods.—Eleven healthy active male volunteers were cooled during a 40-min period using three different methods: ice packs to the neck, axillae, and groin (ICE); water spray and fan (FAN); and 2 L of chilled (20°C) intravenous saline administered during a 20-min period (IV). Rate of decrease in T_c, cardiovascular responses, and any incidence of reported adverse effects were investigated. Trials were presented in a counterbalanced order with the volunteers' body core temperature being elevated to 40.0°C on three occasions via an intermittent walk–run (2 min at 6 $km \cdot h^{-1}$ and 4 min at 10 $km \cdot h^{-1}$) protocol conducted within a climate-controlled chamber (34.2 ± 0.5°C and 62.3 ± 3.1% relative humidity).

Results.—Rate of T_c reduction during the first 20 min of ooling was greater for FAN compared with ICE (0.09 ± 0.02°$C \cdot min^{-1}$ vs 0.07 ± 0.02°$C \cdot min^{-1}$, $P < 0.05$), whereas IV did not differ with the other trials (0.08 ± 0.01°$C \cdot min^{-1}$, $P > 0.05$). Three participants complained of numbness or paresthesia in their arm or hand during administration of the chilled saline, although these symptoms resolved within 5 min of ceasing the infusion.

Conclusions.—All three cooling techniques reduced T_c and would be suitable for first aid application in a field setting during transportation

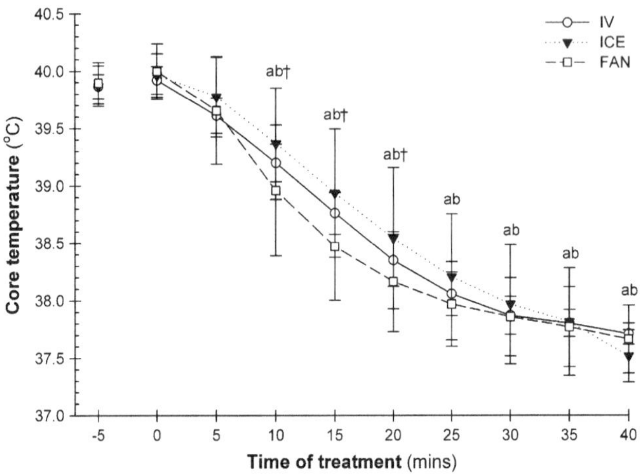

FIGURE 1.—Mean ± SD core temperature at the end of exercise (5 min), start (0 min), and during IV, ICE, and FAN cooling techniques. $^{a}P < 0.05$ versus exercise (5 min); $^{b}P < 0.05$ versus start of treatment (0 min); †$P < 0.05$ ICE versus FAN. (Reprinted from Sinclair WH, Rudzki SJ, Leicht AS, et al. Efficacy of field treatments to reduce body core temperature in hyperthermic subjects. *Med Sci Sports Exerc.* 2009;41:1984-1990.)

to adequate medical facilities. Chilled IV saline did not produce any contraindications, providing a suitable alternative for T_c cooling (Fig 1).

▶ Methods for the hospital treatment of a hyperthermic patient are well established, but cellular damage, inflammatory and coagulatory responses, and the resultant morbidity and mortality[1,2] depend on the time for which the body temperature has been elevated. Unless the hospital is very near at hand, it is important to initiate treatment in the field, preferably bringing the core temperature below 40°C within 30 minutes.[3] Unfortunately, optimal methods of treatment are rarely available in the field. The present small-scale trial brought a panel of 11 volunteers to a level of hyperthermia that many committees of Human Experimentation might have criticized (40°C; the maximum allowed in our laboratory is 39.5°C). The study found that 3 potential methods of field treatment (a powerful industrial fan, ice packs, and cooled intravenous saline) were all effective and had the best response to the fan (Fig 1). Concerns about arrhythmias from the cold infusion[4,5] cannot really be dismissed on the basis of these tests, as the average age of the subjects was only 23 years; evaluation of this risk would require trials on a much larger sample of older adults.

R. J. Shephard, MD (Lond), PhD, DPE

References

1. Casa DJ, Maresh CM, Armstrong LE, et al. Intravenous versus oral rehydration during a brief period: responses to subsequent exercise in the heat. *Med Sci Sport Exerc.* 2000;32:124-133.
2. Shibolet S, Coll R, Gilat T. Heatstroke: its clinical picture and mechanism in 36 cases. *Quart J Med.* 1967;36:525-548.

3. Bynum GD, Pandolf KB, Schuette WH, et al. Induced hyperthermia in sedated humans and the concept of critical thermal maximum. *Am J Physiol.* 1978;235: R228-R236.
4. Proulx CI, Ducharme MB, Kenny GP. Effect of water temperature on cooling efficiency during hyperthermia in humans. *J Appl Physiol.* 2003;94:1317-1323.
5. Proulx CI, Ducharme MB, Kenny GP. Safe cooling limits from exercise-induced hyperthermia. *Eur J Appl Physiol.* 2006;96:434-445.

Comparisons of Cubed Ice, Crushed Ice, and Wetted Ice on Intramuscular and Surface Temperature Changes

Dykstra JH, Hill HM, Miller MG, et al (Calvin College, Grand Rapids, MI; Palm Beach Atlantic Univ, FL; Western Michigan Univ, Kalamazoo; et al)
J Athl Train 44:136-141, 2009

Context.—Many researchers have investigated the effectiveness of different types of cold application, including cold whirlpools, ice packs, and chemical packs. However, few have investigated the effectiveness of different types of ice used in ice packs, even though ice is one of the most common forms of cold application.

Objective.—To evaluate and compare the cooling effectiveness of ice packs made with cubed, crushed, and wetted ice on intramuscular and skin surface temperatures.

Design.—Repeated-measures counterbalanced design.

Setting.—Human performance research laboratory.

Patients or Other Participants.—Twelve healthy participants (6 men, 6 women) with no history of musculoskeletal disease and no known pre-existing inflammatory conditions or recent orthopaedic injuries to the lower extremities.

Intervention(s).—Ice packs made with cubed, crushed, or wetted ice were applied to a standardized area on the posterior aspect of the right gastrocnemius for 20 minutes. Each participant was given separate ice pack treatments, with at least 4 days between treatment sessions.

Main Outcome Measure(s).—Cutaneous and intramuscular (2 cm plus one-half skinfold measurement) temperatures of the right gastrocnemius were measured every 30 seconds during a 20-minute baseline period, a 20-minute treatment period, and a 120-minute recovery period.

Results.—Differences were observed among all treatments. Compared with the crushed-ice treatment, the cubed-ice and wetted-ice treatments produced lower surface and intramuscular temperatures. Wetted ice produced the greatest overall temperature change during treatment and recovery, and crushed ice produced the smallest change.

Conclusions.—As administered in our protocol, wetted ice was superior to cubed or crushed ice at reducing surface temperatures, whereas both cubed ice and wetted ice were superior to crushed ice at reducing intramuscular temperatures.

▶ The authors hypothesize that creating a greater temperature change more quickly may result in more effective treatment. They found that wetted ice packs lowered surface temperature more than either cubed or crushed ice. Also, wetted ice and cubed ice lowered intramuscular temperature more than crushed ice. Based on this, they conclude that wetted ice packs may be more effective than cubed or crushed ice packs. This study was done on persons who had no injuries or musculoskeletal problems. The next step would be to test persons with an injury to determine whether there is a clinically significant difference between these 3 types of ice packs. At this point it is impossible to state whether wetted ice is more effective for treating injuries and inducing analgesia. Nevertheless, the study does imply that if "colder is better" then wetted ice may be more effective. Also, as the authors state in their discussion, their findings imply that premade ice packs that have begun to melt should not be drained before use or discarded as they may be more effective than a freshly made ice pack.

D. E. Feldman, PT, PhD

Effect of oxygen breathing and perfluorocarbon emulsion treatment on air bubbles in adipose tissue during decompression sickness

Randsoe T, Hyldegaard O (Copenhagen Univ Hosp, Denmark; DAN Europe Res Foundation, Italy)

J Appl Physiol 107:1857-1863, 2009

Decompression sickness (DCS) after air diving has been treated with success by means of combined normobaric oxygen breathing and intravascular perfluorocarbon (PFC) emulsions causing increased survival rate and faster bubble clearance from the intravascular compartment. The beneficial PFC effect has been explained by the increased transport capacity of oxygen and inert gases in blood. However, previous reports have shown that extravascular bubbles in lipid tissue of rats suffering from DCS will initially grow during oxygen breathing at normobaric conditions. We hypothesize that the combined effect of normobaric oxygen breathing and intravascular PFC infusion could lead to either enhanced extravascular bubble growth on decompression due to the increased oxygen supply, or that PFC infusion could lead to faster bubble elimination due to the increased solubility and transport capacity in blood for nitrogen causing faster nitrogen tissue desaturation. In anesthetized rats decompressed from a 60-min hyperbaric exposure breathing air at 385 kPa, we visually followed the resolution of micro-air bubbles injected into abdominal adipose tissue while the rats breathed either air, oxygen, or oxygen breathing combined with PFC infusion. All bubble observations were done at 101.3 kPa pressure. During oxygen breathing with or without combined PFC infusion, bubbles disappeared faster compared with air breathing. Combined oxygen breathing and PFC infusion caused faster bubble disappearance compared with oxygen breathing. The combined effect of oxygen breathing and PFC infusion neither prevented nor increased transient bubble growth time, rate, or growth ratio compared with oxygen breathing alone. We conclude that oxygen breathing in combination with PFC infusion causes faster bubble disappearance and does not exacerbate transient bubble growth. PFC infusion may be a valuable adjunct therapy during the first-aid treatment of DCS at normobaric conditions.

▶ The standard treatment for decompression sickness has consisted of recompression in a pressure chamber combined with hyperbaric oxygen breathing. Recompression is intended to reduce bubble size, while the increased partial pressure of oxygen should improve tissue oxygenation and speed the elimination of dissolved inert gas. However, there is an undesirable initial bubble growth during oxygen breathing because the blood has a higher carrying capacity for oxygen than for nitrogen; oxygen moves into the tissue bubbles faster than nitrogen is removed.[1-3] One possible way of countering this problem is the administration of a polyfluorene hydrocarbon (PFC) infusion because nitrogen dissolves readily in PFCs.[4] The present authors tested this new approach during the decompression of rats; a combination of PFC infusion and oxygen breathing did not speed early bubble growth and it also accelerated ultimate bubble disappearance. It seems time to make some careful trials of this approach in humans suffering from decompression sickness.

R. J. Shephard, MD (Lond), PhD, DPE

References

1. Hyldegaard O, Madsen J. Effect of air, heliox and oxygen breathing on air bubbles in aqueous tissues in the rat. *Undersea Hyperb Med.* 1994;21:413-424.
2. Hyldegaard O, Madsen J. Influence of heliox, oxygen and N2O-O2 breathing on N2 bubbles in adipose tissue. *Undersea Biomed Res.* 1989;16:185-193.
3. Hyldegaard O, Møller M, Madsen J. Effect of heliox, oxygen and N2O-O2 breathing on injected bubbles in spinal white matter. *Undersea Biomed Res.* 1991;18:361-371.
4. Dromsky DM, Spiess BD, Fahlman A. Treatment of decompression sickness in swine with intravenous perflurocarbon emulsion. *Aviat Space Environ Med.* 2004;75:301-305.

Increased serum levels of the brain damage marker S100B after apnea in trained breath-hold divers: a study including respiratory and cardiovascular observations

Andersson JPA, Linér MH, Jönsson H (Lund Univ, Sweden)

J Appl Physiol 107:809-815, 2009

The concentration of the protein S100B in serum is used as a brain damage marker in various conditions. We wanted to investigate whether a voluntary, prolonged apnea in trained breath-hold divers resulted in an increase of S100B in serum. Nine trained breath-hold divers performed a protocol mimicking the procedures they use during breath-hold training and competition, including extensive preapneic hyperventilation and glossopharyngeal insufflation, in order to perform a maximum-duration apnea, i.e., "static apnea" (average: 335 s, range: 281–403 s). Arterial blood samples were collected and cardiovascular variables recorded. Arterial partial pressures of O_2 and CO_2 (Pa_{O_2} and Pa_{CO_2}) were 128 Torr and 20 Torr, respectively, at the start of apnea. The degree of asphyxia at the end of apnea was considerable, with Pa_{O_2} and Pa_{CO_2} reaching 28 Torr and 45 Torr, respectively. The concentration of S100B in serum transiently increased from 0.066 µg/l at the start of apnea to 0.083 µg/l after the apnea ($P < 0.05$). The increase in S100B is attributed to the asphyxia or to other physiological responses to apnea, for example, increased blood pressure, and probably indicates a temporary opening of the blood-brain barrier. It is not possible to conclude that the observed increase in S100B levels in serum after a maximal-duration apnea reflects a serious injury to the brain, although the results raise concerns considering negative long-term effects. At the least, the results indicate that prolonged, voluntary apnea affects the integrity of the central nervous system and do not preclude cumulative effects (Fig 1).

▶ Repeated exposure to hypoxia is known to have adverse effects on cerebral function. I still recall a very successful RAF fighter pilot who (in the days of rather primitive oxygen systems) had downed many Luftwaffe planes by flying above his antagonists at an altitude where he became quite hypoxic. When I

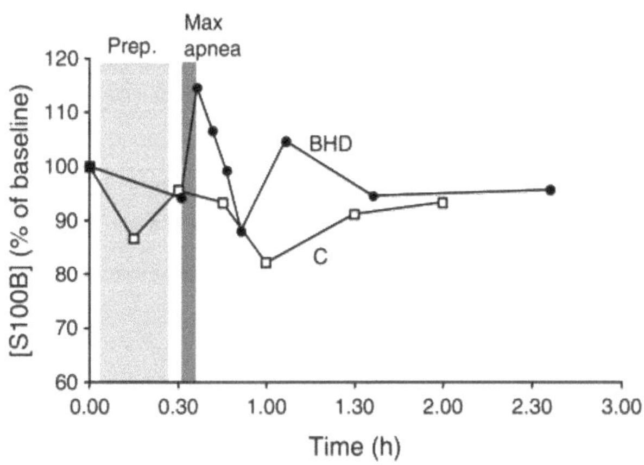

FIGURE 1.—Concentration of S100B in serum, in % of baseline, before apnea and up to 120 min after maximal-duration apnea. Values are means from 9 breath-hold divers (BHD; ●) and 6 resting control subjects (C; □). Bars indicating SD have been omitted for clarity. Vertical gray bars indicate the period for preparations and the maximal-duration apnea performed by the breath-hold divers. (Reprinted from Andersson JPA, Linér MH, Jönsson H. Increased serum levels of the brain damage marker S100B after apnea in trained breath-hold divers: a study including respiratory and cardiovascular observations. *J Appl Physiol*. 2009;107:809-815, with permission from the American Physiological Society.)

knew him, some 10 years later, the effects on his reasoning powers had become all too obvious. More recently, several articles have drawn attention to similar problems in mountaineers. Breath-hold diving is another pursuit where partial pressures of arterial oxygen can drop to exceedingly low values; the world record breath-hold is now for longer than 10 minutes. Potential symptoms ranging from a loss of motor control to a total loss of consciousness are well documented, and indeed have led to a disqualification of some 10% of competitors.[1,2] Blood concentrations of the cerebral protein S100B are now used clinically as a marker of cerebral ischemia and resulting brain damage.[3,4] It is disquieting to see that breath-hold diving also leads to some increases in this marker (Fig 1), with arterial oxygen saturation falling to 54%. However, the changes seem quite transient and are much smaller than in some of the clinical reports. Further research is thus needed to determine whether the observed peak concentration of the marker reflects cerebral injury or is simply an indication of a temporary weakening of the blood-brain barrier.

R. J. Shephard, MD (Lond), PhD, DPE

References

1. Fitz-Clarke JR. Adverse events in competitive breath-hold diving. *Undersea Hyperb Med.* 2006;33:55-62.
2. Lindholm P. Loss of motor control and/or loss of consciousness during breath-hold competitions. *Int J Sports Med.* 2007;28:295-299.
3. Jönsson H, Johnsson P, Birch-Iensen M, Alling C, Westaby S, Blomquist S. S100B as a predictor of size and outcome of stroke after cardiac surgery. *Ann Thorac Surg.* 2001;71:1433-1437.
4. Rothermundt M, Peters M, Prehn JHM, Arolt V. S100B in brain damage and neurodegeneration. *Microsc Res Tech.* 2003;60:614-632.

Exaggerated Pulmonary Hypertension During Mild Exercise in Chronic Mountain Sickness

Stuber T, Sartori C, Schwab M, et al (Univ Hosp of Bern, Switzerland; Univ Hosp, Lausanne, Switzerland; et al)
Chest 137:388-392, 2010

Background.—Chronic mountain sickness (CMS) is an important public health problem and is characterized by exaggerated hypoxemia, erythrocytosis, and pulmonary hypertension. While pulmonary hypertension is a leading cause of morbidity and mortality in patients with CMS, it is relatively mild and its underlying mechanisms are not known. We speculated that during mild exercise associated with daily activities, pulmonary hypertension in CMS is much more pronounced.

Methods.—We estimated pulmonary artery pressure by using echocardiography at rest and during mild bicycle exercise at 50 W in 30 male patients with CMS and 32 age-matched, healthy control subjects who were born and living at an altitude of 3,600 m.

Results.—The modest, albeit significant difference of the systolic right-ventricular-to-right-atrial pressure gradient between patients with CMS and controls at rest (30.3 ± 8.0 vs 25.4 ± 4.5 mm Hg, $P = 5.002$) became more than three times larger during mild bicycle exercise (56.4 ± 19.0 vs 39.8 ± 8.0 mm Hg, $P < .001$).

Conclusions.—Measurements of pulmonary artery pressure at rest greatly underestimate pulmonary artery pressure during daily activity in patients with CMS. The marked pulmonary hypertension during mild exercise associated with daily activity may explain why this problem is a leading cause of morbidity and mortality in patients with CMS.

▶ It is well known that hypoxia increases the pulmonary arterial pressure in an attempt to boost perfusion of the upper part of the lungs and thus increase oxygen intake. It also has long been recognized that the prime candidate for a severe acute attack of mountain sickness is the High Andes mine worker who visits a big city on the coast, catching the last bus back to work, just in time to join his or her shift.[1-3] This study was undertaken at a relatively modest altitude from the viewpoint of mountain sickness (3600 m), but it makes the important point that in individuals with chronic mountain sickness, the modest pulmonary hypertension demonstrable by echocardiography under resting conditions is tripled by light cycle ergometer exercise (a work rate of only 50 W [Fig 1 in the original article], comparable with quite modest daily activities). The exercise response reflects in part an increase in pulmonary blood flow and in part a further decrease in arterial oxygen saturation during physical activity. This study was limited to individuals who were born and living at an altitude of 3600 m and had developed chronic mountain sickness. Acute effects at the same altitude might conceivably be more marked in groups normally resident at sea level, but taking a skiing holiday at 3600 m. However, this is not necessarily the case since chronic mountain sickness may have led to structural changes in the pulmonary vessels of the individuals studied in this report. During acute exposures, any hypertension reflects simply a spasm of the pulmonary arterioles.

R. J. Shephard, MD (Lond), PhD, DPE

References

1. Peñaloza D, Sime F. Chronic cor pulmonale due to loss of altitude acclimatization (chronic mountain sickness). *Am J Med.* 1971;50:728-743.
2. Pak O, Aldashev A, Welsh D, Peacock A. The effects of hypoxia on the cells of the pulmonary vasculature. *Eur Respir J.* 2007;30:364-372.
3. Kato M, Staub NC. Response of small pulmonary arteries to unilobar hypoxia and hypercapnia. *Circ Res.* 1966;19:426-440.

Optic nerve sheath diameter correlates with the presence and severity of acute mountain sickness: evidence for increased intracranial pressure

Fagenholz PJ, Gutman JA, Murray AF, et al (Pheriche Clinic, Spring Season, Nepal; et al)

J Appl Physiol 106:1207-1211, 2009

Increased intracranial pressure is suspected in the pathogenesis of acute mountain sickness (AMS), but no studies have correlated it with the presence or severity of AMS. We sought to determine whether increased optic nerve sheath diameter, a surrogate measure of intracranial pressure, is associated with the presence and severity of AMS. We performed a cross-sectional study of travelers ascending through Pheriche, Nepal (4,240 m), from March 3 to May 14, 2006. AMS was assessed using the Lake Louise score. Optic nerve sheath diameter was measured by ultrasound. Ultrasound exams were performed and read by separate blinded observers. Two-hundred eighty seven subjects were enrolled. Ten of these underwent repeat examination. Mean optic nerve sheath diameter was 5.34 mm [95% confidence interval (CI) 5.18–5.51 mm] in the 69 subjects with AMS vs. 4.46 mm (95% CI 4.39–4.54 mm) in the 218 other subjects ($P < 0.0001$). There was also a positive association between optic nerve sheath diameter and total Lake Louise score (P for trend < 0.0001). In a multivariate logistic regression model of factors associated with AMS, optic nerve sheath diameter was strongly associated with AMS (odds ratio 6.3; 95% CI, 3.7–10.8; $P < 0.001$). In 10 subjects with repeat examinations, change in Lake Louise score had a strong positive correlation with change in optic nerve sheath diameter ($R^2 = 0.84$, $P < 0.001$). Optic nerve sheath diameter, a proxy for intracranial pressure, is associated with the presence and severity of AMS (Fig 2).

► It is widely believed that some of the manifestations of acute mountain sickness, particularly the severe headache, reflect either cerebral edema or dilatation of cerebral blood vessels in an attempt to compensate for hypoxia;[1-3] this view is substantiated by frank cerebral edema in the more severe cases, but the rise of intracranial pressure has not previously had direct and conclusive verification for minor episodes of mountain sickness. This study was conducted at moderate altitude (4240 m). It appears to have been carried out carefully. The sample size was substantial relative to earlier attempts at answering the same question (69 affected subjects and 218 controls). Acute mountain sickness was diagnosed using the standard Lake Louise criteria, and intracerebral pressure was inferred from an ultrasound measurement of optic nerve sheath diameter. The association between acute mountain sickness symptoms and optical sheath diameter was strong (Fig 2), with a clear difference between affected subjects and controls; moreover, the 2 variables moved in parallel as the condition improved or worsened. The study did not differentiate between the 2 previously postulated causes (hypoxic vasodilatation and edema formation), and further laboratory studies (likely using this ultrasonic technique) are needed to set

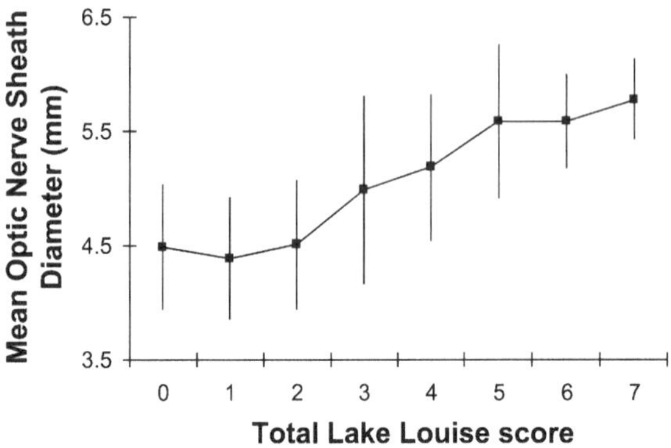

FIGURE 2.—Relationship between Lake Louise score and optic nerve sheath diameter (ONSD). Data from 287 subjects in Pheriche, Nepal. The upward trend in ONSD starts at a Lake Louise score of 3, the threshold for acute mountain sickness (AMS). Whiskers denote the SD. For all data, P for trend < 0.001. (Reprinted from Fagenholz PJ, Gutman JA, Murray AF, et al. Optic nerve sheath diameter correlates with the presence and severity of acute mountain sickness: evidence for increased intracranial pressure. *J Appl Physiol.* 2009;106:1207-1211, with permission from American Physiological Society.)

pharmacological prevention and treatment of acute mountain sickness on a firmer basis.

R. J. Shephard, MD (Lond), PhD, DPE

References

1. Basnyat B, Murdoch D. High altitude illness. *Lancet.* 2003;361:1967-1974.
2. Hackett PH, Roach RC. High altitude illness. *N Engl J Med.* 2001;345:107-114.
3. Roach RC, Hackett PH. Frontiers of hypoxia research: acute mountain sickness. *J Exp Biol.* 2001;204:3161-3170.

Safety of Double-Dose Transdermal Scopolamine

Bar R, Gil A, Tal D (Israel Naval Med Inst, Haifa)
Pharmacotherapy 29:1082-1088, 2009

Study Objective.—To evaluate the safety of double-dose transdermal scopolamine patch therapy.

Design.—Randomized, crossover, double-blind study.

Setting.—Motion sickness clinic in Haifa, Israel.

Participants.—Twenty male sailors aged 18–21 years whose seasickness symptoms improved only slightly or not at all with a single transdermal scopolamine patch.

Intervention.—Subjects received either two transdermal scopolamine patches or one scopolamine patch plus a placebo patch for 24 hours (first session). After at least 1 week from the end of the first session, they received the other treatment for 24 hours (second session).

Measurements and Main Results.—Plasma scopolamine concentrations, physiologic (heart rate and blood pressure), visual, and cognitive function parameters, and adverse effects were assessed before the first session (baseline) and after each 24-hour session. Visual function was tested again 24 hours after patch removal. Subjects also completed an adverse-effects questionnaire immediately after and 24 hours after patch removal for both treatment sessions. A significant difference was found in mean plasma scopolamine concentrations between the single-dose and double-dose treatments (81 vs 127 pg/ml [therapeutic level 100 pg/ml], $p<0.01$). No significant differences were found in heart rate, blood pressure, cognitive function, or visual function measurements. Mild blurred vision was the only adverse effect for which there was a significant difference between the single-dose and double-dose treatments; however, this adverse effect was judged to be not clinically significant.

Conclusion.—Double-dose transdermal scopolamine may improve treatment in patients who fail to respond to a single patch by increasing the plasma scopolamine concentration, without aggravating systemic, visual, or cognitive adverse effects. Thus we recommend that a double dose can be administered safely to these patients (Table 3).

▶ Seasickness remains an important limiting factor in long distance sailing events. In severe weather, up to 60% of even experienced crew members can be seriously incapacitated.[1,2] Scopolamine is generally considered as the most effective remedy for seasickness, and it is commonly applied as a transdermal patch that releases a steady stream of the drug into the blood stream.

TABLE 3.— Results of the 24-Hour Adverse-Effects Questionnaire by Severity Level

	No. (%) of Participants[a]					
	Single-Dose Treatment (n = 18)			Double-Dose Treatment (n = 19)		
Adverse Effect	None	Mild	Moderate-Severe	None	Mild	Moderate-Severe
Near-sighted blurred vision	10 (56)	6 (33)	2 (11)	11 (58)	4 (21)	4 (21)
Far-sighted blurred vision	15 (83)[b]	2 (11)[c]	1 (6)	9 (47)[b]	9 (47)[c]	1 (5)
Dazzle[d]	15 (83)	2 (11)	1 (6)	15 (79)	2 (10)	2 (10)
Eye irritation	13 (72)	4 (22)	1 (6)	15 (79)	3 (16)	1 (5)
Somnolence	6 (33)	4 (22)	8 (44)	7 (37)	3 (16)	9 (47)
Difficulty sleeping	17 (94)	0 (0)	1 (6)	17 (89)	0 (0)	2 (10)
Headache	11 (61)	6 (33)	1 (6)	11 (58)	7 (37)	1 (5)
Constipation	18 (100)	0 (0)	0 (0)	19 (100)	0 (0)	0 (0)
Difficulty urinating	18 (100)	0 (0)	0 (0)	19 (100)	0 (0)	0 (0)
Palpitations	16 (89)	1 (6)	1 (6)	17 (89)	1 (5)	1 (5)
Dyspnea	16 (89)	2 (11)	0 (0)	18 (95)	1 (5)	0 (0)
Depression	16 (89)	2 (11)	0 (0)	16 (84)	1 (5)	2 (10)
Irritability	17 (94)	1 (6)	0 (0)	16 (84)	3 (16)	0 (0)
Difficulty concentrating	9 (50)	6 (33)	3 (17)	6 (32)	7 (37)	6 (32)
Physical weakness	7 (39)	7 (39)	4 (22)	6 (32)	5 (26)	8 (42)
Mental weakness	13 (72)	3 (17)	2 (11)	11 (58)	3 (16)	5 (26)
Skin reaction	17 (94)	0 (0)	1 (6)	17 (89)	0 (0)	2 (10)

[a]Two subjects receiving the single-dose treatment and one subject receiving the double-dose treatment did not complete the questionnaire after 24 hours of therapy.

[b,c]$p<0.05$ for the respective comparisons between treatments; no other significant differences in adverse effects were found between treatments.

[d]Occurs as a result of illumination too intense for adaptation by the eye.

However, about a third of patients fail to show the desired benefit with a single patch, presumably because the drug does not reach the required concentration in the blood stream. It remains unclear whether the problem is slow skin absorption or rapid breakdown and urinary excretion of the scopolamine. This study took a small group of young scopolamine-resistant patients, showing that by using 2 patches simultaneously, blood concentrations could be brought to an effective therapeutic level (this should reach 100 pg/ml at peak, 8-12 hours after application of the patch). Moreover, there was no substantial increase in side effects with use of a second patch (Table 3) other than some increase in blurring of vision. A second patch thus seems a reasonable option for those who fail to respond to a single patch.

R. J. Shephard, MD (Lond), PhD, DPE

References

1. Reason JT, Brand JJ. *Motion Sickness.* London: Academic Press; 1975.
2. Griffin MJ. *Handbook of Human Vibration.* London: Academic Press; 1990. pp. 271-332.

9 Special Considerations: Elderly, Women, and Children

Aerobic Fitness and Mode of Travel to School in English Schoolchildren

Voss C, Sandercock G (Univ of Essex, Colchester, UK)

Med Sci Sports Exerc 42:281-287, 2010

Purpose.—Cycling to school is positively associated with aerobic fitness in Danish schoolchildren and adolescents. The aim of the present study was to determine whether a positive association exists between active travel and aerobic fitness in English schoolchildren, where cycling to school is rare.

Methods.—Participants ($n = 6085$, 47% girls, aged 10.0–15.9 yr) were recruited as part of the East of England Healthy Hearts study. Mass and stature were measured, and body mass index (BMI) was calculated. Aerobic fitness was assessed using the 20-m shuttle run test (20-mSRT); mode of travel to school and physical activity (PA) were assessed by a questionnaire. Differences in BMI, PA, and fitness by travel mode were assessed by ANOVA and ANCOVA. Participants were categorized as "fit" or "unfit" on the basis of existing cutoffs related to adult health. Logistic regression was applied to calculate age, BMI, and PA-adjusted odds of being classified as fit according to travel mode.

Results.—Walking was the most common travel mode to school (50%), and cycling was least frequent (8%). Walkers and cyclists of both sexes were significantly fitter than passive transport users, even after controlling for PA. Walking and cycling were associated with an increased likelihood of being categorized as fit in boys and girls. After adjustment for PA, this association remained significant only in girls. No association was observed between travel mode and BMI.

Conclusions.—These data confirm findings from countries where cycling is very common in showing that cycling to school is positively associated with aerobic fitness. This study adds to the existing literature by showing that walkers and cyclists are more likely to be classified as fit using recognized cut points. Those who walk and cycle to school may, therefore, be at reduced risk for developing chronic diseases in adulthood.

▶ This is a particularly interesting study. When one visits Denmark, one is struck with the commonplace use of the bicycle for public transportation, and studies from that country have demonstrated what one might suspect—greater aerobic fitness levels in youth who cycle to school. It would seem to be an important message, but the next question is, would this hold true for other countries? So here are data supporting this finding in Great Britain, where cycling to school is relatively uncommon. Cycling is an activity that almost all children enjoy (even the obese, in its nonweight-bearing nature), and these data provide ammunition for those promoting cycling to school, or building safe bike paths, or emphasizing cycling education in schools. There is one concern about such findings, though: can one confidently assume that the results of the study indicate that cycling to school will improve physical fitness? Could it be that youth who are more physically fit are more likely to bike? Who knows?

T. Rowland, MD

A 3-year longitudinal analysis of changes in fitness, physical activity, fatness and screen time

Aires L, Andersen LB, Mendonça D, et al (Univ of Porto, Portugal; Univ of Southern Denmark, Odense)

Acta Paediatr 99:140-144, 2010

Aim.—To analyse whether changes in physical activity index (PAI), screen time (ST: television, computer) and body mass index (BMI) made a contribution to longitudinal changes in fitness of children and adolescents. Additionally, we analysed the interaction between baseline fitness level and changes in fitness.

Methods.—This is a 3-year longitudinal study of 345 high school students aged 11–19 years. Students performed curl-ups, push-ups and 20-m shuttle run tests from Fitnessgram. PA and ST were evaluated using a standard questionnaire. Standardized scores of fitness tests were summed. Changes over time were calculated as Δ_1 (2007 minus 2006), Δ_2 (2008 minus 2007) and Δ_3 (2008 minus 2006).

Results.—Changes in PAI were positively and independently associated with changes in fitness in Δ_1, Δ_2 and Δ_3. Changes in BMI were negatively associated with changes in fitness in Δ_3. Participants highly fit at baseline were those who showed positive changes in PAI over Δ_3, decreased changes in ST and had the lowest increase in BMI over 3 years compared with those low-fit at baseline.

Conclusions.—Changes in BMI were associated with changes in fitness over 3 years. However, changes in PAI were the best predictor for changes in fitness in each year and over the 3 years of evaluation in youth.

▶ It is generally considered that sedentary time spent in front of a television or computer screen is a major culprit in the current trends for increasing obesity and lower fitness among youth. These issues are, in fact, complex, and cause and effect relationships have not been firmly established. For instance, if in a cross-sectional study fatness and physical activity are negatively associated, does it mean limited activity is a cause of obesity? Or that obese children exercise less? The same problem occurs with screen time and obesity. Which comes first? And then there is the problem that measures typically used to indicate physical fitness, such as the shuttle run, are negatively related to body fat itself. This study is one of the few that looks at these questions in a longitudinal fashion and tries to tease out separate independent factors. We need more investigations like this. One interesting finding here is that changes in screen time were not associated with those in measures of physical fitness. This supports someone's intriguing suggestion that a child could theoretically watch a great deal of television and still have time to train for a marathon race.

T. Rowland, MD

High Exercise Levels are Related to Favorable Sleep Patterns and Psychological Functioning in Adolescents: A Comparison of Athletes and Controls

Brand S, Gerber M, Beck J, et al (Psychiatric Hosp of the Univ of Basel, Switzerland; Univ of Basel, Switzerland)
J Adolesc Health 46:133-141, 2010

Purpose.—To investigate whether chronic vigorous exercising is related to improved sleep and psychological functioning, and whether this association varies with gender. Both lay and scientific opinions hold that physical activity is an efficient remedy and preventative measure for poor sleep. However, empirical evidence on adolescents is very limited.

Methods.—A total of 434 adolescents (258 athletes, 176 controls; mean age 17.2 years) took part in the study. Weekly hours spent exercising were 17.69 hours and 4.69 hours, respectively. To assess sleep patterns and psychological functioning, participants completed a sleep log for 7 consecutive days and several self-rating questionnaires.

Results.—Compared with controls, athletes reported better sleep patterns including higher sleep quality, shortened sleep onset latency, and fewer awakenings after sleep onset, as well as less tiredness and increased concentration during the day. Athletes reported significantly lower anxiety and fewer depressive symptoms. Compared with males, females reported fewer variations in sleep. Male controls had particularly unfavorable scores related to sleep and psychological functioning.

Conclusions.—Findings suggest that chronic vigorous exercising is positively related to adolescents' sleep and psychological functioning. Results also indicate that males with low exercise levels are at risk for increased sleep complaints and poorer psychological functioning.

▶ As time goes along we are encountering increasing documentation of the positive effects of regular exercise on well-being, and that goes for youth as well as adults. Most of the emphasis in the past has been on physical and physiological health, but there are now an impressive amount of data indicating that emotional health is equally benefited by physical activity. Such studies are difficult to perform, and many lack adeqaute methdology. Taken as a whole, though, the salutary effects of exercise on mental health in youth have been supported. In this study, the emphasis is on sleep patterns and associated emotional markers. And, commonly, the limiting question here is one of causality. This is a cross-sectional study that does not tell us what direction the arrow might go (if it "goes" at all). Does regular exercise allow one to sleep better and thus be more mentally refreshed? Or does sleeping well permit the mental and physical sharpness needed for sports play? Both interpretations are, in fact, feasible.

T. Rowland, MD

Physical Fitness and Physical Activity at Age 13 Years as Predictors of Cardiovascular Disease Risk Factors at Ages 15, 25, 33, and 40 Years: Extended Follow-up of the Oslo Youth Study

Kvaavik E, Klepp K-I, Tell GS, et al (Univ of Oslo, Norway; Univ of Bergen, Norway; et al)

Pediatrics 123:e80-e86, 2009

Objective.—Few studies have examined the association of childhood physical activity and physical fitness with cardiovascular disease risk factors in adulthood. Furthermore, interpretation of these findings is hampered by methodologic shortcomings. In a population-based cohort study, we explored the influence, if any, of childhood physical activity and physical fitness on later cardiovascular disease risk factors.

Methods.—Data were taken from the Oslo Youth Study, a prospective cohort study that began in 1979, when 1016 students (mean age: 13 years;range: 11–15 years) who were attending 6 schools were invited to participate in a health education intervention. Cardiovascular disease risk factor data were collected at baseline and again in 1981 (mean age: 15 years; range: 13–17 years), 1991 (mean age: 25; range: 23–27 years), 1999 (mean age: 33; range: 31–35 years), and 2006 (mean age: 40; range: 38–42 years).

Results.—At baseline, physical fitness was inversely related to BMI, triceps skinfold thickness, and blood pressure (systolic and diastolic; $N = 716$). These associations were also present in prospective analyses at ages 15 ($N = 472$), 25 ($N = 280$; except for systolic blood pressure), and 33 years ($N = 410$, only BMI measured)—albeit with progressively diminishing magnitude—but were lost at 40 years ($N = 294$). There were fewer relationships with cardiovascular disease risk factors when physical activity was the exposure of interest. Controlling for educational attainment of both the parent and the study member had little impact on these associations.

Conclusions.—Although childhood physical fitness seems to reveal some inverse associations with obesity and blood pressure in early adulthood, these effects diminished markedly into middle age.

▶ This longitudinal study revealed that measures of both physical activity and fitness during adolescence lost their predictive value for cardiovascular risk factors as the subjects achieved the middle years of adulthood. This is surprising, because both activity and fitness are linked to such risk factors, as well as specific health outcomes (eg, myocardial infarction) within adult populations. One obvious means of explaining these findings is that the subjects experienced a decline in both participation in physical activities and level of physical fitness as they became older. This would reinforce the use of one rationale for promoting activity and fitness in youth for their future health outcomes as adults: create regular exercise habits in children that will persist as a life-style habit as they grow older. The efficacy of this approach is difficult to prove, but maybe the findings in this study could serve to support such a strategy.

T. Rowland, MD

Sustained participation in youth sport decreases metabolic syndrome in adulthood

Yang X, Telama R, Hirvensalo M, et al (LIKES Res Ctr for Sport and Health Sciences, Jyväskylä, Finland; Univ of Jyväskylä, Finland; et al)

Int J Obes 33:1219-1226, 2009

Objective.—To explore the effect of organized youth sport on metabolic syndrome (MetS) in adulthood.

Design.—Longitudinal study data from the cardiovascular risk in young Finns study.

Subjects.—A total of 1493 males ($n = 704$) and females ($n = 789$) aged 3, 6, 9, 12, 15 and 18 years were randomly selected from five university towns and their rural surroundings in 1980. They were followed up for 21 years. In 2001 they were 24, 27, 30, 33, 36 and 39 years old.

Measurements.—Youth sports participation data (participation in sport-club training and competitions) were assessed in 1980 and 1983 using a self-report questionnaire completed in connection with a medical examination. Participants were divided into athletes and non-athletes at each measurement point, and then classified into four groups: Persistent athlete, Starter, Leaver and Non-athlete. A mean score of youth sport was assessed by calculating the average of four consecutive measurements (1980–1989). MetS risk in 2001 was defined as a categorical variable based on the guidelines of the European Group for the Study of Insulin Resistance (EGIR) and as a continuous MetS-score variable by summing the *z*-scores of individual metabolic variables.

Results.—In males and females, intense participation in youth sports over 3 years was inversely and significantly associated with clustered MetS score and prevalence of MetS defined by EGIR in adulthood ($P < 0.05$). The association remained significant after adjustment for age, baseline clustered MetS score, smoking and total caloric intake and after additional adjustments for adult leisure-time physical activity. Starters during 3 years were less likely to have MetS than non-athletes. Leavers were at a higher risk for MetS than persistent athletes. These associations were attenuated in males by adjustment for all potential confounders. Similar associations were found using EGIR MetS as an outcome.

Conclusions.—Sustained participation in organized sport lasting at least 3 years in youth is associated with reduced risk for developing MetS in adulthood (Fig 1).

▶ Youth who were active for 3 years in organized sports in Finland had a strongly reduced risk of metabolic syndrome during adulthood, as summarized in Fig 1. The authors admit that the mechanisms explaining this relationship are not well understood, especially as the results were found to be independent of adult physical activity. Youth sport could decrease the prevalence of metabolic syndrome while young and then track into adulthood. Participation in organized youth sport may have established lifelong habits for good health, including diet and avoidance of smoking that in turn reduced risk for metabolic syndrome. Youth active in sports, speculated the authors, may have improved their cardiovascular function and physical fitness to such an extent that this carried over into adulthood. This is doubtful. More likely is that self-selection and genetic factors had a direct bearing on the positive association between youth sport and adult health. Nonetheless, the results are interesting and are one more

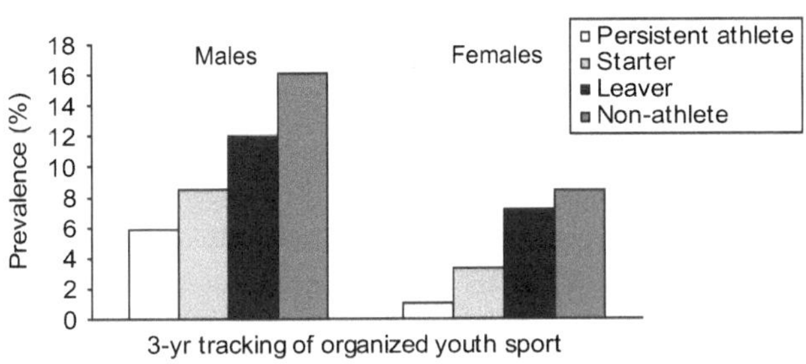

FIGURE 1.—Prevalence of European group for the study of insulin resistance (EGIR) MetS by four youth sport groups over a 3-year period (significance differences between groups tested by χ^2-test: $P < 0.05$ for both sexes). (Reprinted from Yang X, Telama R, Hirvensalo M, et al. Sustained participation in youth sport decreases metabolic syndrome in adulthood. *Int J Obes.* 2009;33:1219-1226.)

reason to encourage parents to support sustained sport activity by their teenagers.

D. C. Nieman, DrPH

The impact of urinary stress incontinence in young and middle-age women practising recreational sports activity: an epidemiological study

Salvatore S, Serati M, Laterza R, et al (Univ of Insubria, Varese, Italy; et al)
Br J Sports Med 43:1115-1118, 2009

Objectives.—To evaluate the prevalence of urinary stress incontinence (USI) in menstruating women practising recreational sports activity, to detect specific sports with a stronger association with urinary incontinence (UI) and to evaluate risk factors possibly related to this condition.

Design.—Epidemiological study.

Setting.—Non-competitive sports organisations in the province of Varese, Italy.

Participants.—679 women of fertile age, practising recreational sports activity.

Intervention.—Anonymous questionnaire on UI.

Main Outcome Measurements.—The questionnaire included questions about patients' general characteristics, occurrence of UI in relation to sport or daily general activities, time of onset of this condition, frequency of leakage episodes, correlation of incontinence with types of movements or sports, subjective impression of being limited on such occasions and/or necessity to modify the type of sport.

Results.—UI was reported by 101 women (14.9%). Of these, 32 (31.7%) complained of UI only during sports activity, 48 (47.5%) only during daily life and 21 (20.8%) in both circumstances. Body mass index and parity were significantly associated with the risk of UI. Looking at the different sports activities, a higher rate of incontinence was found in women participating in basketball (16.6%), athletics (15%), and tennis or squash (11%). 10.4% of women abandoned their favourite sport, because of USI, and a further 20% limited the way they practised their favourite sport to reduce leakage episodes.

Conclusions.—Female UI affects a significant proportion of young women practising non-competitive sports activity; it can cause abandonment of the sport or limitation of its practice.

▶ Despite the fact that an estimated 13% to 46% of women experience urinary incontinence (UI), studies of UI and physical performance had been limited to competitive athletes until this report by Salvatore and colleagues. In their study of nearly 700 premenopausal women, 15% reported UI and half of this cohort complained of urinary leakage during sports activity. Movements that are very common in fitness classes, such as jumping, abdominal exercises, and jogging, were most strongly associated with urinary leakage. About 30% of women with UI modified or discontinued exercise as a result of leakage, but very few

(7 of 101) sought medical treatment for the condition. The authors recommend pelvic floor exercises as the first line of treatment for UI. Clinicians may consider using the UI questionnaire provided in the appendix of the article to ascertain the severity of a patient's incontinence and the impact on her physical activity. This information could then be used to determine strategies to mitigate UI in physically active women and prevent dropout from physical activity due to UI.

C. M. Jankowski, PhD

Physical activity and fertility in women: the North-Trøndelag Health Study

Gudmundsdottir SL, Flanders WD, Augestad LB (Norwegian Univ of Science and Technology (NTNU), Trondheim, Norway; Emory Univ, Atlanta, GA)

Hum Reprod 24:3196-3204, 2009

Background.—Changes in the state of energy balance owing to changes in physical activity may affect the reproductive system. We evaluated the association between physical activity (PA) and fertility and parity in healthy women.

Methods.—A population-based health survey (HUNT 1) was conducted during 1984–1986 in Nord-Trøndelag county, Norway, with follow-up from 1995 to 1997 (HUNT 2). The study included 3887 women, <45 years old in HUNT 2. PA was assessed by baseline questionnaire, and fertility and parity by questionnaire at follow-up. Data focused on overall occurrence of infertility in the population (without biological confirmation).

Results.—Increased frequency, duration and intensity of PA were associated with increased subfertility, and frequency of PA was associated with voluntary childlessness ($P < 0.01$). After adjusting for age, parity, smoking, and marital status, women who were active on most days were 3.2 times more likely to have fertility problems than inactive women. Exercising to exhaustion was associated with 2.3 times the odds of fertility problems versus low intensity. Women with highest intensity of PA at baseline had the lowest frequency of continuing nulliparity and highest frequency of having three or more children during follow-up ($P < 0.05$). Sensitivity analysis including body mass index as confounder did not alter the results. No associations were found between lower activity levels and fertility or parity.

Conclusion.—Increased risk of infertility was only found for the small group of women reporting the highest levels of intensity and frequency of PA. Awareness of the possible risks of infertility should be highlighted among non-athletic women who exercise vigorously (Table 2).

▶ This is a large-scale population study of the problem of infertility, defined as failure to conceive within 1 year of attempting to do so.[1] The problem is important clinically because of the psychological problems induced by infertility,[2] the high costs of efforts at in vitro fertilization,[3] and the increased risks of breast and ovarian cancer[4] among infertile women. An association between infertility and

TABLE 2.—Unadjusted and Adjusted ORs from Logistic Regression for Fertility Problems (Subfertility or Involuntary Childlessness)

PA	Unadjusted OR (95% CI)	Adjusted OR# (95% CI)
Frequency		
Never*	1.0	1.0
<Once a week	2.2 (1.0–4.8)	2.1 (0.9–4.7)
Once a week	2.1 (1.0–4.7)	2.0 (0.9–4.5)
2–3 times a week	2.6 (1.2–5.9)	2.0 (0.9–4.6)
Almost every day	4.3 (1.9–10.1)	3.2 (1.3–7.6)
Intensity		
Easy*	1.0	1.0
Sweating and out of breath	1.3 (1.1–1.9)	1.1 (0.8–1.6)
Exhaustion	3.3 (1.8–6.2)	2.3 (1.2.–4.5)
Duration		
<15 min*	1.0	1.0
16–30 min	0.3 (0.2–0.6)	0.3 (0.2–0.5)
30–60 min	0.6 (0.3–1.0)	0.5 (0.3.–0.9)
>60 min	0.9 (0.5–1.6)	0.6 (0.3–1.2)
PA index		
Low*	1.0	1.0
Medium	1.0 (0.7–1.7)	0.9 (0.6–1.5)
High	2.1 (1.5–3.2)	1.5 (1.0–2.3)

PA, physical activity.
#Adjusted for age, parity, smoking and marital status.
*Reference category OR, odds ratio; CI, confidence interval.

involvement in high performance athletics has been described previously.[5] This article notes that in the general population, also, the practice of frequent and exhausting physical activity is associated with failure to conceive (Table 2), although given the cross-sectional nature of this cohort study, it cannot prove a causal relationship; other characteristics of the active individuals may have contributed to the infertility (including very active husbands with a reduced sperm count!). Previous studies in the general population have suggested that regular exercise has a beneficial effect upon fertility up to a certain level of physical activity,[6] but that a negative response is seen beyond this point.[7] One likely mediator of any change in fertility is an alteration of energy balance and associated changes in hormone profile;[8] it is a pity that this study did not include any information on energy balance, other than body mass index. Although the high incidence of infertility among the most active women is worth noting, the infertility does not seem to have been permanent because those who were most active at baseline, but subsequently reduced their activity, had several subsequent births.

R. J. Shephard, MD (Lond), PhD, DPE

References

1. Kumar A, Ghadir S, Eskandari N, et al. Infertility. In: DeCherney AH, Nathan L, Goodwin TM, et al., eds. *Current Diagnosis and Treatment. Obstetrics & Gynecology.* New York, NY: McGraw Hill; 2007.
2. Greil AL. Infertility and psychological distress: a critical review of the literature. *Soc Sci Med.* 1997;45:1679-1704.

3. Jain T, Hornstein MD. To pay or not to pay. *Fertil Steril.* 2003;80:27-29.
4. Jensen A, Sharif H, Olsen JH, Kjaer SK. Risk of breast cancer and gynecologic cancers in a large population of nearly 50,000 infertile Danish women. *Am J Epidemiol.* 2008;168:49-57.
5. Otis CL, Drinkwater B, Johnson M, Loucks A, Wilmore J. American College of Sports Medicine position stand. The Female Athlete Triad. *Med Sci Sports Exerc.* 1997;29:i-ix.
6. Chavarro JE, Rich-Edwards JW, Rosner BA, Willett WC. Diet and lifestyle in the prevention of ovulatory disorder infertility. *Obstet Gynecol.* 2007;110: 1050-1058.
7. Morris SN, Missmer SA, Cramer DW, Powers RD, McShane PM, Hornstein MD. Effects of lifetime exercise on the outcome of in vitro fertilization. *Obstet Gynecol.* 2006;108:938-945.
8. Redman L. Symposium: diet, nutrition and exercise in reproduction. Physical activity and its effects on reproduction. *Reprod BioMed Online.* 2006;12: 579-586.

Hyperandrogenism May Explain Reproductive Dysfunction in Olympic Athletes

Hagmar M, Berglund B, Brismar K, et al (Karolinska Institutet, Stockholm, Sweden)
Med Sci Sports Exerc 41:1241-1248, 2009

Purpose.—Female athletes are known to be at risk for reproductive dysfunction and osteopenia because of energy deficiency. Although endocrine balance and an optimal body composition are essential for top elite performance, these parameters have not yet been explored fully in Olympic sportswomen. The objective of this study, therefore, was to characterize the menstrual status, body composition, and endocrine balance in female Olympic athletes participating in different disciplines.

Methods.—Ninety Swedish female Olympic athletes underwent a gynecologic examination that included vaginal examination by ultrasound and determination of body composition. In addition, blood samples were collected for the analysis of reproductive hormones and biomarkers of energy availability.

Results.—Of all the athletes, 47% were using hormonal contraception (HC). Menstrual dysfunction (MD) was common (27%) among those not using HC and, particularly, in endurance athletes. However, the proportion of body fat and biomarkers of energy availability were within the normal ranges and none exhibited osteopenia. On the contrary, bone mineral density was generally high, particularly in the power athletes. The most common diagnosis associated with MD was polycystic ovary syndrome (PCOS) and not hypothalamic inhibition because of energy deficiency.

Conclusions.—Female Olympic athletes participating in different sports were found to have an anabolic body composition and biomarkers of energy availability within the normal ranges. Most cases of menstrual disturbances observed were due to PCOS. These findings challenge the

TABLE 4.—Serum Levels of Biomarkers of Energy Availability in Our Power, Endurance, and Technical Athletes

Marker (unit)	Power	Endurance	Technical
Insulin ($mU \cdot L^{-1}$)	4.2 (3.2–6.2)	4.9 (3.6–5.6)	4.2 (2.4–7.2)
IGF-I ($\mu g \cdot L^{-1}$)	248.3 (195.0–322.4)^{b**}	263.9 (211.9–301.0)^{c**}	200.2 (163.8–237.9)
IGFBP-1 ($\mu g \cdot L^{-1}$)	37.0 (25.0–49.0)	29.5 (22.0–66.0)	32.0 (23.0–45.0)
IGF-I/S-IGFBP-1	6.6 (4.7–11.6)	8.0 (4.6–12.1)	5.8 (4.2–7.4)
Cortisol ($nmol \cdot L^{-1}$)	504.5 ± 212.9	414.8 ± 181.4	515.9 ± 160.2
Glucose ($mmol \cdot L^{-1}$)	4.0 ± 0.4	4.1 ± 0.4	3.9 ± 0.4

The values given are means ± SD or medians (Q25–Q75).
For an explanation of the abbreviations, see the text.
Statistically significant differences are indicated by * $P < 0.05$, ** $P < 0.01$, or *** $P < 0.001$, preceded by a letter:
[a]Power versus endurance athletes.
[b]Power versus technical athletes.
[c]Endurance versus technical athletes.

contemporary concept that reproductive dysfunction in sportswomen is typically a consequence of chronic energy deficiency (Table 4).

▶ Many mammals become pregnant only when nutrition is adequate, and this seems true of humans; in underdeveloped societies, prolonged lactation is often a relatively effective method of spacing births. It has thus been hypothesized that in sports where a low body fat is important (prolonged endurance events, aesthetic activities, and weight-categorized competitions) a negative energy balance is responsible for menstrual disorders and infertility. The present report is based on quite a wide range of Swedish female athletes (although none from aesthetic disciplines). It challenges the traditional view, at least as far as endurance sport is concerned, showing disturbed menstrual function despite what were judged to be normal biomarkers of energy availability (Table 4). The chosen markers of poor energy availability included a low concentration of insulin-like growth factor, and high concentrations of insulin growth factor-binding protein and cortisol; together, such a hormonal profile would indicate a catabolic state. The suggested alternative explanation is the development of hyperandrogenic polycystic ovary syndrome. Ultrasound diagnosed this in 37% of the present subjects, as compared with a normal prevalence of 20%, and it is argued that hyperandrogenism gave the competitors a competitive edge. The hypothesis is an interesting one, although it is difficult to reconcile with reports of impaired fertility in male endurance competitors. Most of the endurance competitors had a normal body fat content, but it would have been more convincing to see also data for nitrogen balance in those who were showing menstrual disturbances. The distinction between hyperandrogenic and nutritional menstrual disturbances may have practical value, as the latter is commonly associated with osteopenia (as in the athletic triad).

For further reading on this subject I suggest an article by Lowe et al.[1]

R. J. Shephard, MD (Lond), PhD, DPE

Reference

1. Lowe P, Kovacs G, Howlett D. Incidence of polycystic ovaries and polycystic ovary syndrome amongst women in Melbourne, Australia. *Aust N Z J Obstet Gynaecol.* 2005;45:17-19.

Resistance exercise training during pregnancy and newborn's birth size: a randomised controlled trial

Barakat R, Lucia A, Ruiz JR (Universidad Politécnica de Madrid, Spain; Universidad Europea de Madrid, Spain; Karolinska Institutet, Huddinge, Sweden)

Int J Obes 33:1048-1057, 2009

Objective.—We examined the effect of light intensity resistance exercise training performed during the second and third trimester of pregnancy on the newborn's birth size. We also studied the association between maternal body weight prior to pregnancy and newborn's birth size.

Design.—Randomised controlled trial.

Subjects.—We randomly assigned 160 sedentary gravidae to either a training ($n = 80$) or a control ($n = 80$) group. The training programme focused on light resistance and toning exercises (three times per week, 35–40 min per session). We recorded the Apgar score, birth weight, birth length, and head circumference of the newborn, as well as gestational age at time of delivery from hospital perinatal records. We also measured maternal weight and height before parity and gestational weight gain.

Results.—Maternal characteristics neither differed between groups (all $P > 0.1$) nor newborn characteristics (all $P > 0.1$). Maternal body weight was positively and significantly associated with newborn's birth weight and length only in the control group ($\beta = 19.20$ and 0.065, respectively, $P < 0.01$).

Conclusion.—Light intensity resistance training performed over the second and third trimester of pregnancy does not have a negative impact on the newborn's body size or overall health. Exercise interventions might attenuate the adverse consequences of maternal body weight before pregnancy on the newborn's birth size.

▶ Barakat and colleagues completed a large National Institutes of Health (NIH) funded, randomized controlled trial of the effects of resistance exercise training during pregnancy on many health outcomes of newborns. Here, the primary outcome is newborn birth size. The potential maternal benefits of increased muscle strength include a reduced cardiovascular load as pregnancy progresses due to greater physical reserve, improved posture, prevention of gestational low back pain and diastasis recti, and strengthening of the pelvis floor. The women in this trial were sedentary before pregnancy, but were otherwise healthy. They had singleton pregnancies and were not at high risk for preterm delivery. The prepregnancy body weight and body mass index (BMI), as well as the prevalence of gestational diabetes, miscarriage, and parity, were not different between the exercise and control groups. The overall conclusion of this investigation was that resistance exercise during the second and third trimesters of pregnancy had no adverse effects on newborn birth size or other health characteristics (eg, Apgar score). There were some benefits of the resistance exercise, including less maternal weight gain compared with nonexercising controls. A very interesting finding was that the relation between maternal prepregnancy body weight and newborn body weight changed in response to exercise. In the controls, heavier women had heavier newborns. However, among women who exercised during pregnancy, newborn body weight was not significantly related to maternal prepregnancy body weight. Exercise during pregnancy also disassociated 2-hour glucose of the mother (measured at weeks 24-25 gestation) and newborn body weight. Thus, exercise may reduce the risk of macrosomia associated with maternal body weight or gestational diabetes. It must be noted that this was a low intensity exercise intervention. The warm up and cool down comprised aerobic exercise at ≤60% of estimated maximal heart rate. The main portion of the exercise sessions comprised toning and joint mobilization exercises of the major muscle groups. The resistance exercises were accomplished with <3 kg barbells per exercise, or with resistance bands. All exercise sessions were supervised and heart rate was monitored. Exercises involving extreme stretching and joint overextension, ballistic movements, jumps, and supine postures were avoided. The interested reader is encouraged to read other publications by Dr Barakat.

C. M. Jankowski, PhD

Leisure-Time Physical Activity in Pregnancy and Risk of Postpartum Depression: A Prospective Study in a Large National Birth Cohort

Strøm M, Mortensen EL, Halldorson TI, et al (Statens Serum Institut, Denmark; Univ of Copenhagen, Denmark; et al)

J Clin Psychiatry 70:1707-1714, 2009

Objective.—To explore the association between physical activity during pregnancy and postpartum depression (PPD) in a large, prospective cohort.

Method.—Exposure information from the Danish National Birth Cohort, a large, prospective cohort with information on more than 100,000 pregnancies (1996–2002), was linked to the Danish Psychiatric Central Register and the Danish Register for Medicinal Product Statistics for data on clinically identified cases of depression up to 1 year postpartum. A total of 70,866 women from the Danish National Birth Cohort were included in the analyses. Duration, frequency, and type of physical activity were assessed by a telephone interview at approximately week 12 of gestation. Admission to hospital due to depression (PPD-admission) and prescription of an antidepressant (PPD-prescription) were treated as separate outcomes.

TABLE 4.—Distribution of Participants, OR for PPD-Admission, and OR for PPD-Prescription by Measures of Physical Activity in Gestation Weeks 12 and 30 Combined (N = 70,866)

				PPD-Admission					PPD-Prescription			
				Crude		Adjusted[b]			Crude		Adjusted[b]	
Measure	N	%[a]	No. of Cases	OR	95% CI	OR	95% CI	No. of Cases	OR	95% CI	OR	95% CI
Physical activity, weeks 12 and 30												
Not physically active	33,802	48	75	Reference	...	Reference	...	680	Reference	...	Reference	...
Active	12,536	18	23	0.83	0.52–1.32	0.92	0.57–1.49	177	0.70	0.59–0.82	0.84	0.71–1.01
Changed activity level, weeks 12–30	24,528	35	59	1.08	0.77–1.53	1.09	0.77–1.54	448	0.91	0.80–1.02	0.94	0.82–1.06
Intensity, weeks 12 and 30												
Not physically active	33,802	48	75	Reference	...	Reference	...	680	Reference	...	Reference	...
Moderately active[c]	5,591	8	16	1.29	0.75–2.22	1.43	0.82–2.48	84	0.74	0.59–0.93	0.86	0.68–1.10
Vigorously active[d]	3,700	5	3	0.37	0.12–1.16	0.41	0.13–1.31	41	0.55	0.40–0.75	0.67	0.48–0.93
Changed activity level, weeks 12–30	27,773	39	63	1.02	0.73–1.43	1.04	0.74–1.46	500	0.89	0.80–1.00	0.94	0.83–1.07

Abbreviations: OR = odds ratio, PPD = postpartum depression.
[a]Percentage within variable.
[b]Adjusted for maternal age, parity, pre-pregnant body mass index, alcohol intake, smoking, occupation, education, home ownership, marital status, social support, and history of previous depression.
[c]*Moderately active* defined as reporting less than 25% of total time in physical activity as vigorous activity.
[d]*Vigorously active* defined as reporting at least 25% of total time in physical activity as vigorous activity.

Results.—Through linkage to national registers, we identified 157 cases of PPD-admission and 1,305 cases of PPD-prescription. Women engaging in vigorous physical activity during pregnancy had a lower risk of PPD-prescription compared to women who were not physically active (adjusted odds ratio, 0.81; 95% CI, 0.66–0.99). No association was observed between physical activity and PPD-admission; but, in women who were underweight prior to pregnancy, physical activity was associated with increased risk of PPD-admission.

Conclusions.—Our data are compatible with a protective effect of vigorous physical activity, but not for other measures of physical activity, against postpartum depression requiring antidepressant therapy. No protective effect could be detected on PPD leading to hospitalization.

▶ Postpartum depression is a relatively common problem for the family physician, affecting 5% to 15% of births,[1] and it can have important consequences for the relationship between the mother and her child,[2-4] although there are those who question whether it is a distinct clinical entity.[5] This very large cross-sectional study shows an association between vigorous physical activity during pregnancy and a need for medication against postpartum depression (Table 4). This finding is in keeping with various trials of exercise and physical activity in the general population;[6] the mechanism might be endorphin release or an enhancement of self-image. The present findings may suggest another reason for encouraging physical activity during pregnancy. However, there are several important caveats. The association was seen only for vigorous physical activity, which is not every woman's choice during pregnancy; moreover, this benefit was seen only in terms of the prescription of antidepressant medication and did not include severe cases of depression requiring hospital admission. It is unclear how well the registry of antidepressant use provided unequivocal evidence of postpartum depression. Benefit was also associated with white-collar employment, and thus presumably a higher socioeconomic status that may have reduced the practical problems that poorer women face following delivery.

R. J. Shephard, MD (Lond), PhD, DPE

References

1. O'Hara MW, Swain AM. Rates and risk of postpartum depression-a meta-analysis. *Int Rev Psychiatry.* 1996;8:37-54.
2. Cooper PJ, Murray L. Postnatal depression. *BMJ.* 1998;316:1884-1886.
3. Reck C, Hunt A, Fuchs T, et al. Interactive regulation of affect in postpartum depressed mothers and their infants: an overview. *Psychopathology.* 2004;37: 272-280.
4. Wolkind S. Mothers' depression and their children's attendance at medical facilities. *J Psychosom Res.* 1985;29:579-582.
5. Brockington I. Postpartum psychiatric disorders. *Lancet.* 2004;363:303-310.
6. Stathopoulou G, Powers MB, Berry AC, Smits JAJ, Otto MW. Exercise interventions for mental health: a quantitative and qualitative review. *Clin Psychol Sci Pract.* 2006;13:179-193.

Associations of diet and physical activity during pregnancy with risk for excessive gestational weight gain

Stuebe AM, Oken E, Gillman MW (Brigham and Women's Hosp, Boston MA; Harvard Med School/Harvard Pilgrim Health Care, MA; et al)

Am J Obstet Gynecol 201:58.e1-58.e8, 2009

Objective.—We sought to identify modifiable risk factors for excessive gestational weight gain (GWG).

Study Design.—We assessed associations of diet and physical activity with excessive GWG among 1388 women from the Project Viva cohort study.

Results.—Three hundred seventy-nine women (27%) were overweight (body mass index $\geq$ 26 kg/m^2) and 703 (51%) experienced excessive GWG, according to Institute of Medicine guidelines. In multivariable logistic regression models, we found that intake of total energy (odds ratio [OR], 1.10; 95% confidence interval [CI], 1.00-1.22, per 500 kcal/d), dairy (OR, 1.08; 95% CI, 1.00-1.17, per serving per day), and fried foods (OR, 3.47; 95% CI, 0.91-13.24, per serving per day) were directly associated with excessive GWG. First trimester vegetarian diet (OR, 0.46; 95% CI, 0.28-0.78) and midpregnancy walking (OR, 0.92; 95% CI, 0.83-1.01, per 30 minutes per day) and vigorous physical activity (OR, 0.76; 95% CI, 0.60-0.97, per 30 minutes per day) were inversely associated with excessive GWG.

Conclusion.—A healthful diet and greater physical activity are associated with reduced risk for excessive GWG.

▶ An excessive weight gain during pregnancy is undesirable on several counts: such patients are more likely to require deliver by cesarean section.[1-4] Their risk of pre-eclampsia is also increased[3] and the excessive weight is liable to be retained after delivery.[5-7] The infants born to women who show an excessive weight gain face the risk of being born preterm,[8] and of themselves developing obesity as a child or as an adolescent.[9,10] Plainly, it is thus important to prevent excessive weight gain during pregnancy, if at all possible. This study is cross-sectional in type, but it does suggest the value of regular exercise as one component of prevention. Activity was estimated using a physical activity questionnaire initially designed for the elderly. Thirty minutes of mid-pregnancy walking per day was associated with a small reduction in risk, and the benefit was much larger with 30 minutes of vigorous activity per day (Table 2); however, it is a little puzzling that no benefit was associated with moderate activity. Given that the study was correlational, it is possible that the most active women engaged in other favorable health practices, and that these were responsible for the favorable outcomes. A randomized controlled trial is thus "desirable."

R. J. Shephard, MD (Lond), PhD, DPE

TABLE 2.—Levels of Dietary Intake and Physical Activity Among 1388 Women Enrolled in Project Viva, Comparing Those With and Without Excessive Weight Gain

Variable	GWG Inadequate or Adequate n = 685) Mean or Median	(SD) or [IQR]	Excessive GWG (n = 703) Mean or Median	(SD) or [IQR]	Bivariate *P* value[a]	Multivariate Adjusted Odds of Excessive GWG[b] OR (95% CI)
FOOD AND FOOD GROUPS, SERVINGS/d						
Sugar-sweetened beverages, median [IQR][c]	0.36	[0.11-0.75]	0.37	[0.12-0.75]	.42[d]	0.93 (0.78-1.11)
Fried foods, median [IQR][c]	0.11	[0.07-0.14]	0.11	[0.07-0.14]	.007[d]	3.68 (0.96-14.13)
Dairy	2.90	(1.52)	3.04	(1.49)	.08	1.08 (1.00-1.17)
Low fat dairy	1.49	(1.31)	1.59	(1.34)	.17	1.08 (0.98-1.18)
Whole milk dairy	1.41	(1.01)	1.46	(0.97)	.42	1.06 (0.94-1.20)
Fruits and vegetables	5.84	(2.60)	5.90	(2.71)	.68	1.03 (0.98-1.07)
Red and processed meats	0.53	(0.40)	0.56	(0.39)	.19	1.00 (0.74-1.34)
Whole grains	1.25	(1.03)	1.27	(1.04)	.63	1.06 (0.95-1.19)
NUTRIENTS AND DIETARY PATTERNS, g						
Kcal/d	2060.01	(593.76)	2131.40	(570.36)	.02	1.11 (1.00-1.23)
Fiber (g/d)	19.97	(5.75)	19.50	(5.04)	.10	0.98 (0.87-1.09)
Glycemic index	754.24	(120.92)	746.08	(115.09)	.20	0.98 (0.88-1.08)
Glycemic load	14,597.52	(1940.93)	14,516.26	(1930.13)	.43	1.00 (0.88-1.13)
VEGETARIAN DIET						
First trimester, n (%)	55	(8.0)	27	(3.9)	.001[e]	0.45 (0.27-0.76)
Second trimester, n (%)	42	(6.2)	28	(4.0)	.06[e]	0.70 (0.40-1.20)
MACRONUTRIENT COMPOSITION (% ENERGY)						OR[f]
Carbohydrates	54.95	(6.41)	54.67	(6.30)	.41	1.0 (ref)
Protein	17.53	(2.56)	17.62	(2.46)	.53	1.10 (0.86-1.42)
Total fat	28.94	(5.12)	29.16	(4.93)	.41	
Monounsaturated fat	10.96	(2.33)	10.98	(2.22)	.87	0.63 (0.40-0.99)
Polyunsaturated fat	6.18	(1.40)	6.25	(1.41)	.40	1.32 (0.80-2.18)
Saturated fat	10.78	(2.32)	10.94	(2.21)	.20	1.33 (0.87-2.02)
Trans fat	0.97	(0.29)	0.99	(0.28)	.13	1.27 (0.39-4.13)
PHYSICAL ACTIVITY, min/d[c]						OR per 30 min/d
Walking	34	[17-60]	34	[17-43]	.03[d]	0.92 (0.83-1.01)
Moderate activity	0	[0-17]	0	[0-17]	.53[d]	1.00 (0.85-1.17)
Vigorous activity	0	[0-9]	0	[0-0]	.005[d]	0.76 (0.60-0.96)
Total activity	34	[17-60]	34	[17-43]	.03[d]	0.95 (0.89-1.01)
TV watching	86	[43-129]	86	[51-129]	.11[d]	0.98 (0.93-1.02)
Sedentary lifestyle (< 2.5 h/wk total activity), n (%)	132	(19.3)	165	(23.5)	.06[a]	1.26 (0.95-1.69)

CI, confidence interval; *GWG*, gestaional weight gain; *IQR*, interquartile range; *OR*, odds ratio; *SD*, standard deviation. Stuebe. Excessive gestational weight gain. Am J Obstet Gynecol 2009.

[a]*t* test with equal variance, not excessive vs excessive gain;

[b]adjusted for prepregnancy body mass index (in 5 percentile categories), maternal age (14-20, 20-25, 25-30, 30-35, 35-40, 40+ y) race/ethnicity, smoking status, gestational age at delivery (wks), and nausea in the first trimester of pregnancy;

[c]median and interquartile range presented for exposures that were not normally distributed;

[d]Wilcoxon rank sum test, not excessive vs excessive gain;

[e]χ^2 test;

[f]multivariate nutrient density model. Total energy intake and percent energy from protein, monounsaturated fat, polyunsaturated fat, saturated fat, and trans fat were entered simultaneously into the model, so OR estimates the effect of intake of the macronutrient compared with an equivalent amount of energy from carbohydrates. We present OR per 2% energy for trans fat, per 5% for all other macronutrients; g. We present OR for energy intake per 500 kcal/d; fiber per 5 g/d; glycemic index per 100 u/d; glycemic load per 2000 u/d.

References

1. Stotland NE, Hopkins LM, Caughey AB. Gestational weight gain, macrosomia, and risk of cesarean birth in nondiabetic nulliparas. *Obstet Gynecol.* 2004;104: 671-677.
2. Bianco AT, Smilen SW, Davis Y, Lopez S, Lapinski R, Lockwood CJ. Pregnancy outcome and weight gain recommendations for the morbidly obese woman. *Obstet Gynecol.* 1998;91:97-102.
3. Rosenberg TJ, Garbers S, Lipkind H, Chiasson MA. Maternal obesity and diabetes as risk factors for adverse pregnancy outcomes: differences among 4 racial/ethnic groups. *Am J Public Health.* 2005;95:1545-1551.
4. Stuebe AM, Zera C, Ecker JL, McElrath TM. A prospective assessment of metabolic function, compliance with gestational weight gain guidelines, and associated pregnancy outcomes. *Am J Obstet Gynecol.* 2006;195:S82.
5. Gunderson E, Abrams B, Selvin S. The relative importance of gestational gain and maternal characteristics associated with the risk of becoming overweight after pregnancy. *Int J Obes Relat Metab Disord.* 2000;24:1660-1668.
6. Rooney B, Schauberger C. Excess pregnancy weight gain and long-term obesity: one decade later. *Obstet Gynecol.* 2002;100:245-252.
7. Rooney BL, Schauberger CW, Mathiason MA. Impact of perinatal weight change on long-term obesity and obesity-related illnesses. *Obstet Gynecol.* 2005;106: 1349-1356.
8. Schieve LA, Cogswell ME, Scanlon KS. Maternal weight gain and preterm delivery: differential effects by body mass index. *Epidemiology.* 1999;10: 141-147.
9. Oken E, Tavares EM, Kleinman KP, Rich-Edwards JW, Gillman MW. Gestational weight gain and child adiposity at age 3 years. *Am J Obstet Gynecol.* 2007;196: 322.e1-322.e8.
10. Oken EM, Rifas-Shiman SL, Field AE, Frazier AL, Gillman MW. Maternal gestational weight gain and offspring weight in adolescence. *Obstet Gynecol.* 2008;112:999-1006.

Association between aerobic fitness in late pregnancy and duration of labor in nulliparous women

Kardel KR, Johansen B, Voldner N, et al (Oslo Univ Hosp – Rikshospitalet, Norway)
Acta Obstet Gynecol Scand 88:948-952, 2009

It is established that the level of physical activity in the population generally is too low, and data indicate that pregnant women are no exception. Studies of the effects of aerobic fitness on delivery outcomes are limited. In this observational study, we investigated the effect of aerobic fitness on duration of labor in nulliparous women who started labor spontaneously. Maximal oxygen uptake was measured in 40 nulliparous women at 35–37 weeks of gestation. Duration of labor was defined as the time between 3 cm cervical dilation with regular uterine contractions and delivery. The mean (SD) maximal oxygen uptake was 2.1 (0.3) L/min and duration of labor 583 (317) minutes. Duration of labor was inversely associated with maximal oxygen uptake after adjusting for birthweight ($p = 0.034$). We conclude that measurement of maximal oxygen uptake is safe in pregnancy at 35–37 weeks and that increased aerobic fitness

TABLE 2.—Factors Affecting Duration of Labor

Linear Regression Models	R^2	*B*	Adjusted 95% CI for *B*	*n*	*p*
Duration of labor					
Model 1: maximal VO2 (L/min)	0.26	−326.8	−627.2 to −26.4	39	0.034
Birthweight (g)		0.3	0.1–0.6	39	0.003
Model 2: maximal VO2 (L/min)	0.43	−283.0	−542.8 to −3.3	39	0.047
Birthweight (g)		0.3	0.1–0.5	39	0.006
Any stimulation during labor		274.8	100.0–449.6	39	0.003
Duration of first stage					
Model 1: birthweight (g)	0.15	0.3	0.0–0.5	34	0.026
Model 2: birthweight (g)	0.41	0.2	0.0–0.4	34	0.050
Any stimulation during labor		322.9	141.9–503.9	34	0.001
Duration of second stage					
Birthweight (g)	0.27	0.03	0.01–0.05	34	0.010
Maternal height (cm)		−1.9	−3.6–0.1	34	0.039

Note: Association between aerobic fitness (VO_{2max}) and duration of labor, first, and second stage estimated from multiple linear regression models adjusted for birthweight, stimulation during labor and maternal height. R^2: amount of variation in the data that is explained by the regression model. *B*: regression coefficient (min).

was associated with shorter labor in nulliparous women who started labor spontaneously (Table 2).

▶ There can be little disagreement on the advantages of a short labor, with a reduced risk of fetal asphyxia,[1] and fewer maternal complications such as infections[2] and fistulae.[3] An increased level of physical fitness could theoretically facilitate labor, not only because of a greater ability to push during the second stage of labor, but also because of metabolic and hormonal changes enhancing uterine contractility and endurance. Some previous reports have found a longer second stage of labor[4] and a much higher incidence of Caesarean section[5] among sedentary women. However, others have reported a longer labor, particularly during the first stage, among highly active women.[6,7] Conflicting results may reflect failure to consider parity and imprecise estimates of habitual physical activity. The present authors argued that measurements of peak oxygen intake might provide a clearer indicator of fitness and thus the effects of fitness on labor. Tests were conducted successfully at a late stage of pregnancy without harm to the fetus. Effort during a progressive treadmill test was halted by symptoms such as dyspnea, leg, or general fatigue. The peak heart rate is not stated, but as the average peak oxygen intake was relatively low, it is unclear how successful the test of aerobic power was in reaching maximal aerobic power. The data showed no univariate relationship to the duration of labor, but there was a modest inverse relationship, due mainly to the first stage of labor, after allowing for the birth weight of the child (Table 2). The authors suggest that the mechanism may be an adverse effect of obesity on uterine contractility,[8] rather than an effect from oxygen transport per se; however, if this were the case, one would expect a stronger relationship to oxygen intake per kg of body mass than to absolute oxygen intake. This aspect of the data needs re-examining.

R. J. Shephard, MD (Lond), PhD, DPE

References

1. Neilson JP, Lavender T, Quenby S, Wray S. Obstructed labour. *Br Med Bull.* 2003; 67:191-204.
2. Cheng YW, Hopkins LM, Caughey AB. How long is too long: Does a prolonged second stage of labor in nulliparous women affect maternal and neonatal outcomes? *Am J Obstet Gynecol.* 2004;191:933-938.
3. Creanga AA, Genadry RR. Obstetric fistulas: a clinical review. *Int J Gynaecol Obstet.* 2007;99:S406.
4. Rice PL, Fort IL. The relationship of maternal exercise on labor, delivery and health of the newborn. *J Sports Med Phys Fitness.* 1991;31:95-99.
5. Bungum TJ, Peaslee DL, Jackson AW, Perez MA. Exercise during pregnancy and type of delivery in nulliparae. *J Obstet Gynecol Neonatal Nurs.* 2000;29:258-264.
6. Kardel KR, Kase K. Training in pregnant women: effects on fetal development and birth. *Am J Obstet Gynecol.* 1998;178:280-286.
7. Magann EF, Evans SF, Weitz B, Newnham J. Antepartum, intrapartum, and neonatal significance of exercise on healthy low-risk pregnant working women. *Obstet Gynecol.* 2002;99:466-472.
8. Zhang J, Bricker L, Wray S, Quenby S. Poor uterine contractility in obese women. *BJOG.* 2007;114:343-348.

Effect of Exercise Training on Loss of Bone Mineral Density during Lactation

Lovelady CA, Bopp MJ, Colleran HL, et al (Univ of North Carolina at Greensboro)

Med Sci Sports Exerc 41:1902-1907, 2009

Purpose.—During lactation, women transfer approximately 200 mg of calcium per day to breast milk. For 6 months, this is equivalent to 3%–9% of bone mineral density (BMD) loss at trabecular-rich sites. Bone mass usually returns to prepregnancy levels with cessation of lactation but not in all women. Therefore, the purpose of this study was to determine whether exercise slows bone loss from 4 to 20 wk postpartum (PP).

Methods.—At 4 wk PP, women were randomized to either an exercise group [EG, $n = 10$, weight bearing aerobic exercise ($3\ d \cdot wk^{-1}$, $45\ min \cdot d^{-1}$) and $3\ d \cdot wk^{-1}$ of resistance exercise] or a control group (CG, $n = 10$, no exercise) for 16 wk. Body composition and BMD were measured by dual-energy x-ray absorptiometry at the lumbar spine (LS), hip, and total body. Maximal strength and predicted maximal oxygen consumption ($\dot{V}O_{2max}$) were determined by 1-repetition maximum and submaximal treadmill test, respectively. Repeated-measures ANOVA was used to test for time and time by group differences.

Results.—EG lost significantly less LS BMD than CG (−4.8 ± 0.6% vs −7.0 ± 0.3%, $P < 0.01$). There were no significant differences in total body and hip BMD. Both groups lost fat mass (EG = −2.9 ± 0.7 kg, CG = −1.8 ± 0.4 kg); however, EG lost less lean body mass (−0.7 ± 0.3

TABLE 2.—BMD at Baseline and End Point and Percent Change After the Intervention*

	CG ($n = 10$)			EG ($n = 10$)		
	Baseline	End Point	% Change	Baseline	End Point	% Change
Whole body						
BMD ($g \cdot cm^{-2}$)	1.07 ± 0.03	1.06 ± 0.03	−0.8 ± 0.3	1.09 ± 0.02	1.09 ± 0.02	−0.6 ± 0.4
Lumbar spine						
BMD ($g \cdot cm^{-2}$)	1.07 ± 0.04	1.00 ± 0.03	−7.02 ± 0.6	1.05 ± 0.04	1.00 ± 0.04	−4.8 ± 0.3†
Total hip						
BMD ($g \cdot cm^{-2}$)	0.95 ± 0.04	0.93 ± 0.03	−2.2 ± 0.9	0.96 ± 0.03	0.93 ± 0.03	−2.8 ± 0.8

Values are means ± SEM.
*Significantly different over time, $P < 0.05$.
†Significantly different from CG, $P < 0.01$.

vs −1.6 ± 0.3 kg, $P = 0.05$). Maximal strength increased by 34% to 221% for all exercises in EG, whereas CG changed −5.7% to 12%. Predicted $\dot{V}O_{2max}$ increased in both groups (EG = 11.4 ± 2.0, CG = 6.9 ± 1.7%).

Conclusions.—These results suggest that resistance and aerobic exercise may slow bone loss during lactation (Table 2).

▶ The nutrient demands of the newborn during lactation are substantial, and reports from areas of food shortages have sometimes commented on the deterioration in the teeth of the mother while feeding her child. In terms of calcium, the total demand over 6 months of lactation amounts to a 3% to 9% loss of trabecular calcium.[1] High prolactin and low estrogen levels promote calcium resorption.[2] In many women, the bone mineral normalizes after lactation is completed, but this is not always the case; particular concerns are impoverished adolescents, women with multiple births, and older mothers.[3] The present small scale controlled trial appears to underline the value of weight-bearing physical activity at least 3 times per week over the period of lactation as a means of reducing (but not abolishing) bone mineral loss (Table 2). However, one important weakness in the proof is that the exercise group had a substantially larger daily calcium intake than the controls (+265 mg/d, more than the loss associated with lactation). Moreover, the calcium intake of the control group (944 mg/d) seems less than desirable; further trials are needed in subjects where food intake has been optimized.

R. J. Shephard, MD (Lond), PhD, DPE

References

1. Kalkwarf HJ, Specker BL. Bone mineral changes during pregnancy and lactation. *Endocrine*. 2002;17:49-53.
2. Hayslip CC, Klein TA, Wray HL, Duncan WE. The effects of lactation on bone mineral content in healthy postpartum women. *Obstet Gynecol*. 1989;73: 588-592.
3. Kalkwarf HJ. Hormonal and dietary regulation of changes in bone density during lactation and after weaning in women. *J Mammary Gland Biol Neoplasia*. 1999;4: 319-329.

Effect of Exercise Training on Loss of Bone Mineral Density during Lactation

Lovelady CA, Bopp MJ, Colleran HL, et al (Univ of North Carolina at Greensboro)

Med Sci Sports Exerc 41:1902-1907, 2009

Purpose.—During lactation, women transfer approximately 200 mg of calcium per day to breast milk. For 6 months, this is equivalent to 3%–9% of bone mineral density (BMD) loss at trabecular-rich sites. Bone mass usually returns to prepregnancy levels with cessation of lactation but not in all women. Therefore, the purpose of this study was to determine whether exercise slows bone loss from 4 to 20 wk postpartum (PP).

Methods.—At 4 wk PP, women were randomized to either an exercise group [EG, $n = 10$, weight bearing aerobic exercise ($3\ d \cdot wk^{-1}$, $45\ min \cdot d^{-1}$) and $3\ d \cdot wk^{-1}$ of resistance exercise] or a control group (CG, $n = 10$, no exercise) for 16 wk. Body composition and BMD were measured by dual-energy x-ray absorptiometry at the lumbar spine (LS), hip, and total body. Maximal strength and predicted maximal oxygen consumption ($\dot{V}O_{2max}$) were determined by 1-repetition maximum and submaximal treadmill test, respectively. Repeated-measures ANOVA was used to test for time and time by group differences.

Results.—EG lost significantly less LS BMD than CG (−4.8 ± 0.6% vs −7.0 ± 0.3%, $P < 0.01$). There were no significant differences in total body and hip BMD. Both groups lost fat mass (EG = −2.9 ± 0.7 kg, CG = −1.8 ± 0.4 kg); however, EG lost less lean body mass (−0.7 ± 0.3 vs −1.6 ± 0.3 kg, $P = 0.05$). Maximal strength increased by 34% to 221% for all exercises in EG, whereas CG changed −5.7% to 12%. Predicted $\dot{V}O_{2max}$ increased in both groups (EG = 11.4 ± 2.0, CG = 6.9 ± 1.7%).

Conclusions.—These results suggest that resistance and aerobic exercise may slow bone loss during lactation.

▶ Lovelady and colleagues are the first to publish a randomized controlled study of exercise training as a strategy to mitigate losses of bone mineral density (BMD) during lactation. The lumbar spine, characterized by a high bone turnover rate due to the preponderance of trabecular bone, contributes calcium to support lactation. The 3% to 9% loss of BMD during lactation may not be reversed in all women after the cessation of lactation. It is not clear if lactation contributes to osteoporosis later in life. Twenty women were enrolled in the study 3-weeks postpartum. The intervention focused on the first 5 to 6 months of breastfeeding when the greatest turnover of maternal bone occurs. The 16-week home-based exercise intervention included brisk walking (65%-85% of predicted maximal heart rate up to 45 min per session) 3 days per week and, on alternating days, resistance exercise targeting abdominal and back muscles 3 days per week. The resistance program emphasized the application of direct force through the axial skeleton, such as squats, bench press, and standing military press using handheld weights and exercise balls. Women in the control group were asked not to perform resistance or aerobic exercise, but could walk their babies in strollers at a casual pace. Exclusion criteria included exercising more than twice a week during the previous 3 months and cesarean delivery. Women who fed their infants more than 4 oz of formula daily were disqualified from the study. Four women discontinued the study because they were not able to exclusively breastfeed their infants. Exercisers had significantly less loss of lumbar spine BMD compared with the control group (-4.8 ± 0.3 g/cm^2 vs -7.02 ± 0.6 g/cm^2; $P < .01$). Exercisers also significantly increased muscular strength and endurance and had less loss of lean body mass and a trend for greater loss of body fat. Exercise compliance was >83% due in part to home visits made by research assistants 3 days per week. Although this is a small study that did not include a dietary intervention, it was otherwise well designed and provides compelling evidence for the benefits of weight bearing aerobic and resistance exercise to preserve BMD during lactation.

C. M. Jankowski, PhD

Association Between Regular Exercise and Excessive Newborn Birth Weight

Owe KM, Nystad W, Bø K (Norwegian School of Sport Sciences, Oslo; Norwegian Inst of Public Health, Oslo)
Obstet Gynecol 114:770-776, 2009

Objective.—To estimate the association between regular exercise before and during pregnancy and excessive newborn birth weight.

Methods.—Using data from the Norwegian Mother and Child Cohort Study, 36,869 singleton pregnancies lasting at least 37 weeks were included. Information on regular exercise was based on answers from two questionnaires distributed in pregnancy weeks 17 and 30. Linkage to the Medical Birth Registry of Norway provided data on newborn birth weight. The main outcome measure was excessive newborn birth weight, defined as birth weight at or above the 90th percentile. Logistic regression analyses were used to estimate the associations separately for nulliparous (n = 16,064) and multiparous (n = 20,805) women, and the results are presented as adjusted odds ratios (aORs) with 95% confidence intervals (95% CIs).

Results.—Excessive newborn birth weight was observed in 4,033 (10.9%) newborns, 56.1% (n = 2,263) of whom were born to multiparous women. An inverse association between regular exercise (at least three times per week) and excessive newborn birth weight in pregnancy weeks 17 and 30 was observed in nulliparous women, aOR 0.72 (95% CI 0.56–0.93) and aOR 0.77 (95% CI 0.61–0.96), respectively. Regular exercise performed before pregnancy did not affect the probability of delivering newborns with an excessive birth weight in nulliparous or multiparous women.

TABLE 2.—Regular Exercise and Excessive Birth Weight (90th Percentile or Higher) Stratified by Parity (N = 36,869)

	Nulliparous (n = 16,064)			Multiparous (n = 20,805)		
	% (Frequency)*	cOR (95% CI)	aOR (95% CI)†	% (Frequency)*	cOR (95% CI)	aOR (95% CI)
Model A: prepregnancy exercise						
Never	12.3 (176)	1.00	1.00	10.9 (265)	1.00	1.00
1–3 times per mo	12.8 (339)	1.05 (0.86–1.27)	0.96 (0.75–1.22)	11.0 (471)	1.01 (0.86–1.19)	1.02 (0.88–1.19)
1–2 times per wk	10.6 (484)	0.85 (0.70–1.02)	0.86 (0.68–1.08)	11.4 (752)	1.06 (0.91–1.22)	1.10 (0.95–1.26)
3 or more times per wk	10.3 (706)	0.82 (0.69–0.98)	0.85 (0.68–1.06)	10.6 (697)	0.97 (0.84–1.13)	1.05 (0.91–1.21)
Missing	11.9 (65)	0.96 (0.71–1.30)	1.10 (0.76–1.58)	8.6 (78)	0.77 (0.59–1.01)	0.86 (0.67–1.10)
Model B: exercise wk 17						
Never	12.7 (271)	1.00	1.00	11.2 (398)	1.00	1.00
1–3 times per mo	12.3 (357)	0.96 (0.81–1.14)	0.93 (0.74–1.18)	11.5 (536)	1.02 (0.89–1.18)	1.05 (0.91–1.22)
1–2 times per wk	11.2 (529)	0.86 (0.74–1.01)	0.91 (0.73–1.14)	10.8 (646)	0.96 (0.84–1.09)	0.95 (0.83–1.10)
3 or more times per wk	9.3 (465)	0.70 (0.60–0.82)	0.72 (0.56–0.93)	10.1 (450)	0.88 (0.77–1.02)	0.90 (0.76–1.07)
Missing	11.4 (148)	0.88 (0.71–1.09)	0.93 (0.68–1.28)	11.0 (233)	0.98 (0.82–1.16)	1.12 (0.93–1.37)
Model C: exercise wk 30						
Never	13.1 (511)	1.00	1.00	11.1 (786)	1.00	1.00
1–3 times per mo	11.5 (350)	0.87 (0.75–1.00)	1.04 (0.86–1.27)	11.1 (483)	1.00 (0.89–1.13)	1.02 (0.90–1.15)
1–2 times per wk	10.4 (462)	0.78 (0.68–0.89)	0.90 (0.75–1.09)	11.0 (542)	1.00 (0.88–1.11)	1.00 (0.89–1.13)
3 or more times per wk	8.5 (327)	0.62 (0.53–0.72)	0.77 (0.61–0.96)	9.4 (294)	0.83 (0.72–0.95)	0.96 (0.83–1.12)
Missing	14.2 (120)	1.10 (0.89–1.37)	1.17 (0.87–1.58)	11.9 (158)	1.07 (0.90–1.29)	1.09 (0.90–1.32)

cOR, crude odds ratio; aOR, adjusted odds ratio; CI, confidence interval.

*The proportion of newborns weighing above the 90th percentile within each response category.

†Model A: Adjusted for maternal age, education, body mass index (BMI) prepregnancy, and smoking status. Excluding women with preeclampsia or preexisting diabetes/gestational diabetes mellitus (GDM) did not change the effect estimates. Model B: Adjusted for maternal age, education, BMI prepregnancy, smoking status week 17, prepregnancy exercise, gestational weight change, energy intake (MJ), preexisting diabetes/GDM. Model C: Adjusted for maternal age, BMI prepregnancy, smoking status week 30, exercise week 17, prepregnancy exercise, energy intake (MJ), preeclampsia, preexisting diabetes/GDM, total gestational weight change.

Conclusion.—Regular exercise during pregnancy reduces the odds of giving birth to newborns with excessive birth weight by 23–28% (Table 2).

▶ There is now general agreement that regular moderate physical activity is desirable during a healthy pregnancy.[1] The main constraints are to avoid hyperthermia and hypoglycemia from an excess of activity, because both of these factors can be harmful to the developing fetus. The present large study from Norway suggests that a continuation of regular physical activity at least 3 times per week during pregnancy is helpful in avoiding an excessive birth weight (Table 2), which can be harmful to both the mother (perineal lacerations, excessive hemorrhage, need for Caesarean section) and her child (low Apgar score, birth trauma, and subsequent high risk of obesity).[2-4] The study also underlines the point that exercise before pregnancy is of no value if it is not maintained. If discomfort is felt during walking or jogging, the answer for the pregnant woman is to switch to weight-supported activities such as swimming or cycling. The probable mechanism of weight control is the improvement of glucose tolerance associated with regular physical activity.

R. J. Shephard, MD (Lond), PhD, DPE

References

1. American College of Obstetricians and Gynecologists. ACOG Committee Opinion. Number, 267, January 2002: exercise during pregnancy and the postpartum period. *Obstet Gynecol.* 2002;99:171-173.
2. Zhang X, Decker A, Platt RW, Kramer MS. How big is too big? The perinatal consequences of fetal macrosomia. *Am J Obstet Gynecol.* 2008;198: 517.e1-517.e6.
3. Heiskanen N, Raatikainen K, Heinonen S. Fetal macrosomia—a continuing obstetric challenge. *Biol Neonate.* 2006;90:98-103.
4. Hardy DS. A multiethnic study of the predictors of macrosomia. *Diabetes Educ.* 1999;25:925-933.

Why do pregnant women stop exercising in the third trimester?

Haakstad LAH, Voldner N, Henriksen T, et al (Norwegian School of Sport Sciences, Oslo, Norway; Rikshospitalet Univ Hosp, Oslo, Norway)

Acta Obstet Gynecol Scand 88:1267-1275, 2009

Current exercise guidelines recommend pregnant women to exercise throughout pregnancy. However, a high percentage of pregnant women are sedentary, and there is an increasing decline of physical activity and exercise, especially in the third trimester.

Objective.—The aim of the present study was to compare demographic and health-related factors in pregnant women exercising and not exercising in the third trimester.

Design.—Cross-sectional design comparing exercisers and non-exercisers.

Setting.—Rikshospitalet University Hospital and Norwegian School of Sport Sciences, Oslo, Norway.

Population.—Healthy pregnant women ($n = 467$) were successively allocated from the application form for birth at Rikshospitalet University Hospital.

Methods.—A questionnaire, including questions about demographic variables, physical activity level, common pregnancy complaints, social modeling, attitudes and barriers towards exercise participation was answered between gestation-week 32 and 36.

Main Outcome Measures.—Demographic variables, pregnancy related health factors and social modeling, including exercise counseling by health care providers, were tested using binary logistic regression analysis.

Results.—Less than 11% were defined as regular exercisers in the third trimester. Having high gestational weight gain and no social role models with respect to exercise behavior during childhood were inversely associated with third trimester exercise. Pre-pregnancy exercise was the strongest predictor of regular exercise at late gestation. Not receiving advice about exercise from health professionals was borderline significant. Pelvic girdle pain and sick-leave were not statistically significant factors.

Conclusions.—Pre-pregnancy exercise was strongly related to exercise at late gestation. This study indicates a need for more information

TABLE 4.—Comparison of Background Variables, Mean (SD) and *n* (%) Between Exercisers and Non-Exercisers in the Third Trimester

	Performing regular exercise ($n = 50$)	Not performing regular exercise ($n = 417$)	p-Value
Age (years)	31.2 (3.9)	31.6 (4.0)	0.47
College/university education	43 (86.0)	343 (82.3)	0.57
Pre-pregnancy BMI (kg/m^2)	23.3 (3.5)	23.6 (3.7)	0.52
Pre pregnancy BMI ≥ 25	13 (26.0)	119 (28.5)	0.70
Weight gain (kg)	11.6 (4.3)	14.1 (5.2)	0.01
Parity	1.3 (0.5)	1.2 (0.5)	0.09
Multiparous	15 (30.0)	199 (47.7)	0.02
Daily smokers	1 (2.0)	11 (2.6)	0.79
Alcohol drinking (≥ once a month)	2 (4.0)	21 (5.0)	0.73
PGP	24 (48.0)	242 (58.0)	0.15
Previous pregnancy PGP	7 (14.0)	81 (19.4)	0.32
Urinary incontinence	12 (24.0)	105 (25.2)	0.85
Fecal incontinence (anal and flatus)	3 (6.0)	39 (9.4)	0.43
Work-related physical activity	5 (10.0)	38 (9.1)	0.83
Pre-pregnancy physical activity	40 (80.0)	77 (18.5)	0.00
Time spent on sedentary activities (e.g. ≥4 hours of TV-watching)	3 (6.0)	25 (6.0)	0.98
Working status*			
100%	12 (24.0)	106 (25.4)	
≥50%	16 (32.0)	92 (22.1)	
<50%	2 (4.0)	39 (9.4)	
Unemployed	–	5 (1.2)	
Sick listed	17 (34.0)	147 (35.3)	
Does not work (i.e. student)	1 (2.0)	16 (3.8)	

Note: BMI, body mass index; SD, standard deviation; PGP, pelvic girdle pain.
*$p = 0.48$.

and motivation for moderate exercise before and throughout pregnancy (Table 4).

▶ There is widespread agreement that women should maintain a reasonable level of physical activity throughout pregnancy to reduce the risks of excessive weight gain and pre-eclampsia.[1-5] However, the sad reality is that only a small minority of women (11% in this survey) maintain physical activity during the third trimester. The only real pointer found to augmenting this percentage seems to inculcate the exercise habit before a woman becomes pregnant (Table 4).

R. J. Shephard, MD (Lond), PhD, DPE

References

1. Dempsey JC, Butler CL, Williams MA. No need for a pregnant pause: physical activity may reduce the occurrence of gestational diabetes mellitus and preeclampsia. *Exerc Sport Sci Rev.* 2005;33:141-149.
2. Kuhlmann AK, Dietz PM, Galavotti C, England LJ. Weight-management interventions for pregnant or postpartum women. *Am J Prev Med.* 2008;34:523-528.
3. Polley BA, Wing RR, Sims CJ. Randomized controlled trial to prevent excessive weight gain in pregnant women. *Int J Obes Relat Metab Disord.* 2002;26: 1494-1502.
4. Weissgerber TL, Wolfe LA, Davies GA, Mottola MF. Exercise in the prevention and treatment of maternal-fetal disease: a review of the literature. *Appl Physiol Nutr Metab.* 2006;31:661-674.
5. Gavard JA, Artal R. Effect of exercise on pregnancy outcome. *Clin Obstet Gynecol.* 2008;51:467-480.

Postmenopausal hormone replacement therapy modifies skeletal muscle composition and function: a study with monozygotic twin pairs

Ronkainen PHA, Kovanen V, Alén M, et al (Univ of Jyväskylä, Finland; et al)
J Appl Physiol 107:25-33, 2009

We investigated whether long-term hormone replacement therapy (HRT) is associated with mobility and lower limb muscle performance and composition in postmenopausal women. Fifteen 54- to 62-yr-old monozygotic female twin pairs discordant for HRT were recruited from the Finnish Twin Cohort. Habitual (HWS) and maximal (MWS) walking speeds over 10 m, thigh muscle composition, lower body muscle power assessed as vertical jumping height, and maximal isometric hand grip and knee extension strengths were measured. Intrapair differences (IPD%) with 95% confidence intervals (CI) were calculated. The mean duration of HRT use was 6.9 ± 4.1 yr. MWS was on average 7% (0.9 to 13.1%, $P = 0.019$) and muscle power 16% (−0.8 to 32.8%, $P = 0.023$) greater in HRT users than in their cotwins. Thigh muscle cross-sectional area tended to be larger (IPD% = 6%, 95% CI: −0.07 to 12.1%, $P = 0.065$), relative muscle area greater (IPD% = 8%, CI: 0.8 to 15.0%, $P = 0.047$), and relative fat area smaller (IPD% = −5%,

CI: −11.3 to 1.2%, $P = 0.047$) in HRT users than in their sisters. There were no significant differences in maximal isometric strengths or HWS between users and nonusers. Subgroup analyses revealed that estrogen-containing therapies (11 pairs) significantly decreased total body and thigh fat content, whereas tibolone (4 pairs) tended to increase muscle cross-sectional area. This study showed that long-term HRT was associated with better mobility, greater muscle power, and favorable body and muscle composition among 54- to 62-yr-old women. The results indicate that HRT is a potential agent in preventing muscle weakness and mobility limitation in older women (Fig 2).

▶ The effects of hormone replacement therapy (HRT) on body composition have been directed primarily at changes in total and regional body fat. However, estrogen receptors have been identified in skeletal muscle, and estrogens may have mild anabolic effects on muscle. Randomized controlled trials of HRT on skeletal muscle composition and function in older women have yielded mixed results, perhaps due to differences in HRT formulations and the long time course of clinically relevant changes in muscle mass, strength, and function. Ronkainen and colleagues provide unique data gathered from 15 monozygotic (MZ) twin pairs of HRT users and nonusers, aged 54 to 62 years. The cotwin analysis adjusts for genetic factors and some environmental factors shared early in life. The users and nonusers were well matched on behaviors and comorbidities that could impact muscle quantity and quality. Estrogen (1 mg effective agent) or estrogen plus progesterone replacement was used

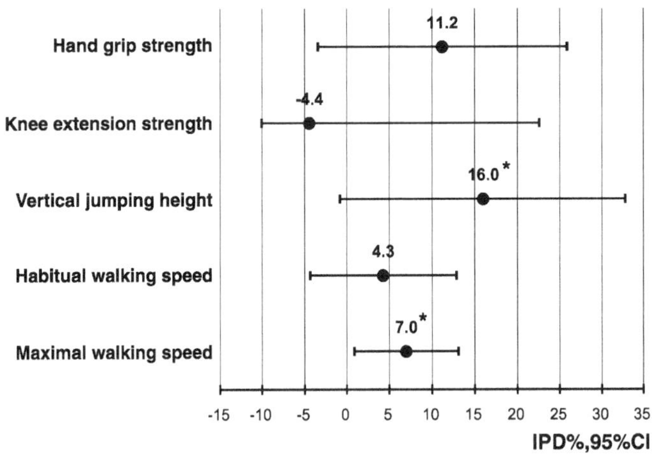

FIGURE 2.—Forest plot presenting muscle performance and mobility of monozygotic (MZ) twin pairs discordant for the long-term use of HRT. The value over each bar represents the intrapair difference (IPD%) calculated as (HRT user − nonuser) ÷ (nonuser) × 100, and the bar itself presents the 95% confidence interval (CI) for IPD%. HRT users had on average 16% better muscle power assessed as vertical jumping height and were also on average 7% faster walkers compared with their cotwins with no HRT history. $^{*}P < 0.05$. (Reprinted from Ronkainen PHA, Kovanen V, Alén M, et al. Postmenopausal hormone replacement therapy modifies skeletal muscle composition and function: a study with monozygotic twin pairs. *J Appl Physiol*. 2009;107:25-33, with permission from the American Physiological Society.)

by all but 5 women who used tibolone. The HRT users had 5-fold greater circulating estrogens than the nonusers, but no difference in testosterone (total or free) or sex hormone-binding globulin (SHBG). The effects of estrogen-based HRT on tissue composition were evidenced by a significantly lower total body fat percent, total thigh fat area, subcutaneous fat, and fat infiltration into muscle (trend only) and larger muscle area relative to the thigh muscle compartment. Regarding muscle function, HRT users had greater walking speed and muscle power, but not strength, than nonusers (Fig 2). The better walking performance in twins using HRT may be attributed to larger thigh muscles, a lower body fat percentage, and/or greater lower body muscle power. The > 20% greater muscle power in estrogen users compared with their twin supports a neuroprotective effect of estrogens on peripheral motor neurons. These results indicate a role for HRT in protecting muscle function in postmenopausal women. Whether HRT would promote or protect muscle quality and quantity in older women with frailty indicators is unknown.

C. M. Jankowski, PhD

When, why and for whom there is a relationship between physical activity and menopause symptoms

McAndrew LM, Napolitano MA, Albrecht A, et al (War Related Illness and Injury Ctr, East Orange, NJ; Temple Univ, Philadelphia, PA; The Miriam Hosp and Brown Med School, Providence, RI; et al)

Maturitas 64:119-125, 2009

Objectives.—The relationship between enhanced physical activity and decreased menopause symptoms is equivocal. In this study we sought to better understand this relationship by examining the association of physical activity to different symptom domains and by examining mediating and moderating variables.

Study Design.—Women participating in a randomized control trial on physical activity were given a menopause symptom measure (MENQOL) at follow-up. Of the 280 women participating, 113 (mean age = 52) reported having symptoms they attributed to menopause. Regression analyses were run to examine if change in physical activity predicted fewer symptoms. Exercise self-efficacy was examined as a mediator and depressive symptoms as a moderator.

Results.—An increase in physical activity from baseline was found to be related to reporting fewer total menopause symptoms ($\beta = -0.22$, $p = .02$). When the total menopause symptoms score was examined by domain, increased physical activity was found to be related to reporting fewer general symptoms attributed to menopause (psychosocial ($\beta = -0.18$, $p = .05$) and physical ($\beta = -0.23$, $p = .01$)), but had no effect on specific symptoms of menopause (vasomotor and sexual). Exercise self-efficacy was found to mediate the relationship between increased physical activity and total, physical and psychosocial menopause symptoms. Finally, for individuals with high depressive symptoms, those who increased physical activity the most reported fewer sexual symptoms of menopause.

Conclusion.—This study suggests that physical activity participation is associated with lower general symptom reporting as opposed to specifically impacting menopause symptoms. Further, exercise self-efficacy mediates the relationship between physical activity and general menopause symptoms, suggesting a psychological pathway.

▶ Physical activity is known to improve the health and well-being of women, but little is known about the effects of physical activity in reducing menopausal symptoms. The study by McAndrew and colleagues takes advantage of a randomized controlled trial of physical activity interventions in middle-aged women to test the hypothesis that increased physical activity would be associated with fewer general menopausal symptoms. A secondary hypothesis was that this association would be mediated by self-efficacy for exercise because self-efficacy is a consistent mediator of behavioral and psychological outcomes. Additional analyses were carried out to determine the associations of physical activity with sexual, physical, psychosocial, and vasomotor symptoms. The sample of 280 women included about equal representation of premenopausal and menopausal women. Hormonal status was not measured; thus, a limitation of the study is self-reported menopausal status. Women who increased their physical activity over 12 months had fewer general and physical menopausal symptoms. However, physical activity was not related to sexual or vasomotor symptoms. Women with a strong self-efficacy for exercise and those with symptoms of depression before starting exercise stand to experience the most relief from general menopausal symptoms. The clear message from this study is that physical activity provides relief from some, but not all, symptoms of menopause. Women who expect that exercise will provide relief from the vasomotor symptoms of menopause may be disappointed and abandon the exercise habit. These women should be encouraged to maintain the regular exercise to their best ability for other health benefits, particularly given the increased risk of cardiovascular disease associated with the menopausal transition.

C. M. Jankowski, PhD

When, why and for whom there is a relationship between physical activity and menopause symptoms

McAndrew LM, Napolitano MA, Albrecht A, et al (War Related Illness and Injury Ctr, East Orange, NJ; Temple Univ, Philadelphia, PA; The Miriam Hosp and Brown Med School, Providence, RI; et al)

Maturitas 64:119-125, 2009

Objectives.—The relationship between enhanced physical activity and decreased menopause symptoms is equivocal. In this study we sought to better understand this relationship by examining the association of physical activity to different symptom domains and by examining mediating and moderating variables.

Study Design.—Women participating in a randomized control trial on physical activity were given a menopause symptom measure (MENQOL) at follow-up. Of the 280 women participating, 113 (mean age = 52) reported having symptoms they attributed to menopause. Regression analyses were run to examine if change in physical activity predicted fewer symptoms. Exercise self-efficacy was examined as a mediator and depressive symptoms as a moderator.

Results.—An increase in physical activity from baseline was found to be related to reporting fewer total menopause symptoms ($\beta = -0.22$, $p = .02$). When the total menopause symptoms score was examined by domain, increased physical activity was found to be related to reporting fewer general symptoms attributed to menopause (psychosocial ($\beta = -0.18$, $p = .05$) and physical ($\beta = -0.23$, $p = .01$)), but had no effect on specific symptoms of menopause (vasomotor and sexual). Exercise self-efficacy was found to mediate the relationship between increased physical activity and total, physical and psychosocial menopause symptoms. Finally, for individuals with high depressive symptoms, those who increased physical activity the most reported fewer sexual symptoms of menopause.

Conclusion.—This study suggests that physical activity participation is associated with lower general symptom reporting as opposed to specifically impacting menopause symptoms. Further, exercise self-efficacy mediates the relationship between physical activity and general menopause symptoms, suggesting a psychological pathway (Fig 1).

▶ Given the positive effects of physical activity upon depression and anxiety, a positive effect upon the symptoms of menopause might be anticipated. However, several previous random controlled trials of moderate exercise in menopausal women have yielded inconsistent results.[1-3] Although designed

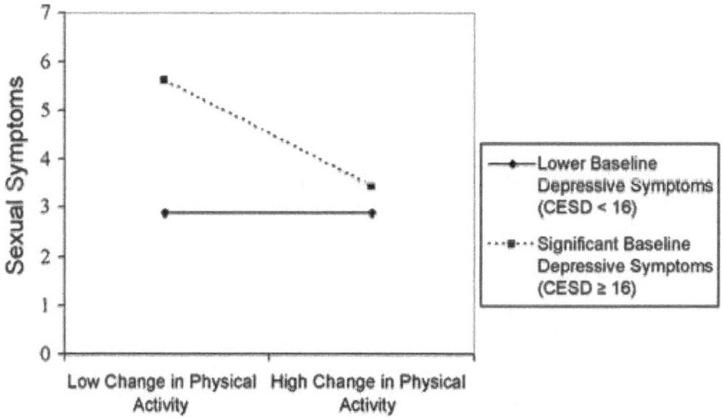

FIGURE 1.—Graph of the interaction of physical activity and depression predicting sexual symptoms. (Reprinted from McAndrew LM, Napolitano MA, Albrecht A, et al. When, why and for whom there is a relationship between physical activity and menopause symptoms. *Maturitas.* 2009;64:119-125.)

as a randomized trial, the present analysis seems based primarily on actual changes in exercise behavior. The study was thus correlational in type. It found associations between a subject's willingness to follow a recommended increase in physical activity, a decrease in depression, and a decrease in sexual symptoms (Fig 1). However, as in an earlier study,[4] the improvement in menopause symptomatology was related more to general manifestations than to specific effects on vascular and sexual symptoms. The authors of this article follow Elavsky and McAuley[4] in attributing the apparent benefits of their program to an increase in self-efficacy for exercise. However, the problem in interpreting the findings is that of most correlational studies: depression can in itself reduce physical activity. Thus, if depression decreases as menopause resolves, this may encourage an individual to increase her physical activity, rather than the converse.

R. J. Shephard, MD (Lond), PhD, DPE

References

1. Elavsky S, McAuley E. Physical activity and mental health outcomes during menopause: a randomized controlled trial. *Ann Behav Med.* 2007;33:132-142.
2. Aiello EJ, Yasui Y, Tworoger SS, et al. Effect of a yearlong, moderate-intensity exercise intervention on the occurrence and severity of menopause symptoms in postmenopausal women. *Menopause.* 2004;11:382-388.
3. Wilbur J, Miller AM, McDevitt J, Wang E, Miller J. Menopausal status, moderate-intensity walking, and symptoms in midlife women. *Res Theory Nurs Pract.* 2005; 19:163-180.
4. Slaven L, Lee C. Mood and symptom reporting among middle-aged women: the relationship between menopausal status, hormone replacement therapy, and exercise participation. *Health Psychol.* 1997;16:203-208.

Performance, Training and Lifestyle Parameters of Marathon Runners Aged 20–80 Years: Results of the PACE-study

Leyk D, Erley O, Gorges W, et al (German Sport Univ Colgone, Germany; Inst of the Federal Armed Forces Med Services, Koblenz, Germany; et al)

Int J Sports Med 30:360-365, 2009

Successful finishing of marathon requires regular endurance training and appropriate lifestyle. Thus, marathon running times and training data from large samples of physically active and fit elderly are ideal for the assessment of age-related performance. In the present study we analyzed 439 278 running times from result lists of 108 marathon competitions and data from a survey via internet questionnaire about training and behavioural factors of marathon finishers. Marathon times and 6992 data sets from the internet questionnaire were separated into groups based on age and sex and analyzed by two-way ANOVA. Our main findings are that 1) there are virtually no relevant running time differences ($p < 0.01$) in marathon finishers from 20 to 55 years and 2) the majority of middle-aged and elderly athletes have training histories of less than seven years of running. With the exception of marathon running times we did not encounter any significant gender related differences ($p > 0.01$). The present findings strengthen the concept that considers aging as a biological process that can be considerably speeded up or slowed down by multiple lifestyle related factors.

▶ In principle, the age-related deterioration in a competitive performance such as marathon running (Fig 1 in the original article) could provide a good indication of functional aging, and a number of studies of masters athletes have been undertaken with a view to defining the rate of loss of aerobic and muscular function. The information obtained has been useful in middle age, but in the older age groups the curve showing the rate of functional loss has been distorted by limitations in the number of participants, and a decrease in training programs even among those who remain involved. This study has been successful in accumulating data on a large number of individuals in their 60s and 70s, although the twin problems of a declining pool of participants and a decrease in training probably continue to exaggerate the true inherent rate of aging. Moreover, many of the subjects only began marathon running relatively recently. It would be interesting to know what the aging curves would look like for individuals who had been running long distances for 60 or more years. The survey was cross-sectional in type, and it could be argued that with aging it became progressively less representative of the population, as those with various health problems dropped out of running programs. Another possible issue is the use of an Internet survey—a larger proportion of the older participants may not have had access to Internet communication. Nevertheless, the survey does show that a proportion of elderly people can sustain a very credible level of physical activity to an advanced age.

R. J. Shephard, MD (Lond), PhD, DPE

Maximal oxygen intake and independence in old age

Shephard RJ (Univ of Toronto, Ontario, Canada)

Br J Sports Med 43:342-346, 2009

This brief review examines the likelihood that a deterioration of aerobic fitness will lead to a loss of independence in old age. The rate of deterioration of maximal aerobic power observed in middle-aged adults continues unabated during the retirement years. Loss of independence seems likely if maximal oxygen intake falls below a threshold of 18 ml/[kg.min] in men and 15 ml/[kg.min] in women, reached at 80–85 years. A regular programme of aerobic exercise can slow or reverse the functional deterioration, reducing the individual's biological age by 10 or more years, and potentially prolonging independence by a similar amount. There remains a need to clarify the importance of decreasing aerobic fitness relative to other potential causes of dependency but, from the practical viewpoint, regular aerobic activity should be commended to elderly people since it can address many of the issues of both functional loss and chronic disease.

▶ In this review, Dr Shephard updates the current knowledge of changes in maximal oxygen consumption during aging, its relation to functional independence, and the role of exercise in preserving aerobic capacity later in life. The lowest maximal oxygen intake values in free living elderly men and women were 18 mL/[kg.min], and 15 mL/[kg.min], respectively. Cross-sectional and longitudinal studies suggest a loss of 5 mL/[kg.min] per decade in women and men from ages 20 to 60 years, a rate that seems to prevail through age 85. This loss may be attenuated to 3 to 4 mL/[kg.min] per decade in physically active adults. For each 1 mL/[kg.min] decrease, the risk of functional dependency increased 14%, suggesting a need to maintain, if not improve, cardiovascular fitness during later life. A review of numerous aerobic training studies involving older adults, published since 1990, indicates that VO_2 peak improves 13% to 17% in response to training of 8 to 52 weeks, with greater improvements seen with longer interventions. Dr Shephard reminds us that the healthy survivor effect remains an important caveat to our current knowledge of both age- and intervention-related changes in VO_2 peak. That is, observational and exercise intervention studies attract those individuals experiencing successful aging. Several important gaps in current knowledge include identifying the relative importance of causes of institutionalization, the fraction of nursing home admissions attributable to a critical decline in aerobic conditioning, and identifying home-based services that are most effective at postponing institutionalization.

C. M. Jankowski, PhD

Effects of Testosterone on Muscle Strength, Physical Function, Body Composition, and Quality of Life in Intermediate-Frail and Frail Elderly Men: A Randomized, Double-Blind, Placebo-Controlled Study

Srinivas-Shankar U, Roberts SA, Connolly MJ, et al (Univ of Manchester, UK; Univ of Auckland, New Zealand)
J Clin Endocrinol Metab 95:639-650, 2010

Context.—Physical frailty is associated with reduced muscle strength, impaired physical function, and quality of life. Testosterone (T) increases muscle mass and strength in hypogonadal patients. It is unclear whether T has similar effects in intermediate-frail and frail elderly men with low to borderline-low T.

Objective.—Our objective was to determine the effects of 6 months T treatment in intermediate-frail and frail elderly men, on muscle mass and strength, physical function, and quality of life.

Design and Setting.—We conducted a randomized, double-blind, placebo-controlled, parallel-group, single-center study.

Participants.—Participants were community-dwelling intermediate-frail and frail elderly men at least 65 yr of age with a total T at or below 12 nmol/liter or free T at or below 250 pmol/liter.

Methods.—Two hundred seventy-four participants were randomized to transdermal T (50 mg/d) or placebo gel for 6 months. Outcome measures included muscle strength, lean and fat mass, physical function, and self-reported quality of life.

Results.—Isometric knee extension peak torque improved in the T group (*vs.* placebo at 6 months), adjusted difference was 8.6 (95% confidence interval, 1.3–16.0; $P = 0.02$) Newton-meters. Lean body mass increased and fat mass decreased significantly in the T group by 1.08 ± 1.8 and 0.9 ± 1.6 kg, respectively. Physical function improved among older and frailer men. Somatic and sexual symptom scores decreased with T treatment; adjusted difference was −1.2 (−2.4 to −0.04) and −1.3 (−2.5 to −0.2), respectively.

Conclusions.—T treatment in intermediate-frail and frail elderly men with low to borderline-low T for 6 months may prevent age-associated loss of lower limb muscle strength and improve body composition, quality of life, and physical function. Further investigations are warranted to extend these results.

▶ The study of exogenous testosterone (T) therapy conducted by Srinivas-Shankar and colleagues is unique because enrollment was limited to hypogonadal (serum total testosterone < 12 nmol/L) older men who were frail or intermediate frail. Frailty was adequately defined using the criteria of Fried et al,[1] which includes unintentional weight loss, self-reported exhaustion, low physical activity, slow walking time, and low handgrip strength. Men with 1 or 2 criteria were categorized as intermediate frail ($n = 224$), whereas those with 3 or more criteria were considered frail ($n = 38$). Participants were randomly assigned to transdermal T (50 mg/d) or placebo for 6 months. Serum T was monitored in all men, and dose adjustments were made to maintain a serum total T in the range of 18 to 30 nmol/L in the active treatment group. Changes in isometric and isokinetic knee extensor and flexor peak torque were greater in the T-treated men, although only isometric knee extension was significantly different from placebo. It is clinically relevant to know whether strength development in the legs translates to improved physical function. In this study, there was some evidence for improved walking time and overall function (physical performance test) in response to T therapy, although changes between groups did not reach statistical significance. A subgroup analysis revealed significantly better physical function in older (≥75 years) or frail men treated with T. Interestingly, the change in knee extensor strength was not different in the T- and placebo-treated frail or older men, indicating a disconnection between isometric strength and physical function changes. The expected body composition changes were found with T therapy, that is, a significant increase in lean mass and a decrease in fat mass compared with placebo. Sexual and somatic symptoms also improved significantly with T therapy. These findings suggest that T replacement therapy may be most appropriate to improve or mitigate the further loss of physical function in frail hypogonadal older men. A future study that restricts enrollment to frail men would be suited to test this assertion.

C. M. Jankowski, PhD

Reference

1. Fried LP, Tangen CM, Walston J, et al. Frailty in older adults: evidence for a phenotype. *J Gerontol A Biol Sci Med Sci.* 2003;56:M146-M156.

Testosterone and Growth Hormone Improve Body Composition and Muscle Performance in Older Men

Sattler FR, Castaneda-Sceppa C, Binder EF, et al (Univ of Southern California, Los Angeles; Tufts Univ, Boston, MA; Washington Univ, St. Louis, MO; et al)
J Clin Endocrinol Metab 94:1991-2001, 2009

Context.—Impairments in the pituitary-gonadal axis with aging are associated with loss of muscle mass and function and accumulation of upper body fat.

Objectives.—We tested the hypothesis that physiological supplementation with testosterone and GH together improves body composition and muscle performance in older men.

Design, Setting, and Participants.—One hundred twenty-two community-dwelling men 70.8 ± 4.2 yr of age with body mass index of 27.4 ± 3.4 kg/m^2, testosterone of 550 ng/dl or less, and IGF-I in lower adult tertile (≤167 ng/dl) were randomized to receive transdermal testosterone (5 or 10 g/d) during a Leydig cell clamp plus GH (0, 3, or 5 μg/kg·d) for 16 wk.

Main Outcome Measures.—Body composition by dual-energy x-ray absorptiometry, muscle performance, and safety tests were conducted.

Results.—Total lean body mass increased (1.0 ± 1.7 to 3.0 ± 2.2 kg) as did appendicular lean tissue (0.4 ± 1.4 to 1.5 ± 1.3 kg), whereas total fat mass decreased by 0.4 ± 0.9 to 2.3 ± 1.7 kg as did trunk fat (0.5 ± 0.9 to 1.5 ± 1.0 kg) across the six treatment groups and by dose levels for each parameter ($P \leq 0.0004$ for linear trend). Composite maximum voluntary strength of upper and lower body muscles increased by 14 ± 34 to 35 ± 31% ($P < 0.003$ in the three highest dose groups) that correlated with changes in appendicular lean mass. Aerobic endurance increased in all six groups (average 96 ± 137sec longer). Systolic and diastolic blood pressure increased similarly in each group with mean increases of 12 ± 14 and 8 ± 8 mm Hg, respectively. Other predictable adverse events were modest and reversible.

Conclusions.—Supplemental testosterone produced significant gains in total and appendicular lean mass, muscle strength, and aerobic endurance

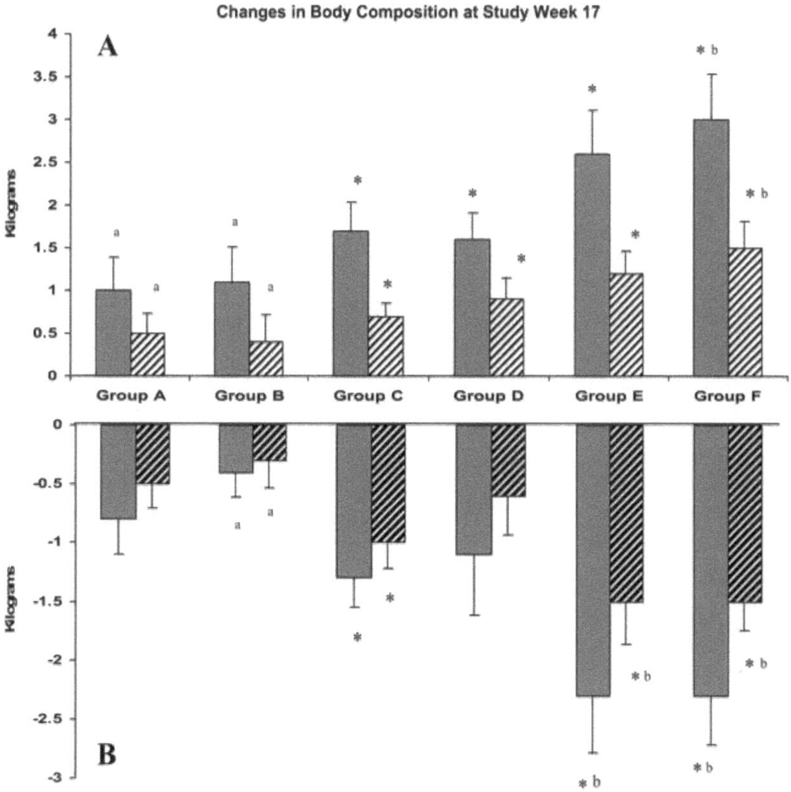

FIGURE 3.—DEXA-derived changes (mean ± 1 SE) in LBM and fat mass for each treatment group from baseline to wk 17. A, Increases in total LBM (*solid bars*) and appendicular lean mass (*hatched bars*). Changes across groups are significant for linear trend for total lean mass ($P = 0.0002$) and appendicular lean ($P = 0.0002$). B, Decreases in total body fat mass (*solid bars*) and trunk fat (*hatched bars*). Changes across groups are significant for linear trend for total fat mass ($P = 0.0004$) and trunk fat ($P = 0.0003$). *, Bonferoni adjusted within group changes ($P < 0.008$). Pairs of treatment groups with *different letters* (*e.g.* a *vs.* b) are significantly different by one-way ANCOVA with pairwise comparison (Tukey adjusted; $P < 0.05$). (Reprinted from Sattler FR, Castaneda-Sceppa C, Binder EF, et al. Testosterone and growth hormone improve body composition and muscle performance in older men. *J Clin Endocrinol Metab*. 2009;94:1991-2001. Copyright 2009, The Endocrine Society.)

with significant reductions in whole-body and trunk fat. Outcomes appeared to be further enhanced with GH supplementation (Fig 3).

▶ This is the first study to investigate the combined effect of testosterone and growth hormone therapy over 16 weeks on the body composition and physical fitness levels of older men (ages 65-90 years). The results were striking, with mean increases in total lean mass of up to 3 kg (maximum increase of 7.5 kg) and mean decreases in fat of up to 2.3 kg (maximum decrease of 7.1 kg) (Fig 3). Strength measures increased by about 23%, with small increases in aerobic endurance also recorded. These changes occurred with few adverse outcomes (eg, increases in hematocrit and blood pressure). The aging process is associated with dramatic decreases in muscle mass and strength, and gains in body fat, especially for the 1 in 3 men with low endogenous testosterone.[1,2] These data support the role of combined testosterone and growth hormone therapy, especially in those in the lowest tertile for plasma levels of these anabolic hormones.

D. C. Nieman, DrPH

References

1. Srinivas-Shankar U, Wu FC. Frailty and muscle function: role for testosterone? *Front Horm Res.* 2009;37:133-149.
2. Nass R, Johannsson G, Christiansen JS, Kopchick JJ, Thorner MO. The aging population—is there a role for endocrine interventions? *Growth Horm IGF Res.* 2009;19:89-100.

Effects of aging on human skeletal muscle after immobilization and retraining

Suetta C, Hvid LG, Justesen L, et al (Univ of Copenhagen, Denmark; et al)
J Appl Physiol 107:1172-1180, 2009

Inactivity is a recognized compounding factor in sarcopenia and muscle weakness in old age. However, while the negative effects of unloading on skeletal muscle in young individuals are well elucidated, only little is known about the consequence of immobilization and the regenerative capacity in elderly individuals. Thus the aim of this study was to examine the effect of aging on changes in muscle contractile properties, specific force, and muscle mass characteristics in 9 old (61–74 yr) and 11 young men (21–27 yr) after 2 wk of immobilization and 4 wk of retraining. Both young and old experienced decreases in maximal muscle strength, resting twitch peak torque and twitch rate of force development, quadriceps muscle volume, pennation angle, and specific force after 2 wk of immobilization ($P < 0.05$). The decline in quadriceps volume and pennation angle was smaller in old compared with young ($P < 0.05$). In contrast, only old men experienced a decrease in quadriceps activation. After retraining, both young and old regained their initial muscle strength, but old had smaller gains in quadriceps volume compared with young, and pennation angle increased in young only ($P < 0.05$). The present study is the first to demonstrate that aging alters the neuromuscular response to short-term disuse and recovery in humans. Notably, immobilization had a greater impact on neuronal motor function in old individuals, while young individuals were more affected at the muscle level. In addition, old individuals showed an attenuated response to retraining after immobilization compared with young individuals.

▶ Very little is known about the physiological responses of unloading, and subsequent recovery, on muscle mass and function in older adults. Suetta and colleagues addressed this knowledge gap by measuring the changes in muscle strength, mass, and architecture as well as neuromuscular activation and twitch characteristics in 11 young and 9 older healthy men (aged 24 and 67 years, respectively) in response to lower limb immobilization and recovery. All participants were moderately active but not engaged in resistance exercise training. For 2 weeks, 1 leg was casted from the ankle to the upper thigh and participants walked with crutches. A 4-week recovery phase featuring resistance training of the legs followed cast removal. Muscle and neuromuscular outcomes were measured before and after immobilization and following recovery. Muscle strength was measured using maximal voluntary contraction (MVC) and central activation (electrically evoked muscle force) of the quadriceps muscle. Young and old men lost 16% to 20% of MVC during immobilization but made a full recovery. An age difference was found for central activation, whereby only the older men had a significantly reduced activation after immobilization, followed by complete restoration after retraining. The changes in quadriceps muscle volume (via MRI) were intriguing. The younger men had a larger loss of muscle volume compared with the older men during immobilization but made a complete recovery during retraining. Muscle volume of the older men remained significantly lower than baseline following retraining (Fig 2 in the original article). Regardless of the age, the loss of muscle volume during immobilization was associated with greater baseline muscle volume (Fig 3 in the original article). Pennation angle of the vastus lateralis, a measure of muscle architecture, decreased more in younger than older men during immobilization (−9.3% vs −6.1%) but was fully recovered only in the young men. The contractile properties, peak twitch torque and rate of force development, significantly decreased after immobilization and increased with retraining but did not differ by age group. These findings led the authors to conclude that immobilization has adverse effects on muscle size and structure in younger men and neuronal function in older men. Furthermore, age attenuates the capacity to recover muscle mass and architecture following immobilization.

C. M. Jankowski, PhD

Effects of Power Training on Muscle Thickness of Older Men

Nogueira W, Gentil P, Mello SNM, et al (Catholic Univ of Brasilia, Taguatinga, Brazil; Univ of Brasilia, Brazil)
Int J Sports Med 30:200-204, 2009

The present study aimed at comparing the effects of traditional resistance training (TRT) and power training (PT) in inducing muscle hypertrophy in older men. Twenty older men (aged between 69 and 76 years) were divided in two groups: TRT training (n = 9) and PT training (n = 11). The volunteers trained twice a week, during 10 weeks. Both groups performed an equal work output and the same exercises with loads between 40% and 60% of 1 RM. Three sets of eight repetitions of each exercise were performed with rest intervals of 90s between sets. Muscle thickness was measured by ultrasound at the biceps brachii (BIC) and rectus femoris (RF), using a 12 MHz high resolution scanning probe. An ANCOVA was used to compare post training muscle thickness values between TRT and PT, using baseline values as covariates. According to the results, RF muscle thickness increased only in PT, while BIC muscle thickness increased in both groups, but with larger increases in PT. In conclusion, ten weeks of PT induced muscle hypertrophy of the upper and lower limb muscles in older men. PT training may yield better results in muscle hypertrophy when compared with TRT.

▶ Power training is a form of resistance exercise that is characterized by a very fast concentric (shortening) phase and a slow eccentric (lengthening) phase. With aging, muscular power is lost to a much greater extent than strength, and thus the benefits of power training have been investigated in a growing number of exercise intervention studies in older adults. Nogueira and colleagues measured changes in muscle thickness in older men in response to a 10-week, twice weekly, intervention that compared power training with traditional resistance training. Muscle thickness of the biceps brachii and rectus femoris, measured by ultrasound, was used to indicate hypertrophy in the upper and lower body, respectively. Importantly, both exercise groups performed the same total work. Muscular strength increased significantly in both groups. The power training group had greater increases in muscle power than the traditional resistance training group, which is in accordance with the principal of specificity of training. The thickness of the rectus femoris increased significantly only in the power trainers. Biceps thickness increased significantly in both groups, but the increase was greater in the power trainers. Therefore, in a relatively short period of time (10 weeks and 20 exercise sessions), lower and upper body muscles exhibited greater hypertrophy with power training than traditional resistance training. One of the many potential mechanisms underlying power training is the preservation of fast-twitch, type II muscle fibers. Aging is associated with the preferential loss of type II fibers, which likely contributes to the decline in muscle power. The ability to generate force quickly is an important component of maintaining physical function. For example, rapid generation of force in the lower limbs is necessary to recover from a stumble without falling. Thus, power training may be an efficient and effective intervention to protect physical function and prevent falls.

C. M. Jankowski, PhD

Fear of Moving Outdoors and Development of Outdoor Walking Difficulty in Older People

Rantakokko M, Mänty M, Iwarsson S, et al (Univ of Jyväskylä, Finland; Lund Univ, Lund, Sweden)

J Am Geriatr Soc 57:634-640, 2009

Objectives.—To study which individual characteristics and environmental factors correlate with fear of moving outdoors and whether fear of moving outdoors predicts development of mobility limitation.

Design.—Observational prospective cohort study and cross-sectional analyses.
Setting.—Community and research center.
Participants.—Seven hundred twenty-seven community-living people aged 75 to 81 were interviewed at baseline, of whom 314 took part in a 3.5-year follow-up.
Measurements.—Fear of moving outdoors and its potential individual and environmental correlates were assessed at baseline. Perceived difficulties in walking 0.5 km and 2 km were assessed twice a year over a 3.5-year period.
Results.—At baseline, 65% of the women and 29% of the men reported fear of moving outdoors. Poor socioeconomic status; musculoskeletal diseases; slow walking speed; and the presence of poor street conditions, hills in the nearby environment, and noisy traffic correlated with fear of moving outdoors. At the first 6-month follow-up, participants with fear of moving outdoors had more than four times the adjusted risk (odds ratio (OR) = 4.6, 95% confidence interval (CI) = 1.92–11.00) of developing difficulties in walking 0.5 km and a three times greater adjusted risk (OR = 3.10, 95% CI = 1.49–6.46) for developing difficulty in walking 2 km compared with those without fear. The difference in the prevalence of walking difficulties remained statistically significant over the 3.5-year follow-up (P = .02 and P = .009, respectively).
Conclusion.—Fear of moving outdoors is common in older adults and increases the risk of developing self-reported difficulties in walking 0.5 km and 2 km. Knowledge about individual and environmental factors underlying fear of moving outdoors and finding ways to alleviate fear of moving outdoors are important for community planning and prevention of disability (Table 2).

▶ It is important that the elderly participate regularly in 30 to 60 minute bouts of deliberate walking. For this age group, walking is one of the most common and effective methods of maintaining the health of the cardiovascular system, the strength of the leg muscles, and functional independence.[1] Some seniors enjoy distance walking, but others are inhibited by a variety of fears (Table 2), and as the present cross-sectional analysis shows, there is a substantial relationship between such fears and self-reported difficulties in walking 0.5 or 2 km. Previous studies have emphasized fears of crime[2] and of falling.[3,4] To this list, the present study adds female sex, muscular diseases, noisy traffic, hills, and poor road or sidewalk conditions. In previous studies it has generally been unclear whether the fear is a cause or an effect of difficulty in walking. The present study is thus important in showing that people who initially have no problem in walking are likely to develop limitations sooner if they are initially afraid of walking outside. The fears show socioeconomic gradients, in part because those who are wealthy can more easily find pleasant and crime-free places to walk. The present observations were made in the fall and in the spring, but in northern countries ice is also an important deterrent during the winter months, and in Canada icy conditions can persist for long enough to allow

TABLE 2.—Factors Associated with Fear of Moving Outdoors in Logistic Regression Analysis at Baseline in People Aged 75 to 81 (N = 654–727)

Factor	Bivariate*	Multivariate†
	Odds Ratio (95% Confidence Interval)	
Living alone	0.94 (0.67–1.32)	0.77 (0.52–1.14)
Education in years	0.94 (0.90–0.98)	0.96 (0.91–1.01)
Financial situation bad or moderate versus good or very good	1.49 (1.09–2.04)	1.13 (0.77–1.65)
Cardiovascular disease	1.21 (0.87–1.68)	1.19 (0.83–1.72)
Lung disease	0.99 (0.65–1.49)	0.83 (0.51–1.35)
Musculoskeletal disease	1.94 (1.42–2.66)	1.90 (1.33–2.73)
Center for Epidemiologic Studies Depression Scale score	1.02 (0.99–1.04)	1.00 (0.98–1.03)
Mini-Mental State Examination score	0.96 (0.90–1.02)	0.93 (0.85–1.02)
10 m walking speed, m/s	0.58 (0.36–0.94)	0.87 (0.48–1.56)
Difficulties versus no difficulties walking 0.5 km	1.01 (0.48–2.15)	0.84 (0.29–2.38)
Difficulties versus no difficulties walking 2 km	1.19 (0.75–1.82)	0.91 (0.50–1.67)
Environmental factors		
Poor street condition	1.71 (1.13–2.58)	1.31 (0.80–2.12)
Hills	1.59 (1.08–2.32)	1.28 (0.81–2.04)
Long distances	1.36 (0.81–2.31)	1.14 (0.62–2.11)
Lack of resting places	1.36 (0.84–2.22)	1.04 (0.56–1.90)
Noisy traffic	2.67 (1.57–4.56)	2.40 (1.32–4.39)
Dangerous crossroads	1.43 (0.90–2.29)	1.12 (0.65–1.95)

*Age- and sex-adjusted bivariate odds ratios.
†Age- and sex-adjusted multivariate full model with all variables included in the model simultaneously.

a substantial deterioration of physical condition. The authors offer no easy solution to the problem, but in many North American communities one possibility for restoring confidence in walking would be to organize sessions in large, air-conditioned shopping centers.

R. J. Shephard, MD (Lond), PhD, DPE

References

1. Simonsick EM, Guralnik JM, Volpato S, Balfour J, Fried LP. Just get out the door! Importance of walking outside the home for maintaining mobility: findings from the women's health and aging study. *J Am Geriatr Soc.* 2005;53:198-203.
2. Green G, Gilbertson JM, Grimsley MF. Fear of crime and health in residential tower blocks. A case study in Liverpool, UK. *Eur J Public Health.* 2002;12:10-15.
3. Friedman SM, Munoz B, West SK, Rubin GS, Fried LP. Falls and fear of falling: which comes first? A longitudinal prediction model suggests strategies for primary and secondary prevention. *J Am Geriatr Soc.* 2002;50:1329-1335.
4. Fletcher PC, Hirdes JP. Restriction in activity associated with fear of falling among community-based seniors using home care services. *Age Ageing.* 2004;33:273-279.

Relative Effects of Weight Loss and Strength Training on Balance Recovery

Matrangola SL, Madigan ML (Virginia Tech–Wake Forest School of Biomedical Engineering and Sciences, Blacksburg, VA; et al)

Med Sci Sports Exerc 41:1488-1493, 2009

Obesity is associated with an increased risk of falls and injury. Weight loss and strength training can be beneficial to balance, but knowing which is more beneficial would lead to interventions designed for maximal benefit in balance.

Purpose.—The goal of this study was to investigate the relative effects of weight loss and strength training on balance recovery using an ankle strategy.

Methods.—We used a combination of experimental testing and forward dynamic simulations. Nine male subjects (body mass index = 30.1–36.9 $kg \cdot m^{-2}$) were released from a forward lean and attempted to recover balance using an ankle strategy. Lean angle was increased until subjects required a step or hip flexion to recover balance. The maximum lean angle, θ_{max}, was used as the measure of balance recovery capability. Experimental data served as inputs to an inverted pendulum model of balance recovery. Multiple simulations were performed to determine the effects of weight and strength on θ_{max}.

Results.—Both strength training and weight loss increased θ_{max}. Comparing the percent changes in weight and strength required to increase θ_{max}, a targeted amount revealed differences in intervention potency. For example, to increase θ_{max} by 1°, an 8.6 ± 0.8% decrease in weight or 15.3 ± 1.1% increase in strength was required. The differences in efficacy between the interventions became more apparent as larger increases in θ_{max} were targeted.

Conclusions.—Balance recovery can improve with weight loss or strength gain, but a smaller amount of weight loss is needed than strength gain for a targeted improvement in balance recovery. This suggests that weight loss is a more potent intervention than strength training in improving balance recovery using an ankle strategy (Fig 6).

▶ Falls are a major source of both morbidity and death in elderly patients. Previous reports have shown that recovery of balance is improved by an increase of muscle strength.[1-3] Likewise, postural sway in the obese can be reduced by a reduction in body mass,[4,5] with a probable reduction in the risk of falls. The present investigation sought to determine which of the 2 approaches was the most effective in enhancing balance, and concluded that, for a given percentage change from baseline values, a loss of body mass was a more effective tactic than an increase of muscle strength (Fig 6). Most people would probably want to use both approaches, particularly as each carries benefits other than simply an enhancement of balance. There also is an inherent weakness in the argument favoring weight loss because it is usually easier to induce a large percentage increase in muscle strength than a large decrease in body mass; in one recent study, body mass decreased by 5%, but strength increased

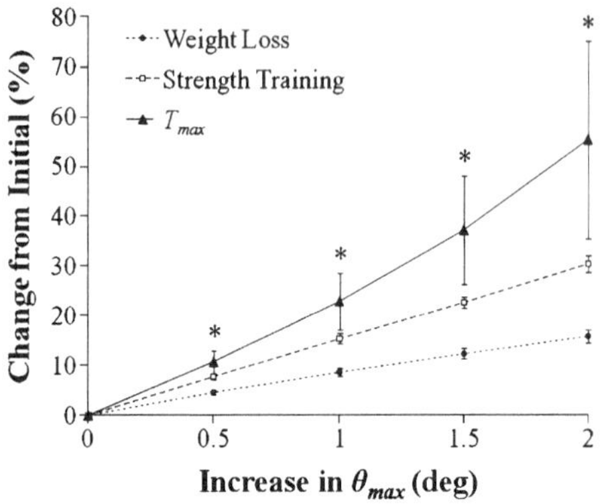

FIGURE 6.—Average changes in the three interventions that were necessary to attain 0°–2° improvements in θ_{max}. The x-axis quantifies the targeted increase in θ_{max}, and the y-axis quantifies the percent change of each intervention necessary to attain this targeted increase. All three interventions were different from each other at each increase in θ_{max} investigated. Also, differences in the three interventions increased as larger increases in θ_{max} were targeted. An excursion of 2° corresponds to a forward COM displacement of 3.1 cm. *Significant difference, $P < 0.05$. (Reprinted from Matrangola SL, Madigan ML. Relative effects of weight loss and strength training on balance recovery. *Med Sci Sports Exerc.* 2009;41: 1488-1493.)

by 32%.[6] Another point to underline is that although poor balance is a problem of the elderly, this study was conducted on young men. The technique of examining balance (release from a forward lean) was also very different from the type of disturbance accounted in the normal life of an elderly person (for example, regaining dynamic balance after tripping over the edge of a carpet).

R. J. Shephard, MD (Lond), PhD, DPE

References

1. Corbeil P, Simoneau M, Rancourt D, Tremblay A, Teasdale N. Increased risk for falling associated with obesity: mathematical modeling of postural control. *IEEE Trans Neural Syst Rehabil Eng.* 2001;9:126-136.
2. Robinovitch SN, Heller B, Lui A, Cortez J. Effect of strength and speed of torque development on balance recovery with the ankle strategy. *J Neurophysiol.* 2002; 88:613-620.
3. Whipple RH, Wolfson LI, Amerman PM. The relationship of knee and ankle weakness to falls in nursing home residents: an isokinetic study. *J Am Geriatr Soc.* 1987;35:13-20.
4. Teasdale N, Hue O, Marcotte J, et al. Reducing weight increases postural stability in obese and morbid obese men. *Int J Obes.* 2007;31:153-160.
5. Maffiuletti NA, Agosti F, Proietti M, et al. Postural instability of extremely obese individuals improves after a body weight reduction program entailing specific balance training. *J Endocrinol Invest.* 2005;28:2-7.
6. Sartorio A, Maffiuletti NA, Agosti F, Lafortuna CL. Gender-related changes in body composition, muscle strength and power output after a short-term multidisciplinary weight loss intervention in morbid obesity. *J Endocrinol Invest.* 2005;28: 494-501.

Improvements in whole muscle and myocellular function are limited with high-intensity resistance training in octogenarian women

Raue U, Slivka D, Minchev K, et al (Ball State Univ, Muncie, IN)

J Appl Physiol 106:1611-1617, 2009

Advanced sarcopenia is prevalent among octogenarian women; yet little is known about myocellular quality and plasticity in this cohort. The aim of this investigation was to examine single muscle fiber contractile function and whole muscle characteristics before and after 12 wk of high-intensity progressive resistance training (PRT) in very old (85 ± 1 yr) women (OW, $n = 6$). Young women [YW (21 ± 2 yr old), $n = 9$] were included as a control group. Whole muscle strength [1 repetition maximum (RM)] and size (CT scans) were assessed before and after PRT. Functional experiments (size, peak force, velocity, and power) were performed on vastus lateralis myosin heavy chain (MHC) I and IIa muscle fibers before and after PRT. With PRT, 1-RM strength increased ($P < 0.05$) in YW (36%) and OW (26%). Thigh muscle cross-sectional area increased (5%) in YW ($P < 0.05$), but thigh muscle did not hypertrophy in OW. Before PRT, there were no differences in single-fiber parameters between YW and OW. With PRT, MHC IIa fiber size (28%), peak force (31%), and power (28%) improved, but no changes were observed in MHC I fibers, in YW ($P < 0.05$). There were no improvements in MHC I or IIa single-fiber function in OW. These data show that the myocellular functional profile in OW is similar to that in YW but that OW have a blunted hypertrophic response to PRT at the whole muscle and myocellular level. The limited myocellular plasticity in OW with PRT contrasts with that in YW and previous PRT studies in elderly women only a decade younger. These data suggest that attempts to greatly enhance skeletal muscle mass and function should begin before 80 yr of age (Table 4).

▶ Waning muscle strength is commonly an important source of functional limitation among the very old, limiting their ability to carry small amounts of shopping, to rise from a chair, or even to get out of bed or rise from a toilet seat without assistance. Thus, there was considerable interest some 20 years ago when reports were published suggesting that an appropriately adapted program of high-intensity training could do much to restore the muscle function of nonagenarians.[1] The authors of the present report previously studied people in their mid-70s, reaching similar conclusions to Fiatarone and associates.[2,3] However, this report cautions that the ability to restore lost muscle does not appear to extend beyond the age of 80, and the findings must earn some respect, for although the sample size was small (9 subjects), the authors obtained muscle fiber biopsies before and after 12 weeks of high-intensity progressive resistance training. Young control subjects showed the anticipated muscle hypertrophy, gains of peak force, and power being mirrored by a 28% increase in the size of myosin heavy-chain type IIa fibers. However, the elderly women showed no improvement in the size or functional properties of type IIa fibers (Table 4). The lack of cell plasticity in the older subjects may reflect

TABLE 4.—Comparison of Vastus Lateralis MHC I and IIa Single Muscle Fiber Size and Contractile Function Changes with 12 wk of High-intensity PRT in 21-, 74-, and 85-yr-old Women

	21-Year-Old Women		74-Year-Old Women		85-Year-Old Women	
	MHC I	MHC IIa	MHC I	MHC IIa	MHC I	MHC IIa
CSA, μm^2	⇆	↑28%	↑55%	⇆	⇆	⇆
P_o, mN	⇆	↑31%	↑32%	↑14%	⇆	⇆
V_o, FL/s	⇆	⇆	⇆	⇆	⇆	⇆
Power, $\mu N \cdot FL^{-1} \cdot s^{-1}$	⇆	↑28%	↑51%	↑25%	⇆	⇆

Values are percentages. Data for 74-yr-old women are from Ref. 51. ↑, $P < 0.05$, pre- to posttraining. ⇆, No change pre- to posttraining.

changes in cell signaling,[4] gene expression,[5] protein expression,[6] or satellite cell count.[7] Although the octogenarians did make some practical gains in strength, presumably mainly through improved coordination, the important lesson from these observations seems that it is important to build up an adequate reserve of muscle tissue before reaching the age of 80 years.

R. J. Shephard, MD (Lond), PhD, DPE

References

1. Fiatarone MA, Marks EC, Ryan ND, Meredith CN, Lipsitz LA, Evans WJ. High-intensity strength training in nonagenarians. Effects on skeletal muscle. *JAMA.* 1990;263:3029-3034.
2. Trappe S, Godard M, Gallagher P, Carroll C, Rowden G, Porter D. Resistance training improves single muscle fiber contractile function in older women. *Am J Physiol Cell Physiol.* 2001;281:C398-C406.
3. Trappe S, Williamson D, Godard M, Porter D, Rowden G, Costill D. Effect of resistance training on single muscle fiber contractile function in older men. *J Appl Physiol.* 2000;89:143-152.
4. Funai K, Parkington JD, Carambula S, Fielding RA. Age-associated decrease in contraction-induced activation of downstream targets of Akt/mTOR signaling in skeletal muscle. *Am J Physiol Regul Integr Comp Physiol.* 2006;290: R1080-R1086.
5. Hameed M, Orrell RW, Cobbold M, Goldspink G, Harridge SD. Expression of IGF-I splice variants in young and old human skeletal muscle after high resistance exercise. *J Physiol.* 2003;547:247-254.
6. Bamman MM, Ragan RC, Kim JS, et al. Myogenic protein expression before and after resistance loading in 26-and 64-yr-old men and women. *J Appl Physiol.* 2004;97:1329-1337.
7. Kadi F, Charifi N, Denis C, Lexell J. Satellite cells and myonuclei in young and elderly women and men. *Muscle Nerve.* 2004;29:120-127.

Baseline and Follow-Up Characteristics of Participants and Nonparticipants in a Randomized Clinical Trial of Multifactorial Fall Prevention in Denmark

Vind AB, Andersen HE, Pedersen KD, et al (Glostrup Univ Hosp, Denmark)

J Am Geriatr Soc 57:1844-1849, 2009

Objectives.—To address the external validity of a trial of multifactorial fall prevention through an analysis of differences between participants and nonparticipants regarding socioeconomic and morbidity variables.

Design.—Analysis of nonresponse in a randomized clinical trial.

Setting.—Geriatric outpatient department.

Participants.—One thousand one hundred five community-dwelling adults aged 65 and older who had sustained at least one injurious fall.

Measurements.—Marital status, housing tenure, income, comorbidity, hospitalization, fractures, and drug use before invitation to participate in the trial. Fractures, hospitalization and death were measured for 6 months of follow-up.

Results.—Four hundred forty-seven responding nonparticipants and 266 nonresponding nonparticipants were compared with 392 participants in the trial. Lower income (odds ratio (OR) = 2.38, 95% confidence interval (CI) = 1.28–4.28) and more days of hospitalization during the previous 5 years (OR = 1.96, 95% CI = 1.15–3.33) predicted responding nonparticipation; independent predictors of being a nonresponding nonparticipant were unmarried status (OR = 2.0, 95% CI = 1.36–2.94), lower income (OR = 4.74, 95% CI = 2.30–9.78), more days of hospitalization (OR = 3.49, 95% CI = 1.99–6.11), and prior fractures (OR = 1.56, 95% CI = 1.02–2.38). Nonresponding nonparticipants were significantly more likely to die (OR = 12.99, 95% CI = 1.6–105.6) or be hospitalized (OR = 2.66, 95% CI = 1.7–4.1) than participants during 6 months of follow-up.

Conclusion.—Nonresponding nonparticipants of a trial of multifactorial fall prevention differed significantly from participants in terms of socioeconomic and morbidity variables and were more likely to be hospitalized or die during 6 months of follow-up. Because of the differences between the two populations, it is questionable whether results from this randomized trial can be generalized to people potentially eligible for participation.

▶ One of the areas where the health benefits of exercise are well proven is fall prevention in seniors. Strength and balance training has proven particularly effective in some settings. The Cochrane systematic review advocates strength and balance training as a first-line strategy to prevent falls. Note that despite the many studies of strength and balance training proving effective, there are exercise studies that have failed to reduce falls.

The importance of this article is that it raises the question, "Do the results of randomized control trials (RCTs) generalize to broad populations?" It is a fundamental question within research methodology as one of the main applications of the research is to drive evidence-based treatment.

The strength of this study was that the authors had population-based registry data on the individuals who did not respond to the invitation to join a fall-prevention RCT. Thus, they were able to compare 3 groups: those who agreed to participate in the RCT, those who responded to the invitation but declined participation, and those who did not even respond.

The details of the differences are not hugely important in the sports medicine setting—interested readers will follow up this article. However, what raises issues across all RCTs is that there were significant differences!

Clinicians, researchers, and sports medicine fellows can use this article to keep in mind the issue that RCTs have limitations. We must always strive to undertake RCTs with the most generalizability we can. Often our treatment will be based on suboptimal evidence.

For those working to undertake exercise trials in seniors, the following points are worth keeping in mind. Improved recruitment is likely to follow from (1) face-to-face contact, (2) recommendation by community leaders, (3) having trained personnel, (4) study-provided transportation, and (5) a positive and accessible environment for participants. Telephone prompting improved recruitment into RCTs in older people.

K. M. Khan, MD, PhD

Biopsychosocial Characteristics of Community-Dwelling Older Adults with Limited Ability to Walk One-Quarter of a Mile

Hardy SE, McGurl DJ, Studenski SA, et al (University of Pittsburgh, PA; et al)

J Am Geriatr Soc 58:539-544, 2010

Objectives.—To establish nationally representative estimates of the prevalence of self-reported difficulty and inability of older adults to walk one-quarter of a mile and to identify the characteristics independently associated with difficulty or inability to walk one-quarter of a mile.

Design.—Cross-sectional analysis of data from the 2003 Cost and Use Medicare Current Beneficiary Survey.

Setting.—Community.

Participants.—Nine thousand five hundred sixty-three community-dwelling Medicare beneficiaries aged 65 and older, representing an estimated total population of 34.2 million older adults.

Measurements.—Self-reported ability to walk one-quarter of a mile, sociodemographics, chronic conditions, body mass index, smoking, functional status.

Results.—In 2003, an estimated 9.5 million older Medicare beneficiaries had difficulty walking one-quarter of a mile, and 5.9 million were unable to do so. Of the 20.2 million older adults with no difficulty in activities of daily living (ADLs) or instrumental activities of daily living (IADLs), an estimated 4.3 million (21%) had limited ability to walk one-quarter of a mile. Having difficulty or being unable to walk one-quarter of a mile was independently associated with older age, female sex, non-Hispanic

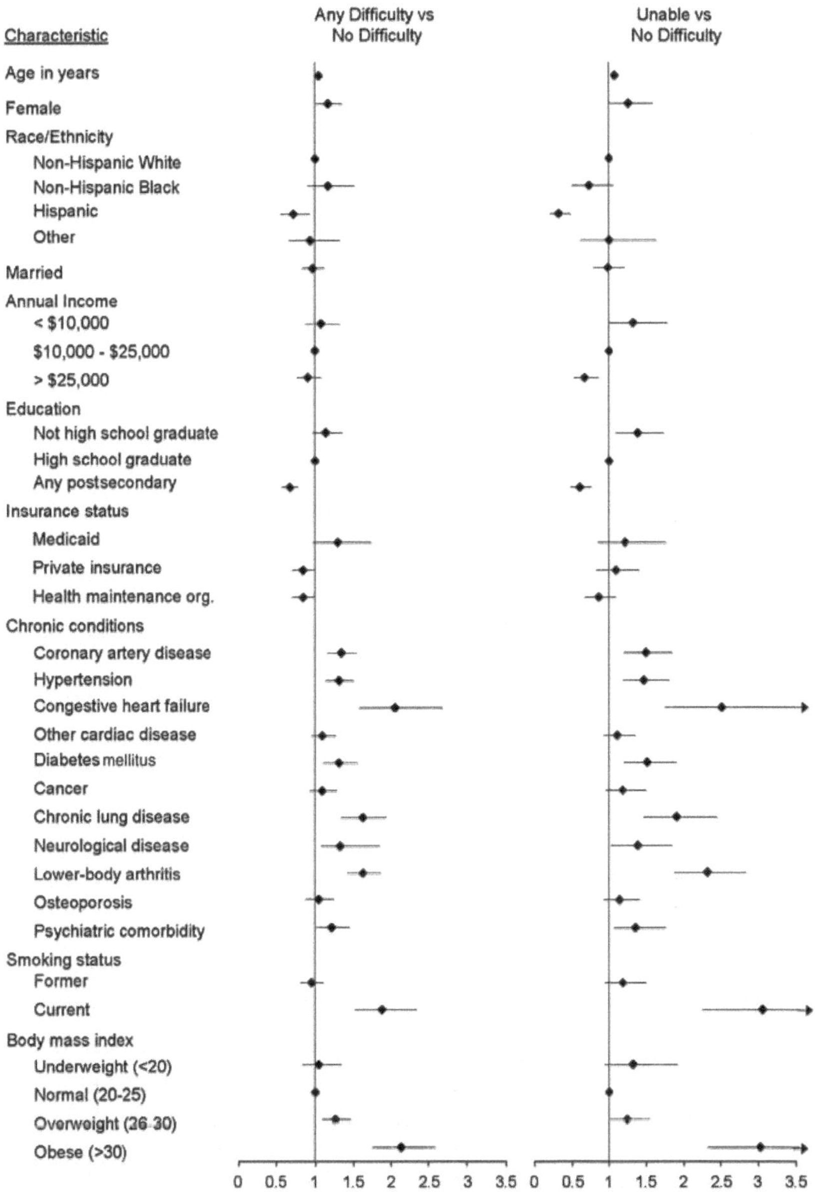

FIGURE 1.—Association in community-dwelling older adults between biopsychosocial characteristics and difficulty walking or inability to walk one-quarter of a mile. The analytical sample included 9,563 participants representing an estimated 34.2 million beneficiaries. Diamonds represent adjusted odds ratios (OR) and lines 95% confidence intervals. ORs represent the relative odds of having difficulty walking and being unable to walk one-quarter of a mile (vs no difficulty) associated with each characteristic, adjusted for all other characteristics listed plus activities of daily living and instrumental activities of daily living. (Reprinted from Hardy SE, McGurl DJ, Studenski SA, et al. Biopsychosocial characteristics of community-dwelling older adults with limited ability to walk one-quarter of a mile. *J Am Geriatr Soc.* 2010;58:539-544, with permission from The American Geriatrics Society, John Wiley and Sons.)

ethnicity, lower educational level, Medicaid entitlement, most chronic medical conditions, current smoking, and being overweight or obese.

Conclusion.—Almost half of older adults and 20% of those reporting no ADL or IADL limitations report limited ability to walk one-quarter of a mile. For functionally independent older adults, reported ability to walk one-quarter of a mile can identify vulnerable older adults with greater medical problems and fewer resources and may be a valuable clinical marker in planning their care. Future work is needed to determine the association between ability to walk one-quarter of a mile walk and subsequent functional decline and healthcare use (Fig 1).

▶ Old age is marked by a progression of physical problems—difficulty in walking up a slope, problems in carrying a bag of groceries, and a gradual shortening of potential walking distance. It is thus logical that such measures should provide useful indicators of an individual's biological (as opposed to chronological) age and overall state of health. Those who maintain a reasonable level of daily physical activity should be able to continue to walk a quarter of a mile or further till the age of 85 or even 90 years; I am now nearly 81 years of age, and a 5-km walk still presents no challenge to me. It is a sad commentary on the inadequate level of physical activity taken by many North Americans that more than 40% of the United States population older than 65 years of age who were eligible for Medicaid entitlement reported difficulty walking a quarter of a mile. The issue is important not only for the individual but also for the National treasury, since those who cannot walk have greater needs for medical treatment and institutional care.[1-6] Two of the most important correlates of the difficulty in walking—obesity and smoking—are plainly open to preventive measures (Fig 1).

R. J. Shephard, MD (Lond), PhD, DPE

References

1. Harrow BS, Tennstedt SL, McKinlay JB. How costly is it to care for disabled elders in a community setting? *Gerontologist.* 1995;35:803-813.
2. Manton KG. A longitudinal study of functional change and mortality in the United States. *J Gerontol.* 1988;43:S153-S161.
3. Wolinsky FD, Callahan CM, Fitzgerald JF, Johnson RJ. Changes in functional status and the risks of subsequent nursing home placement and death. *J Gerontol.* 1993;48:S94-S101.
4. Shephard RJ, Montelpare WM. Geriatric benefits of exercise as an adult. *J Gerontol.* 1988; 1988;M86-M90.
5. Fried LP, Guralnik JM. Disability in older adults: evidence regarding significance, etiology, and risk. *J Am Geriatr Soc.* 1997;45:92-100.
6. Newman AB, Simonsick EM, Naydeck BL, et al. Association of long-distance corridor walk performance with mortality, cardiovascular disease, mobility limitation, and disability. *JAMA.* 2006;295:2018-2026.

The Effect of a High-Intensity Functional Exercise Program on Activities of Daily Living: A Randomized Controlled Trial in Residential Care Facilities

Littbrand H, Lundin-Olsson L, Gustafson Y, et al (Umeå Univ, Sweden; et al)

J Am Geriatr Soc 57:1741-1749, 2009

Objectives.—To evaluate whether a high-intensity functional weight-bearing exercise program reduces dependency in activities of daily living (ADLs) in older people living in residential care facilities, focusing on people with dementia.

Design.—Randomized, controlled trial.

Setting.—Nine residential care facilities.

Participants.—One hundred ninety-one older people dependent in ADLs and with a Mini-Mental State Examination score of 10 or greater. One hundred (52.4%) of the participants had dementia.

Intervention.—A high-intensity functional weight-bearing exercise program or a control activity consisting of 29 sessions over 3 months.

Measurements.—The Barthel ADL Index; follow-up at 3 months (directly after the intervention) and 6 months with intention-to-treat analyses.

Results.—There were no statistically significant differences between the groups regarding overall ADL performance. Analyses for each item revealed that a smaller proportion of participants in the exercise group had deteriorated in indoor mobility at 3 months (exercise 3.5% vs control 16.0%, $P = .01$) and 6 months (7.7% vs 19.8%, $P = .03$). For people with dementia, there was a significant difference in overall ADL performance in favor of the exercise group at 3 months (mean difference 1.1, $P = .03$) but not at 6 months.

Conclusion.—A high-intensity functional weight-bearing exercise program seems to reduce ADL decline related to indoor mobility for older people living in residential care facilities. The program does not appear to have an overall effect on ADLs. In people with dementia, the exercise program may prevent decline in overall ADL performance, but continuous training may be needed to maintain that effect.

▶ I have previously argued the importance of regular physical activity in avoiding the institutionalization of the elderly,[1] a point confirmed by both cross-sectional comparisons and longitudinal studies of elderly populations.[2,3] Benefit accrues from both aerobic exercise and resistance training.[4] However, it is less clear how far benefits can be realized once the person has been institutionalized. It is difficult to get disabled patients with dementia to undertake an effective amount of exercise, and some of the programs claiming benefit have been uncontrolled, with apparent improvements stemming from greater attention rather than the added exercise. Even if there are gains in strength, balance and gait, these changes do not necessarily translate into a greater ability to undertake the activities of daily living. This controlled study included a substantial sample of the institutionalized elderly and was based on 29 45-minute exercise sessions performed over 13 weeks. The exercise sessions mimicked the activities of daily life, including walking, stepping, squatting, and standing without support, and control subjects met as a group for seated activities such as watching films or group games. Although the program did not appear to change the overall ability to undertake the activities of daily living, it did increase indoor mobility even in those with dementia, which probably reduced their risk of future health complications.

R. J. Shephard, MD (Lond), PhD, DPE

References

1. Shephard RJ. *Aging, Physical Activity & Health*. Champaign, IL: Human Kinetics; 1997.
2. Paterson DH, Cunningham DA, Koval JJ, St Croix CM. Aerobic fitness in a population of independently living men and women aged 55–86 years. *Med Sci Sports Exerc*. 1999;31:1813-1820.
3. Paterson DH, Govindasamy D, Vidmar M, Cunningham DA, Koval JJ. Longitudinal study of determinants of independence in an elderly population. *J Am Geriatr Soc*. 2004;52:1632-1638.
4. Paterson DH, Jones GR, Rice CL. Aging and physical activity: evidence to develop exercise recommendations for older adults. *Appl Physiol Nutr Metab*. 2007;32: S69-S108.

The Effect of a High-Intensity Functional Exercise Program on Activities of Daily Living: A Randomized Controlled Trial in Residential Care Facilities

Littbrand H, Lundin-Olsson L, Gustafson Y, et al (Umeå Univ, Sweden; et al)

J Am Geriatr Soc 57:1741-1749, 2009

Objectives.—To evaluate whether a high-intensity functional weight-bearing exercise program reduces dependency in activities of daily living (ADLs) in older people living in residential care facilities, focusing on people with dementia.

Design.—Randomized, controlled trial.

Setting.—Nine residential care facilities.

Participants.—One hundred ninety-one older people dependent in ADLs and with a Mini-Mental State Examination score of 10 or greater. One hundred (52.4%) of the participants had dementia.

Intervention.—A high-intensity functional weight-bearing exercise program or a control activity consisting of 29 sessions over 3 months.

Measurements.—The Barthel ADL Index; follow-up at 3 months (directly after the intervention) and 6 months with intention-to-treat analyses.

Results.—There were no statistically significant differences between the groups regarding overall ADL performance. Analyses for each item revealed that a smaller proportion of participants in the exercise group had deteriorated in indoor mobility at 3 months (exercise 3.5% vs control 16.0%, $P = .01$) and 6 months (7.7% vs 19.8%, $P = .03$). For people with dementia, there was a significant difference in overall ADL performance in favor of the exercise group at 3 months (mean difference 1.1, $P = .03$) but not at 6 months.

Conclusion.—A high-intensity functional weight-bearing exercise program seems to reduce ADL decline related to indoor mobility for older people living in residential care facilities. The program does not appear to have an overall effect on ADLs. In people with dementia, the exercise program may prevent decline in overall ADL performance, but continuous training may be needed to maintain that effect.

▶ This randomized controlled trial (RCT) assessed the effect of a specific high-intensity functional exercise program in a population of elderly persons living in residential care facilities. The study is well described and supports the use of such exercise for reduction in decline of indoor mobility, however, there was no effect regarding overall performance of activities of daily living as measured by the Barthel index score. This may indicate that other strategies may be needed to ensure improvement in activities of daily living and not only physical function and balance. Among those who had dementia, the exercise program was beneficial in preventing decline in activities of daily living in the short-term, and the authors explain that the literature has shown that among persons with cognitive impairments living in nursing homes, rehabilitation interventions must be maintained over time to have a beneficial effect. The strength of this study is its design (RCT). The authors express that the Barthel index may not be sensitive to pick up certain differences, such as faster and safer performance of these activities. Although the program may need to be expanded to include other strategies beyond gait and balance, it appears that there are certain benefits to high-intensity functional exercise in this population.

D. E. Feldman, PT, PhD

The effect of group-based exercise on cognitive performance and mood in seniors residing in intermediate care and self-care retirement facilities: a randomised controlled trial

Brown AK, Liu-Ambrose T, Tate R, et al (Westmead Hosp, Sydney, Australia; Centre for Hip Health, Vancouver, Canada; Univ of Sydney, Ryde, Australia; et al)
Br J Sports Med 43:608-614, 2009

Objective.—To determine the effect of a general group-based exercise programme on cognitive performance and mood among seniors without dementia living in retirement villages.

Design.—Randomised controlled trial.

Setting.—Four intermediate care and four self-care retirement village sites in Sydney, Australia.

Participants.—154 seniors (19 men, 135 women; age range 62 to 95 years), who were residents of intermediate care and self-care retirement facilities.

Intervention.—Participants were randomised to one of three experimental groups: (1) a general group-based exercise (GE) programme composed of resistance training and balance training exercises; (2) a flexibility exercise and relaxation technique (FR) programme; or (3) noexercise control (NEC). The intervention groups (GE and FR) participated in 1-hour exercise classes twice a week for a total period of 6 months.

Main Outcome Measures.—Using standard neuropsychological tests, we assessed cognitive performance at baseline and at 6-month re-test in three domains: (1) fluid intelligence; (2) visual, verbal and working memory; and (3) executive functioning. We also assessed mood using the Geriatric Depression Scale (GDS) and the Positive and Negative Affect Schedule (PANAS).

Results.—The GE programme significantly improved cognitive performance of fluid intelligence compared with FR or NEC. There were also significant improvements in the positive PANAS scale within both the GE and FR groups and an indication that the two exercise programmes reduced depression in those with initially high GDS scores.

Conclusions.—Our GE programme significantly improved cognitive performance of fluid intelligence in seniors residing in retirement villages compared with our FR programme and the NEC group. Furthermore, both group-based exercise programmes were beneficial for certain aspects of mood within the 6-month intervention period.

▶ There is increasing recognition of the role of physical activity for maintaining cognitive function. Evidence that this is the case in children is not new. Now studies are showing evidence of "neural plasticity" in seniors. This is a large randomized controlled trial (RCT) for the field and the participants are reasonably frail—they were seniors who were receiving at least some level of care. This is a group where worsening cognitive function is a major concern and was previously thought inevitable. Professor Lord is renowned in the field of seniors and exercise, and this is a well-designed study. Group-based exercise provided benefits in various domains including fluid intelligence and mood. I note that the flexibility training improved mood as well—this may have been due to the socialization. In addition to these data, please note that there are compelling data showing seniors benefit from cardiovascular training with improved executive function. MRI has confirmed these beneficial effects. Most recently, resistance training in senior men and women has proven beneficial. Exercise for your brain, not just your heart!

K. M. Khan, MD, PhD

The Lifestyle Interventions and Independence for Elders Pilot (LIFE-P): 2-Year Follow-up

Rejeski WJ, Marsh AP, Chmelo E, et al (Wake Forest Univ School of Medicine, Winston-Salem, NC)

J Gerontol A Biol Sci Med Sci 64A:462-467, 2009

Background.—It is well recognized that physical activity (PA) is important for older adults; yet, clinicians remain pessimistic about the ability of older adults with compromised function to adhere to long-term treatment and to maintain behavior change once treatment has been terminated.

Methods.—We examined the functional status of older adults at a field center (Wake Forest University) 2 years after completing 12 months of treatment in the Lifestyle Interventions and Independence for Elders Pilot study. At baseline, participants were randomized to either a PA or a successful aging (SA) control group. Outcome measures included an interview assessment of PA, the Short Physical Performance Battery (SPPB), and performance on a 400-m self-paced walking test.

Results.—Two years after the formal intervention had ended, participants who were originally in the PA group continued to engage in more minutes of moderate PA and tended to have better SPPB and walking speed than those in the SA group (effect sizes [ES]: SPPB = 0.40, walking speed = 0.37). Seven (12.7%) participants in the PA group failed the 400-m walk at the 36-month follow-up assessment, whereas this number was 11 (21.6%) in the SA group.

Conclusion.—Older adults who have compromised physical function are able to sustain some of the benefits derived from participating in structured PA 2 years after supervised treatment has been terminated.

▶ The great value of this study is that it provides rare information regarding the extended effects of an intervention to increase physical activity and physical function in older adults with functional limitations. The physical activity intervention of the LIFE-P included aerobic walking, strength, balance, and flexibility training.[1] The authors provided 2-year follow-up data from one of the centers in the LIFE-P multicenter randomized controlled trial. The response rate for 2-year follow-up was an impressive 75%. The 70- to 80-year-old women and men in the physical activity (PA) group engaged in moderate intensity exercise approximately 165 min per week, approximately 60 min per week more than the successful aging group (SA; controls). The PA group also maintained better physical functional performance than SA. The LIFE-P intervention included a group-mediated behavioral component that may be the key to the success reported herein, and also an important component of future physical activity intervention studies in older adults.

C. M. Jankowski, PhD

Reference

1. Pahor M, Blair SN, Espeland M, et al. Effects of a physical activity intervention on measures of physical performance: results of the lifestyle interventions and independence for elders pilot (LIFE-P) study. *J Gerontol Biol Sci Med Sci.* 2006;61: 1157-1165.

Cardiorespiratory fitness and brain atrophy in early Alzheimer disease

Burns JM, Cronk BB, Anderson HS, et al (Univ of Kansas School of Medicine; et al)

Neurology 71:210-216, 2008

Objective.—To examine the correlation of cardiorespiratory fitness with brain atrophy and cognition in early-stage Alzheimer disease (AD).

Background.—In normal aging physical fitness appears to mitigate functional and structural age-related brain changes. Whether this is observed in AD is not known.

Methods.—Subjects without dementia (n = 64) and subjects with early-stage AD (n = 57) had MRI and standard clinical and psychometric evaluations. Peak oxygen consumption (VO_2^{peak}), the standard measure of cardiorespiratory fitness, was assessed during a graded treadmill test. Normalized whole brain volume, a brain atrophy estimate, was determined by MRI. Pearson correlation and linear regression were used to assess fitness in relation to brain volume and cognitive performance.

Results.—Cardiorespiratory fitness (VO_2^{peak}) was modestly reduced in subjects with AD (34.7 [5.0] mL/kg/min) vs subjects without dementia (38.1 [6.3] mL/kg/min, $p = 0.002$). In early AD, VO_2^{peak} was associated with whole brain volume (beta = 0.35, $p = 0.02$) and white matter volume (beta = 0.35, $p = 0.04$) after controlling for age. Controlling for additional covariates of sex, dementia severity, physical activity, and physical frailty did not attenuate the relationships. VO_2^{peak} was associated with performance on delayed memory and digit symbol in early AD but not after controlling for age. In participants with no dementia, there was no relationship between fitness and brain atrophy. Fitness in participants with no dementia was associated with better global cognitive performance ($r = 0.30$, $p = 0.02$) and performance on Trailmaking A and B, Stroop, and delayed logical memory but not after controlling for age.

Conclusions.—Increased cardiorespiratory fitness is associated with reduced brain atrophy in Alzheimer disease (AD). Cardiorespiratory fitness may moderate AD-related brain atrophy or a common underlying AD-related process may impact both brain atrophy and cardiorespiratory fitness.

▶ There is increasing concern about the growing prevalence of Alzheimer's disease as the population ages in most developed countries. In the last few years, there has been tantalizing evidence that regular physical activity can slow the normal aging of cerebral structure and function,[1,2] but studies of the value of physical activity in patients with Alzheimer's disease have yielded conflicting results. This study is based in part on a cross-sectional comparison between the normal elderly and those with Alzheimer's disease, and in part on correlational studies within the group affected by Alzheimer's disease. Most previous reports have relied on questionnaire assessments of physical activity, which are notoriously unreliable in the elderly, particularly if mental function is impaired. Burns and associates reasoned that measurements of maximal oxygen intake would give a more reliable measure of physical activity, although again questions arise as to whether the mentally impaired can be motivated to give an all out treadmill effort, and the lower peak heart rate in the Alzheimer group lends some support to such a criticism. Keeping this qualification in mind, Burns et al showed a modest correlation between maximal oxygen intake and brain volumes (Fig 1 in the original article). Even if the difficulty of motivation is overcome it remains arguable that the disease has limited the patient's interest in habitual physical activity rather than activity playing a causal role. However, there are convincing reports that physical activity enhances neurogenesis and learning in aging mice,[3] and it would be worthwhile endeavoring to confirm the present findings using other objective measures of physical activity such as accelerometers, preferably adopting a prospective experimental design where the activity of experimental patients is increased for a substantial time.

R. J. Shephard, MD (Lond), PhD, DPE

References

1. Colcombe SJ, Erickson KI, Raz N, et al. Aerobic fitness reduces brain tissue loss in aging humans. *J Gerontol Ser A Biol Sci Med Sci.* 2003;58:M176-M180.
2. Colcombe SJ, Kramer AF, Erickson KI, et al. Cardiovascular fitness, cortical plasticity, and aging. *Proc Natl Acad Sci.* 2004;101:3316-3321.
3. van Praag H, Shubert T, Zhao C, Gage FH. Exercise enhances leaning and hippocampal neurogenesis in aged mice. *J Neurosci.* 2005;25:8680-8685.

Stability of Kyphosis, Strength, and Physical Performance Gains 1 Year After a Group Exercise Program in Community-Dwelling Hyperkyphotic Older Women

Pawlowsky SB, Hamel KA, Katzman WB (Univ of California; San Francisco State Univ, CA)

Arch Phys Med Rehabil 90:358-361, 2009

Objective.—To determine if subjects maintained improvements in kyphosis, spinal extensor strength, and physical performance 1 year after a 12-week multidimensional group exercise program.

Design.—Follow-up data compared with posttest outcome measures.

Setting.—Outpatient academic medical center.

Participants.—Nineteen of the initial 21 women, ages 65 to 80, with thoracic kyphosis of 50° or greater at the onset of the study completed follow-up testing.

Interventions.—Initial intervention included multidimensional group exercise performed 2 times a week for 12 weeks, consisting of spinal extensor strengthening, flexibility exercises, and integrated spinal proprioception training. Subjects exercised independently during the following year.

Main Outcome Measures.—Primary measures at the 1-year follow-up were usual and best kyphosis. Secondary measures included spinal extensor strength, modified Physical Performance Test (PPT), and the Jug Test.

Results.—Subjects maintained gains at the 1-year follow-up ($P > .05$). Best kyphosis improved by 3° during the follow-up year ($P = .022$). There were no significant declines in usual kyphosis ($P = .302$), spinal extensor strength ($P = .999$), PPT ($P = .087$), and the Jug Test ($P = .999$) at follow-up.

Conclusions.—Hyperkyphotic women maintained gains in usual kyphosis, spinal extensor strength, and physical performance 1 year after a group exercise program. Improvement in best kyphosis in the year after the intervention was also observed. Detraining effects may be minimized by multidimensional exercises.

▶ Kyphosis may be a significant risk factor for future vertebral fractures and has been associated with greater difficulty in performing activities of daily living and functional performance. This is a 1-year follow-up of an exercise intervention to improve kyphosis in women aged 65 and older with kyphosis of 50° (Cobb angle) or greater. The 12-week intervention included strengthening, range of motion, and proprioceptive postural alignment training in twice weekly supervised sessions and home-based exercise. Kyphosis and physical function improved significantly in response to the training. Physical function was measured using a modified physical performance test. The 5° to 6° improvement in usual and best kyphosis in response to the intervention was clinically relevant, given that it exceeded the progression of kyphosis typically seen over a decade in older adults. One year later, 19 of the 21 women in the intervention study returned for follow-up testing. Two women had changed their exercise habits since the intervention study, with one continuing to do the home-based intervention exercises. Best kyphosis (best posture) improved by an additional 3°. Physical performance tended to decline. Participants were categorized as "mildly frail" before the intervention, "not frail" immediately after the intervention, and reverted to mildly frail 1 year later. Although this is a small study and did not include a control group, it shows some promising outcomes. The further improvement in kyphosis, even without continuation of the home-based exercise, was surprising and perhaps attributable to the integrated proprioception component of the training. The intervention was relatively short and delivered in a group setting, which would enhance cost-effectiveness. A larger randomized controlled study with a follow-up interval is needed to confirm these preliminary, yet intriguing, results.

C. M. Jankowski, PhD

Article Index

Chapter 1: Epidemiology, Prevention of Injuries, Lesions of Head and Neck

Chapter 2: Other Musculoskeletal Injuries

Chapter 3: Biomechanics, Muscle Strength and Training

Chapter 4: Physical Activity, Cardio-respiratory Physiology and Immune Function

Chapter 5: Metabolism and Obesity, Nutrition and Doping

Chapter 6: Cardiorespiratory Disorders

Chapter 7: Other Medical Conditions

Chapter 8: Environment Factors

Chapter 9: Special Considerations: Elderly, Women, and Children

Author Index

A

B

C

D

E

R

S

T

U

V

W

Y

Z

Kolibri 360 GmbH
Ferdinand-Jühlke-Straße 7
99095 Erfurt, Deutschland
produktsicherheit@kolibri360.de